Low Back Pain

Guest Editor

ALISON STOUT, DO

PHYSICAL MEDICINE AND REHABILITATION CLINICS OF NORTH AMERICA

www.pmr.theclinics.com

Consulting Editor

GEORGE H. KRAFT, MD, MS

November 2010 • Volume 21 • Number 4

SAUNDERS an imprint of ELSEVIER, Inc.

W.B. SAUNDERS COMPANY
A Division of Elsevier Inc.

1600 John F. Kennedy Boulevard • Suite 1800 • Philadelphia, Pennsylvania 19103

http://www.theclinics.com

PHYSICAL MEDICINE AND REHABILITATION CLINICS OF NORTH AMERICA Volume 21, Number 4
November 2010 ISSN 1047-9651, ISBN-13: 978-1-4377-2484-4

Editor: Debora Dellapena
Developmental Editor: Jessica Demetriou

Reprints. For copies of 100 or more of articles in this publication, please contact the Commercial Reprints Department, Elsevier Inc., 360 Park Avenue South, New York, NY 10010-1710. Tel.: 212-633-3812; Fax: 212-462-1935; E-mail: reprints@elsevier.com.

Physical Medicine and Rehabilitation Clinics of North America (ISSN 1047-9651) is published quarterly by Elsevier Inc., 360 Park Avenue South, New York, NY 10010-1710. Months of issue are February, May, August, and November. Business and Editorial Offices: 1600 John F. Kennedy Blvd., Suite 1800, Philadelphia, PA 19103-2899. Customer Service Office: 3251 Riverport Lane, Maryland Heights, MO 63043. Periodicals postage paid at New York, NY and additional mailing offices. Subscription price per year is $230.00 (US individuals), $414.00 (US institutions), $122.00 (US students), $280.00 (Canadian individuals), $540.00 (Canadian institutions), $175.00 (Canadian students), $345.00 (foreign individuals), $540.00 (foreign institutions), and $175.00 (foreign students). Foreign air speed delivery is included in all *Clinics* subscription prices. All prices are subject to change without notice. **POSTMASTER:** Send address changes to *Physical Medicine and Rehabilitation Clinics of North America*, Customer Service Office: Elsevier Health Sciences Division, Subscription Customer Service, 3251 Riverport Lane, Maryland Heights, MO 63043. **Customer Service: 1-800-654-2452 (US). From outside of the United States, call 314-447-8871. Fax: 314-447-8029. E-mail: JournalsCustomer Service-usa@elsevier.com (for print support); JournalsOnlineSupport-usa@elsevier.com (for online support).**

Physical Medicine and Rehabilitation Clinics of North America is indexed in *Excerpta Medica, MEDLINE/ PubMed (Index Medicus), Cinahl, and Cumulative Index to Nursing and Allied Health Literature.*

Printed and bound by CPI Group (UK) Ltd, Croydon, CR04YY

Transferred to Digital Print 2011

Contributors

CONSULTING EDITOR

GEORGE H. KRAFT, MD, MS
Alvord Professor of Multiple Sclerosis Research; Professor, Department of Rehabilitation
Medicine and Adjunct Professor, Department of Neurology, University of Washington
School of Medicine, Seattle, Washington

GUEST EDITOR

ALISON STOUT, DO
Director, Spine and Musculoskeletal Medicine, Rehabilitation Care Services, Veterans
Administration Puget Sound; Department of Rehabilitation, University of Washington,
Seattle, Washington

AUTHORS

DAVID BAGNALL, MD
Amherst, New York

KEVIN A. CARNEIRO, DO
Assistant Professor, Department of Physical Medicine and Rehabilitation, University
of North Carolina, North Carolina

LEIGHTON CHAN, MD, MPH
Chief, Rehabilitation Medicine Department, Clinical Center, National Institutes of Health,
Bethesda, Maryland

EDUARDO J. CRUZ COLON, MD
Resident, University of Medicine and Dentistry of New Jersey, Kessler Rehabilitation
Institute, West Orange, New Jersey

KATHERINE D. DOERR, MD
Department of Physical Medicine and Rehabilitation, Harvard Medical School;
Spaulding Rehabilitation Hospital, Boston, Massachusetts

JANNA FRIEDLY, MD
Acting Assistant Professor, Department of Rehabilitation Medicine, University
of Washington, Seattle, Washington

ARTHUR HARTOG, MD, PhD
DC Pain Center Rotterdam, Rotterdam, The Netherlands

DAVID J. KENNEDY, MD
Assistant Professor, Department of Orthopaedics and Rehabilitation, University of Florida
College of Medicine, Gainesville, Florida

TIMOTHY J. LEE, MD
Internist, Seattle, Washington

GERARD A. MALANGA, MD
Director, Pain Management, Overlook Pain Center, Summit; Director, Physical Medicine and Rehabilitation Sports Medicine Fellowship, Atlantic Health, Morristown; Clinical Professor, Department of Physical Medicine and Rehabilitation, University of Medicine and Dentistry of New Jersey, New Jersey Medical School, Newark, New Jersey

TIMOTHY MAUS, MD
Department of Radiology, Mayo Clinic, Rochester, Minnesota

DAVID A. MAZIN, MD
Assistant Professor, Department of Orthopedics and Physical Rehabilitation, University of Massachusetts Memorial Medical Center, Worcester, Massachusetts

JAMES E. MOORE, PhD
Director, Rehabilitation Institute of Washington; Clinical Assistant Professor, Department of Psychiatry and Behavioral Sciences, University of Washington School of Medicine, Seattle, Washington

NAYNA PATEL, MD
Core Orthopaedic, Encinitas, California

JOSHUA D. RITTENBERG, MD
Department of Physical Medicine and Rehabilitation, Kaiser Permanente Medical Group, Oakland, California

ALEXIUS E.G. SANDOVAL, MD
Multiple Sclerosis Fellow, Department of Rehabilitation Medicine, University of Washington, Seattle, Washington

MAX SHOKAT, DO
Department of Orthopaedics and Rehabilitation, University of Florida College of Medicine, Gainesvllle, Florida

JOSEPH P. SULLIVAN, MD, PhD
Clinical Instructor, Department of Orthopedics and Physical Rehabilitation, University of Massachusetts Memorial Medical Center, Worcester, Massachusetts

CHRISTOPHER STANDAERT, MD
Clinical Associate Professor, University of Washington Sports and Spine Physicians at Harborview Medical Center, Seattle, Washington

ALISON STOUT, DO
Director, Spine and Musculoskeletal Medicine, Rehabilitation Care Services, Veterans Administration Puget Sound; Department of Rehabilitation, University of Washington, Seattle, Washington

CHRISTOPHER J. VISCO, MD
Assistant Professor, Department of Rehabilitation and Regenerative Medicine, Columbia University College of Physicians and Surgeons, New York, New York

ARIANA J. VORA, MD
Department of Physical Medicine and Rehabilitation, Harvard Medical School, Department of Physical Medicine and Rehabilitation, Massachusetts General Hospital; Department of Physical Medicine and Rehabilitation, Spaulding Rehabilitation Hospital, Boston, Massachusetts

LEE R. WOLFER, MD, MS
Spinal Diagnostics and Treatment Center, Daly City, California

Contents

In this article, the epidemiology of back pain and the use of a variety of treatments for back pain in the United States are reviewed. The dilemma faced by medical providers caring for patients with low back pain is examined in the context of epidemiologic data. Back pain is becoming increasingly common and a growing number of treatment options are being used with increasing frequency in clinical practice. However, limited evidence exists to demonstrate the effectiveness of these treatments. In addition, health-related quality of life for persons with back pain is not improving despite the availability and use of an expanding array of treatments. This dilemma poses a difficult challenge for medical providers treating individual patients who suffer from back pain.

Careful consideration of functional lumbosacral anatomy reveals the capacity for pain generation in the disc, zygapophysial joint, sacroiliac joint, and surrounding ligaments. However, the methods used to definitively implicate a particular anatomic structure in axial low back pain have limitations. Anatomically and biomechanically, the discs and posterior elements are inextricably connected to a dynamic biotensegrity network of ligaments, muscles, and fascia. This article examines key lumbosacral anatomic structures and their functional interdependence at the macroscopic, microscopic, and biomechanical level. Particular attention is given to the capacity of each structure to generate low back pain.

Myofascial pain syndrome is a common nonarticular local musculoskeletal pain syndrome caused by myofascial trigger points located at muscle, fascia, or tendinous insertions, affecting up to 95% of people with chronic pain disorders. Clinically, myofascial pain syndrome can present as painful restricted range of motion, stiffness, referred pain patterns, and autonomic dysfunction. The underlying cause is often related to muscular imbalances, and following a thorough physical examination the condition should be treated with a comprehensive rehabilitation program. Additional treatment options include pharmacologic, needling with or without anesthetic agents or nerve stimulation, and alternative medicine treatments such as massage or herbal medicines. Repeated trigger point injections should be avoided, and corticosteroids should not be injected into trigger points.

Timothy Maus

Imaging is an integral part of the clinical examination of the patient with back pain; it is, however, often used excessively and without consideration of the underlying literature. The primary role of imaging is the identification of systemic disease as a cause of the back or limb pain; magnetic resonance imaging (MRI) excels at this. Systemic disease as a cause of back or limb pain is, however, rare. Most back and radiating limb pain is of benign nature, owing to degenerative phenomena. There is no role for imaging in the initial evaluation of the patient with back pain in the absence of signs or symptoms of systemic disease. When conservative care fails, imaging may be undertaken with due consideration of its risks: labeling the patient as suffering from a degenerative disease, cost, radiation exposure, and provoking unwarranted minimally invasive or surgical intervention. Imaging can well depict disc degeneration and disc herniation. Imaging can suggest the presence of discogenic pain, but the lack of a pathoanatomic gold standard obviates any definitive conclusions. The imaging natural history of disc herniation is resolution. There is very poor correlation between imaging findings of disc herniation and the clinical presentation or course. Psychosocial factors predict functional disability due to disc herniation better than imaging. Imaging with MRI, computed tomography (CT), or CT myelography can readily identify central canal, lateral recess, or foraminal compromise. Only when an imaging finding is concordant with the patient's pain pattern or neurologic deficit can causation be considered. The zygapophysial (facet) and sacroiliac joint are thought to be responsible for axial back pain, although with less frequency than the disc. Imaging findings of the structural changes of osteoarthritis do not correlate with pain production. Physiologic imaging, either with single-photon emission CT bone scan, heavily T2-weighted MRI sequences (short-tau inversion recovery), or gadolinium enhancement, can detect inflammation and are more predictive of an axial pain generator.

Alexius E.G. Sandoval

Low back pain with radiating pain to the hip, buttock, or limb is the most common reason for electrodiagnostics referral. Electrodiagnostics is used to assess for lumbosacral radiculopathy potentially underlying low back pain. It serves as an extension of the clinical history and physical examination, and complements neuroimaging. Common low back pathologies amenable to electrodiagnostic evaluation include lumbosacral disk herniation and spinal stenosis. Electrodiagnostics may aid in the decision-making process when considering surgical management, and may aid in patient selection. The usefulness of electrodiagnostics is maximized when performed for the appropriate patient, and when the findings are properly interpreted.

The determination of whether a patient should pursue an active or passive treatment program is often made by medical practitioners. Knowledge about all forms of treatment, including complementary and alternative (CAM) treatments, is essential in the treatment of low back pain. Medical practitioner-directed active treatments that have been shown to be effective for the treatment of low back pain include physical therapy-directed exercise programs such as core stabilization and mechanical diagnosis and therapy (MDT). Based on the current literature, it appears that yoga is the most effective nonphysician-directed active treatment approach to nonspecific low back pain when comparing other CAM treatments. Acupuncture is a medical practitioner-directed passive treatment that has been shown to be a good adjunct treatment. More randomized controlled studies are needed to support both CAM treatments and exercise in the treatment of low back pain.

Analgesic medications are commonly used for low back pain (LBP). Evidence on the efficacy of pharmacologic therapy for LBP comes from clinical trials that have many limitations, including short-term studies and selective trial populations. Evidence currently supports the use of short-term pharmacologic treatment for LBP. However, the safety and efficacy of long-term pharmacologic therapy for LBP is uncertain and therefore best used with caution, monitoring, and as one component of a comprehensive paincare approach emphasizing rehabilitation.

Psychosocial factors are at least as important as biomedical factors in the onset, maintenance, and treatment of chronic low back pain. This article reviews some of the common psychosocial factors that influence the course of pain from acute to chronic status, cognitive behavioral interventions used to alter dysfunctional pain cognitions, and avoidance behaviors and the emotional distress that can accompany pain and pose barriers to recovery. The interplay of cognitive, emotional, behavioral, biomedical, and social factors is described using a fear avoidance model. Interdisciplinary pain rehabilitation is discussed as an effective option for more biopsychosocially complex patients.

The commonly performed spinal procedures, such as epidural injections, spinal nerve blocks, zygapophysial joint (z-joint) interventions, and discography, are reported to be safe. However, diagnostic and therapeutic spinal interventions can lead to serious complications, although their incidence seems to be low. Knowledge of potential complications is still required to minimize risks. This article describes the risks associated with the most commonly performed procedures, precautions that can be taken to minimize these risks, and treatment options available once complications have occurred.

Epidural steroid injection (ESI) has been used as a treatment for low back pain for over 50 years. In the last 10 to 15 years, there has been a significant increase in the use of ESIs for the treatment of low back pain and radicular pain without clear improvements in outcomes. Recent literature has focused on the use of ESIs as treatment for radicular pain associated with low back pain, with some studies showing benefit over control groups for limb symptoms. There is a lack of literature, however, to support the use of ESIs for the treatment of axial low back pain. The theoretical basis for their use, technical considerations, and the literature available for different approaches of access to the epidural space as pertaining to the treatment for low back pain without radiculopathy are reviewed.

The sacroiliac joint and the lumbar zygapophysial joints are both known pain generators with demonstrated pain-referral patterns. They are both amenable to image-guided intraarticular injection of corticosteroids, a procedure that is commonly performed for pain. The literature on the efficacy of intraarticular corticosteroid injections for these joints is currently limited. This article covers the diagnostic dilemmas associated with these joints, the utility of anesthetic blocks, and the literature on the efficacy of intraarticular corticosteroid injections.

Radiofrequency (RF) neurotomy is an interventional procedure used to alleviate certain types of low back pain. RF energy is used to thermally coagulate the specific nerves that transmit pain signals. Recent evidence has shown that this procedure demonstrates significant efficacy in relieving low back pain in lumbar zygapophysial joints, and research is ongoing to determine if pain relief for the sacroiliac joint is also possible. This article provides an evidence-based background for performing RF neurotomy, discusses the relevant anatomy, and highlights the indications and technique for lumbar and sacral RF neurotomy.

Spinal cord stimulation (SCS) and intrathecal drug delivery (IDD) are forms of neuromodulation, meaning that they are reversible and nondestructive. SCS is generally limited to conditions such as radiculopathy and pain of CNS orgin. IDD is primarily effective for nociceptive or mixed pain, and its usage is generally limited to conditions within that realm.

Alison Stout

Discography is a purely diagnostic interventional procedure performed to confirm or refute the hypothesis that a specific lumbar disc is the predominant source of a patient's low back pain. In patients with severe low back pain, unresponsive to conservative care, discography is used when clinical evaluation suggests that the pain is emanating from the intervertebral disc and other sources of pain have been ruled out. The evidence for its use remains controversial. There is variability and subjectivity in discography techniques and diagnostic criteria, making some investigators question its validity. When standardized diagnostic criteria are used, however, the specificity of discography improves dramatically. Recently long-term side effects have been studied, and lumbar discography seems to increase disc degeneration and herniation as detected on magnetic resonance imaging. Although the clinical significance is unclear, it is an important risk to consider prior to performing discography, and changes in discography techniques may be indicated. Discography remains the only technique, however, that can be used to determine whether a patient's low back pain is emanating from the intervertebral disc and is a valid test when coupled with careful patient selection, strict adherence to standardized technique and diagnostic criteria, and consideration of possible long-term sequelae.

Nayna Patel

Osteoporosis is the most common metabolic bone disorder. Vertebral compression fractures (VCFs) are a significant cause of back pain. Pain after VCF can be attributed to incomplete healing and progressive collapse of the bone. Conservative management has been the historical treatment option for patients with painful percutaneous vertebroplasties (PVs). Although seemingly harmless, conservative treatment can be risky for elderly patients suffering from VCFs. PV can be used to treat VCFs in some patients. The exact mechanism of pain relief by vertebroplasty is not understood; the pain relief is probably because of improved vertebral body strength and stiffness and decreasing motion of the vertebral body and periosteal and interosseous nerves. But, PV is not without risks. Therefore, until further studies show that PV is superior to conservative treatment, with equivalent complications profile, PV should be reserved for patients who have failed conservative treatment.

THE CLINICS ARE NOW AVAILABLE ONLINE!
Access your subscription at:
www.theclinics.com

Foreword
Low Back Pain

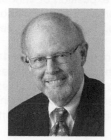

George H. Kraft, MD, MS
Consulting Editor

Who of you reading this issue of *Physical Medicine and Rehabilitation Clinics of North America* has not had low back pain (LBP) at one time or another?

I suspect that the true answer is that all of you have had at least one episode of LBP. You are the lucky ones. There is a strong likelihood that the majority of you have had at least several episodes, and some may even qualify as being in that unfortunate group of chronic LBP sufferers.

For all of you, then, this issue of *Physical Medicine and Rehabilitation Clinics of North America* will have a different meaning than many other *Clinics* issues; contrasted to issues discussing more uncommon medical problems, this issue covers familiar territory. Although familiar, there are many new concepts discussed within this red cover. Indeed, that exemplifies the purpose of these *Clinics*: to present a "living textbook" that can frequently be updated, but yet as easily referenced as is any medical text. The *Physical Medicine and Rehabilitation Clinics of North America* is, in essence, a textbook with many chapters that stay updated.

It is not an easy task to present familiar material in new ways, and I want to thank Dr Allison Stout for taking this on. Not only did she agree to Guest Edit this issue, she excelled in the role. Being a Guest Editor is not an easy job, and I heard from at least one author that she really kept on top of this project. For those of you who may have had some experience in editing or writing for a textbook, you know that the date of publication is typically extended a year or more later than the initial date. Article authors not uncommonly view *Clinics* articles in the same way, so it is no small achievement for a GE to keep a project on time. Dr Stout did a superb job of this, allowing us to bring to you a comprehensive, 16-article issue on LBP that can stand alone as a contemporary manual for the evaluation and conservative management of this common disorder.

This issue is organized into a logical sequence of three sections: first, anatomy and physiology; then, diagnostic techniques; and finally, the last section dealing with nonsurgical treatment. Dr Stout has selected 19 expert practitioners and teachers to contribute to these 16 articles.

Phys Med Rehabil Clin N Am 21 (2010) xi–xii
doi:10.1016/j.pmr.2010.08.004

pmr.theclinics.com

The first section starts with the epidemiology of LBP. It then moves on to discuss the anatomy and pathophysiology of the lumbar discs, posterior elements, and the sacroiliac joints. Following this is an article reviewing current concepts of myofascial pain.

The diagnostic section is next and presents an up-to-date exposition of various imaging and electrodiagnostic techniques. This back-to-back presentation of pathologic anatomy and physiologic dysfunction emphasizes the importance and complementary value of these two important diagnostic tools.

The last two thirds of this issue, dealing with management of LBP, consist of 11 articles. The first article in this section outlines conservative management techniques and details exercises and alternative treatments. Pharmacologic management is then discussed, followed by a discussion of the psychological issues frequently encountered in LBP. Thereafter follows a review of the interplay of psychosocial issues with chronic LBP.

The final part of the treatment section first reviews the attendant risks of interventional techniques. Next, injections are discussed: first epidural and then sacroiliac and zygapophysial joints. Radiofrequency neurotomy is then presented.

The 13th articles then turns to interventional management of chronic LBP, and the next two articles analyze discography and percutaneous vertebroplasty. The issue concludes with a well-balanced article by Dr Stout analyzing the various therapeutic interventions in axial LBP.

I know that readers who treat LBP will find this self-contained issue of *Physical Medicine and Rehabilitation Clinics of North America* a "must-have" for your examining room. My thanks go to Dr Stout and her selected article authors for all of their efforts in creating this valuable issue.

George H. Kraft, MD, MS
Department of Rehabilitation Medicine
University of Washington
1959 NE Pacific Street, RJ-30
Seattle, WA 98195, USA

E-mail address:
ghkraft@uw.edu

Preface
Low Back Pain

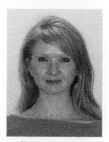

Alison Stout, DO
Guest Editor

Despite advances in science and technology, the incidence and severity of low back pain have not improved and its socioeconomic burden has increased. The number and type of nonsurgical treatments continue to grow with a relative lack of understanding of the best practice and standards for employing these treatments. The utilization of limited health care resources for the treatment of low back pain is of interest to patients, physicians, insurance companies, policymakers, and lawyers; all of whom may have different and competing goals. This Physical Medicine and Rehabilitation Clinics issue aims to help practitioners understand the different etiologies of low back pain and the evidence for various nonsurgical treatments available from a biomechanical model, while considering neuropsychological, behavioral, and sociological influences.

Alison Stout, DO
Rehabilitation Care Services
Veterans Administration Puget Sound HCS
1660 South Columbian Way
Seattle, WA 98108, USA

Department of Rehabilitation
University of Washington
1959 NE Pacific Street
Seattle, WA 98195, USA

E-mail address:
stouta@uw.edu

Phys Med Rehabil Clin N Am 21 (2010) xiii
doi:10.1016/j.pmr.2010.08.005
1047-9651/10/$ – see front matter © 2010 Elsevier Inc. All rights reserved.

pmr.theclinics.com

Epidemiology of Spine Care: The Back Pain Dilemma

Janna Friedly, MD[a],*, Christopher Standaert, MD[b],
Leighton Chan, MD, MPH[c]

KEYWORDS

• Low back pain • Epidemiology • Low back pain treatments
• Low back pain outcomes • Spine interventions

Spine-related disorders are among the most frequently encountered problems in clinical medicine. Low back pain (LBP) alone affects up to 80% of the population at some point in life, and 1% to 2% of the United States adult population is disabled because of LBP.[1,2] The substantial need for care of these patients, coupled with our poor understanding of the fundamental basis of LBP in many individuals, has led to an ever-expanding array of treatment options, including medications, manipulative care, percutaneous interventional spine procedures, and an increasing repertoire of surgical approaches.[3] The estimated total cost of direct medical expenditures in the United States for spine care in 2006 was more than $85 billion, and the data suggest that the use and costs of spine care have been increasing at an alarming rate in recent years.[4,5] Self-reported health status among people with spine problems (including physical functioning, mental health, work, and social limitations) does not seem to be improving, and the overall numbers of people seeking Social Security Disability Insurance for spine-related problems and the percentage of people with disability caused by musculoskeletal pain are increasing.[4] Complication rates, including deaths, associated with treatments for spinal pain are also increasing.[3,4,6,7] The statistics are concerning and raise a fundamental question: are spine problems worsening over time or are we simply using an increasing number of costly treatments that are not effective?

Valuable insights into this question can be obtained by examining the available epidemiologic data on spinal pain and treatment. This article addresses in particular the epidemiologic data on percutaneous and surgical spinal procedures and examines

[a] Department of Rehabilitation Medicine, University of Washington, 325 Ninth Avenue, Seattle, WA 98104, USA
[b] University of Washington Sports and Spine Physicians, Box 359721, 325 Ninth Avenue, Seattle, WA 98104, USA
[c] Rehabilitation Medicine Department, Clinical Center, National Institutes of Health, Building 10, Room 1-1469 10 Center Drive, MSC 1604, Bethesda, MD 20892-1604, USA
* Corresponding author.
E-mail address: friedlyj@uw.edu

Phys Med Rehabil Clin N Am 21 (2010) 659–677
doi:10.1016/j.pmr.2010.08.002
1047-9651/10/$ – see front matter © 2010 Elsevier Inc. All rights reserved.

national trends in the use of noninterventional treatments such as physical therapy and exercise programs, and opioid medications. The costs associated with these treatments, the potential risks, and the overall effect on the quality of care provided to persons with spine problems in the United States are also examined.

PREVALENCE OF LBP

Despite the vast amount of research devoted to LBP, the epidemiology of this condition is not well understood, and the overall prevalence of LBP in the United States is unclear. There are several techniques for estimating the prevalence of spine problems, including survey techniques as well as the use of medical billing claims data. Each method has its strengths and weaknesses. Retrospective surveys obtain information directly from affected individuals but may be subject to recall bias. Claims-based data may avoid this limitation and are not dependent on individual reporting but detect only those subjects whose physicians coded for back pain associated with a given episode of care in the office. Additional challenges arise from heterogeneity in many other aspects of published studies, including the definitions of LBP that are used. The varying methodologies often lead to different patient groups being studied, which can be problematic from clinical and policy perspectives. Based on health care use data (ie, people who present to a health care provider for care for LBP), the prevalence estimates for LBP are as low as 12% to 15%.[8] However, estimates from self-report survey data on the prevalence of LBP range from 28% to 40% of the population depending on the methodology used.[8,9]

Given the difficulty associated with accurately estimating the prevalence of LBP at any specific time, it seems apparent that there are also difficulties with assessing changes in prevalence over time. A recent study reported telephone survey data collected in 1992 and again in 2006 from a sample in North Carolina indicating that the prevalence of chronic, disabling LBP rose significantly during that time frame, increasing from 3.9% of the population in 1992 to 10.2% in 2006.[10] Although this study was not designed to address causation, the investigators suggest that increasing rates of obesity, depression, or other psychosocial factors may explain this increase in LBP prevalence. Claims-based data seem to indicate a smaller increase in prevalence. The percentage of people presenting to physician offices for LBP steadily, but only slightly, increased from 12% in 1998 to 15% in 2004 (**Fig. 1**). Although both sets of data could suggest that the overall prevalence of LBP is increasing, it is difficult to tell to what degree these changes represents a true increase in the proportion of the population suffering from LBP versus a change in the propensity of people to either report or seek care for low back complaints. If it is the latter, this situation may represent evolving societal beliefs about pain rather than a change in the number of people who suffer from LBP.

The uncertainty regarding a potential increase in the prevalence of LBP in the US population becomes relevant when analyzing the array of data indicating escalating rates of use of health care services related to LBP. Is the increase in use due to an increase in the relative number of patients with pain, an increase in the percentage of those with pain seeking and/or receiving care, or, as was suggested in recent data from Martin and colleagues,[4] an increase in the per-patient use of care? These questions are important when considering the policy and care implications because the answers speak to the efficacy of, and hence necessity for, specific treatments. Given the available data, the answer is likely that the increasing use rates represent a combination of factors including an increased prevalence of chronic LBP, changes in the treatments used, and changes in societal beliefs regarding pain.

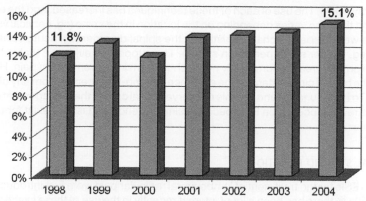

Fig. 1. Percentage of the US population with LBP. (*From* Katz S, editor. The burden of musculoskeletal diseases in the United States. Rosemont (IL): Bone and Joint Decade, American Academy of Orthopaedic Surgeons; 2008. Copyright © 2008 American Academy of Orthopedic Surgeons; *Modified* with permission from The Burden of Musculoskeletal Diseases in the United States. Source of data: National Center for Health Statistics, National Ambulatory Medical Care Survey, 1998–2004.)

THE USE OF INTERVENTIONAL SPINE PROCEDURES

Interventional spine procedures have been used for many decades for a variety of spinal disorders and range from percutaneous injections to surgery. For a variety of reasons, there has been a recent proliferation in the number of techniques available for use and marked increases in the use rates for many of the procedures. Percutaneous interventions include epidural steroid injections (ESIs) via several different approaches, facet/zygapophysial joint (z-joint) procedures, spinal cord stimulation, several intradiscal procedures, and, more recently, procedures intended to remove disc or other material in the spinal canal or to obtain segmental fusion. Surgical procedures range from well-established approaches for discectomy and/or spinal canal decompression to multiple means of addressing segmental fusion using several different approaches, materials, instruments, and indications. However, the evidence to support the use of many of these procedures is limited.

From the surgical perspective, there are sound data on the efficacy of discectomy for acute radicular pain associated with a disc herniation, decompressive laminectomy for symptomatic spinal stenosis, and fusion for degenerative spondylolisthesis in well-selected patients.[11–16] However, selecting appropriate candidates for surgery can be challenging because of variability in diagnosis and characterizing clinical and radiographic characteristics of these conditions. In addition, the clinical benefit of surgery even in well-selected patients can wane, and many patients may do just as well long-term with more conservative options.[17,18] The data on the efficacy of surgery for isolated LBP are more suspect, and there are many additional patients in whom surgical procedures are either not indicated or contraindicated because of other issues.[17,19] Surgical care also may carry significant risks and costs.[11,20,21]

Because the role of surgery is limited for the larger population of patients with low back pain, there is a need for less invasive options. As noted earlier, several percutaneous procedures for spinal disorders have been developed and are frequently used clinically, most with limited scientific evidence of efficacy. The most commonly used and studied procedures of this type are ESIs, followed in frequency by z-joint procedures, which include intraarticular injections, medial branch blocks, and radiofrequency neurotomy (RFN). The use of each of these techniques has increased, and the evidence to support their use varies depending on the location in the spine (eg, cervical vs lumbar spine) as well as specific characteristics of the spinal disorder (eg, acute sciatica) and patient (eg, worker's compensation status). The supportive evidence that is available for these procedures predominantly notes short-term improvements in pain. However, even in the best of circumstances the evidence for long-term benefit from any of these is lacking. To better understand the role of interventional care in the management of spinal pain, this review focuses on ESIs because similar trends and issues exist for the other procedures.

EPIDURAL STEROID INJECTIONS

Although ESIs for the treatment of lumbosacral radicular pain were first introduced in the early 1950s,[22] there has been a lot of interest recently in the use of these injections as an alternative to more invasive surgical procedures for treating spinal pain. Since the introduction pf ESIs, many investigators have examined them for the treatment of lumbosacral radiculopathy as well as axial (nonradicular) spinal pain syndromes.[23–33] Although most studies have addressed the use of ESIs for isolated lumbosacral radiculopathy resulting from discogenic or other causes, some investigators have advocated their use for more diffuse symptoms associated with lumbar spinal stenosis.[34–36] The current literature reports success rates of 18% to 90% for ESIs, depending on methodology, outcome measures, patient selection, and technique.[37] Some studies,[23,32,38] but not all,[30,33,39] have found that ESIs can offer short-term pain reduction to a select group of patients, but there is little evidence of long-term improvement in pain or function.[39–42] Given the overall spectrum of treatment approaches available for spinal pain, short-term pain relief can offer significant clinical benefits in appropriate circumstances, and this seems to be the primary beneficial effect of ESIs advocated by many investigators.

Several studies have attempted to examine the influence of ESIs on the subsequent need for lumbar surgery as an outcome measure. The results have been mixed. An initial prospective randomized controlled trial (RCT) by Riew and colleagues[27] reported that a significantly higher proportion of patients receiving transforaminal ESIs with anesthetic and corticosteroid opted not to have surgery compared with a control group receiving similar procedures with anesthetic alone. This study followed patients for up to 2 years after the first injection. However, in a separate report on 5-year follow-up of the same patients, there were no differences between the treatment and control groups in terms of lumbar surgery.[38] A significant percentage of the treatment group was lost to follow-up for this study, making it difficult to draw any definitive conclusions from these data. A more recent study by Schaufele and colleagues[43] in 2006 compared interlaminar versus transforaminal ESIs for persons with chronic LBP who had failed other conservative treatments. In this retrospective case-control study of 40 patients, the investigators found that 2 (10%) of the patients receiving transforaminal ESIs and 5 (25%) of the patients receiving interlaminar ESIs underwent subsequent lumbar surgery within 1 year after the initial injection. Follow-up beyond 1 year was not reported for these patients. Although the sample size in this study is small, this study is representative of the type of evidence available. Overall, the data indicating a significant effect of ESIs on surgical rates are not robust.

Some limited data are available on the cost-effectiveness of ESIs. Price and colleagues[40] performed an RCT of ESIs in the United Kingdom and concluded that they did not meet the national guidelines for cost-effectiveness, specifically noting that "ESIs do not provide good value for money." The investigators believed that further research is needed to compare alternative treatments for LBP and to identify subgroups of patients who might benefit more from ESIs. One drawback of this study is that it was performed in the United Kingdom, where there is a national health service, so it is unclear how applicable their cost analysis is to the US population. To date, there have been no cost-effectiveness studies of ESIs or other interventional pain procedures in the United States.

Regardless of which outcome is considered, one of the biggest challenges in interpreting the literature regarding the efficacy or effectiveness of ESIs is the paucity of high-quality RCTs. A recent survey of the published literature shows that there have been 18 RCTs of ESIs compared with placebo or control treatment for a variety of LBP conditions in the last 25 years. Most of these studies have serious methodological failings that limit their usefulness, including the lack of routine fluoroscopic guidance for injections in any study published before 2000. During this same period, there have been 78 systematic reviews of ESIs, with divergent conclusions based on critical review of the same studies. Although isolated investigators have believed the data support the use of ESIs for specific populations, several more thorough reviews point to the limited or absent data on long-term pain relief or functional improvement associated with these procedures.[44,45] The most recent Cochrane review on the subject takes issue with the entire spectrum of percutaneous spine procedures, concluding "there is insufficient evidence to support the use of injection therapy in subacute and chronic low-back pain."[45]

Despite the ambiguities in the data supporting ESIs, these procedures have developed widespread acceptance and are used with increasing frequency as a treatment of radiculopathy and other LBP disorders.[46] In the United States, the use rates for ESIs of all types are escalating dramatically. In one analysis of Medicare claims from 1994 to 2001, there was a nearly 3-fold increase in ESI rates (**Fig. 2**) and a 7-fold increase in subsequent reimbursed costs.[47] These rates outpace the growth in the Medicare population in that time frame as well as the estimated increase in the prevalence of persons with LBP.[8] Similar findings were noted in a study by Carrino and colleagues,[46] also using Medicare claims data. The data from these studies do not offer insight into the cause of the increasing rates for ESIs, but this may be related to several possible factors such as expanding clinical usefulness, cultural changes, or socioeconomic issues.

UNDERSTANDING THE INCREASE IN USE

One of the more optimistic explanations available for the disproportionately escalating rate of ESI use could be improvements in health care delivery, including more effective management of spinal pain in the general population. If these improvements are

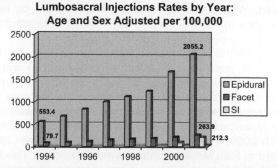

Lumbosacral Injections Rates by Year: Age and Sex Adjusted per 100,000

2055.2

553.4

263.9

79.7

212.3

☐ Epidural
■ Facet
☐ SI

1994   1996   1998   2000

Fig. 2. Cumulative number of ESI systematic reviews and RCTs. (*From* Friedly J, Chan L, Deyo R. Increases in lumbosacral injections in the Medicare population: 1994 to 2001. Spine 2007;32(16):1756.)

occurring, improvements in measures of health or disability or a decrease in rates of surgical intervention for specific spine problems might be expected. The available data do not seem to indicate that this is the case. Paradoxically, measures of spine health in the United States show declines in recent years, and surgical rates for the treatment of degenerative spine problems have been dramatically increasing.[48,49] When specifically looking at the effect of ESIs on surgical rates, Medicare claims data suggest that the performance of these procedures is positively associated with higher surgical rates rather than falling rates. In addition, epidemiologic studies have shown that the total number of people receiving ESIs who subsequently undergo lumbar surgery is increasing, as is the proportion of people undergoing surgery who have received ESIs.[47,50] This particularly seems to be the case in areas of the country that have higher overall rates of injections.[50] A study conducted using national Veteran's Administration (VA) data on more than 13,000 individuals also showed that those who underwent more than 3 ESIs during a 2-year period were at increased risk of undergoing subsequent surgery compared with those who received 3 or fewer.[50] Although none of these data indicate that performing ESIs increases surgical rates, they do not support the argument that ESIs (especially greater than 3 in the same patient) are substituting for lumbar surgery on a large-scale basis. Taken as an aggregate, these studies raise serious questions as to our ability to lower the need for surgery through the use of ESIs, which, along with pain reduction, is one of the prime benefits cited by many advocates of these procedures.

An additional surrogate measure to consider as an indicator of the broader health effect of ESIs is the use of opioid pain medications for those undergoing spinal procedures. As is the case with spinal injections and surgery, epidemiologic data indicate that opioid use in the United States is increasing at an alarming rate and that complications/deaths associated with opioid use (both prescribed and recreational/illicit use) are increasing.[6,7,51,52] Although there are no data to indicate a causal relationship between the increase in interventional procedures for back pain and the use of opioid medications, one might hope that there would be evidence of a reduction in opiate use following ESIs. The data available are not supportive of this idea, either. An epidemiologic study performed within the VA system over a 2-year period showed no reduction in the use of opioids after ESI.[50] Most people in this study were using opioids both before and after the intervention (64% vs 67%).[50] This study did not determine the indication for the use of opioid medications in these patients and was not an RCT, both of which pose limitations on interpretation of the data. However, that there was no evidence of a reduction in opioid use raises the concern that in clinical practice the use of injections may not be associated with a significant decrease in opioid use as would be expected. When considered with the information on health status and surgical rates, the data make it difficult to argue that the expanding use of ESIs is accounting for major improvements in health outcomes.

Other explanations for the changes seen in use rates for ESIs may be found in more socioeconomic factors, such as alterations in the distribution and numbers of the providers who are performing the procedures. In the last 10 years, interventional pain management has blossomed, including a substantial increase in the number of fellowships offered (usually either anesthesiology or physical medicine and rehabilitation [PM&R]). The American Board of Pain Management began board certification in 2000. As of March 2009, more than 2200 physicians had been board certified by the American Board of Pain Medicine (http://www.abpm.org/). This figure represents approximately 16% of the total number of providers board certified in PM&R and anesthesiology in the same period according to statistics from the American Board of Medical Specialties. In one study on geographic variations of ESI use, ESI rates strongly correlated with the number of providers performing these procedures in a given area ($r = 0.79$, $P<.001$), suggesting that the supply of physicians who perform injections may be a significant factor in the increase in ESI use.[53] The influx of specialists board certified in interventional pain care and the increasing role of PM&R in interventional spine care could thus be major contributors to the increase in interventional pain procedures being performed. Some have argued that board certification programs and improved training in pain management have led to improvements in the quality of care provided for persons suffering from chronic pain and that the increase in the number of procedures being performed is partially in response to a previously unmet need. However, given the foregoing discussion it has yet to be shown that the increase in supply of board-certified physicians and the treatments provided has made a substantial difference in the functioning, quality of life, or pain levels of people with chronic LBP.

Another socioeconomic issue potentially affecting the use of ESIs is the growth of physician-owned ambulatory surgical centers (ASCs) in the United States. ASCs are freestanding facilities designed specifically for outpatient surgical procedures that do not require an overnight or inpatient hospital admission. The number of Medicare-certified ASCs increased by more than 60% from 2000 to 2007, totaling nearly 5000 across the United States. During this time, Medicare payments for services provided at ASCs more than doubled, from $1.4 billion to $2.9 billion.[54] Ninety-five percent of Medicare-certified ASCs are privately owned, for-profit businesses, most of which are owned by local physician investors. The Stark self-referral law, established in 1989 to ensure that economic conflicts of interest do not drive up use, does not apply to ASCs, making it possible for physicians to refer their own patients to the ASCs with which they may have financial relationships. By delivering care in these centers, physician investors can increase practice revenues by receiving facility fees that often are larger than the professional fees they receive for the procedures. This type of arrangement may affect physician behavior by creating financial conflicts of interest for physicians practicing in ASCs and potentially increase use rates for various forms of interventional care. In support of this concept, there are data on imaging and spine surgery rates to suggest that financial incentives associated with physician-owned facilities may alter physician practice patterns.[55,56]

In addition to financial interests, there are several legitimate potential reasons why a variety of procedures may be performed in ASCs as opposed to other locations such as hospitals and physician offices. Included in these reasons are the possibility of improved outcomes related to specialized staffing, more efficient protocols, dedicated equipment, better customer service, and the presence of more convenient locations with shorter wait times than hospital settings.[57] Although the Center for Medicare and Medicaid Services (CMS) examines cost and use trends to determine the appropriate reimbursement for procedures performed at ASCs, there have been few published data comparing outcomes for procedures performed in these settings with those in more traditional hospital settings[57,58] and none examining interventional pain procedures for back pain.

These issues are of concern because, although interventional spine procedures can be performed in physician offices, ASCs, or outpatient hospital settings, there are some data to suggest that an increasing percentage are being performed at ASCs.[59] ESIs are one of the most frequently performed procedures at ASCs, outpaced only by colonoscopies/endoscopies and cataract surgeries.[60] This situation may be related to increased physician reimbursement for procedures performed at these sites compared with offices or outpatient hospitals, particularly when accounting for facility fees captured by physician ASC owners as dividends.[61,62] These data leave open the idea that financial incentives for providers performing ESIs in physician-owned facilities may be a significant driver of use rates.

When looking at the totality of the published data on ESIs, a concern is that the increase in their use is more related to economic factors than to clinical ones. Although the rates of ESIs and other interventional spine procedures are expanding rapidly, there is no evidence of broad societal or clinical benefits. There is some literature indicating short-term improvements in pain after ESIs, but the literature base is replete with numerous systematic reviews built on a paucity of well-designed RCTs. More data are needed on indications, patient selection, frequency, route of administration, and cost-effectiveness to establish the true clinical usefulness of these procedures. Considering the state of the literature alongside the societal need and desire to use nonsurgical treatment options and the economic factors related to physician supply and reimbursement, it becomes difficult to argue that the primary impetus behind the recent increased use of ESIs and other spinal procedures is clinical usefulness.

ADDITIONAL PERCUTANEOUS INTERVENTIONAL SPINE PROCEDURES
Z-joint Injections and RFN

There are fewer epidemiologic data examining the use of z-joint intraarticular steroid injections and RFN (ie, radiofrequency ablation of the z-joint medial branch nerve) than there are for ESIs. There is good evidence to indicate that z-joints are potential sources of back pain.[63–66] Injection of these joints with corticosteroids, as is performed for many peripheral joints, is believed to have the potential to transiently relieve pain. In addition, these joints are innervated by the medial branches of the lumbar dorsal rami, and these nerves are targets for nerve blocks using anesthetics, steroid medications, or RFN, the latter of which may result in destruction of the nerves believed to convey pain from the joints.

Similar to the situation for ESIs, the literature on z-joint procedures is underwhelming. Most studies on intraarticular z-joint injections have been unable to convincingly show significant benefit for LBP, although optimizing patient selection is challenging and the overall quality of these studies is limited. There is some evidence to suggest that RFN of the medial branches may provide pain relief in highly selected patients.[67–70] Although there are ardent advocates for these procedures, recent reviews are not supportive, with Chou and colleagues[17] noting that "insufficient evidence exists to reliably validate" RFN. Despite the equivocal evidence to support their use, z-joint procedures are being used with increasing frequency.[46,47] For example, Medicare payments for z-joint injections increased from $141 million in 2003 to $307 million in 2006 (Office of Inspector General report, September 2008) and the number of claims during that period increased by 78%. Because of the lack of evidence to support the use of lumbar z-joint injections as well as concerns regarding the percentage of injections billed inappropriately (including overbilling for bilateral procedures because of coding and documentation errors), there has recently been intensive review of coverage policies for z-joint injections and RFN. There are currently no published epidemiologic data on the use of radiofrequency ablation in the lumbar spine, and this needs to be further examined. The reactive stance of the payers to the data indicates the larger concern over the effectiveness and use of interventional spine procedures.

Emerging Techniques

There are several emerging interventional spine procedures. The role that many of these play in spine care is unclear. Perhaps the best way to address the future is to examine the past. A cautionary note on the broader spectrum of spinal procedures may be seen in the example of intradiscal electrothermal therapy (IDET). This procedure was developed and introduced in the 1990s as a less invasive alternative to fusion for discogenic back pain. The intent was to introduce a thermal coil into the annulus fibrosis of a painful lumbar disc and, through heating of the thermal coil, achieve pain relief via either collagenous remodeling or anular denervation (the exact mechanism of action was still theoretic at the time of clinical release).[71] The device used in this procedure (SpineCath produced by ORATEC, Inc, Menlo Park, CA) was approved as a 510-K device with only limited safety data to show its equivalence to a cautery probe previously approved by the US Food and Drug Administration (FDA). Once FDA approval was obtained for the device and preliminary data from small nonrandomized cohort studies funded by the manufacturer were published, IDET quickly gained popularity as a percutaneous spine intervention for discogenic pain. There was a great deal of enthusiasm for this procedure based on early studies, and its use increased dramatically in the 1990s and early 2000s. After these initial positive reports were published, the company that developed IDET and the SpineCath used for the procedure was sold to Smith & Nephew for considerable profit, and Smith & Nephew began a marketing campaign to advance the sales of the SpineCath used in IDET procedures. However, subsequently published RCTs on IDET were not so encouraging and failed to show anything other than perhaps a narrow benefit from the procedure.[72,73] Despite the increasing RCT evidence that IDET was not effective, 2 subsequent industry-sponsored systematic reviews were published that concluded that IDET was safe and effective for discogenic pain.[74,75] However, a nonindustry-sponsored systematic review did not identify any significant benefit of IDET. After a review of the available data and input from multiple medical specialty societies, CMS issued a noncoverage decision regarding IDET (http://www.cms.gov/). Consequently, the use of IDET has decreased and insurance coverage and reimbursement for this procedure have been limited dramatically. Despite the lack of evidence to show effectiveness and the resultant limitations on coverage for IDET, some providers still strongly advocate for the use of this procedure.[74,76]

The penetration of IDET into the clinical marketplace and its continued use despite lack of substantial evidence of benefit and lack of coverage by many insurers speaks both to the perceived need for effective and less invasive alternatives to surgical care for LBP and to some of the potential problems with patient expectations, financial incentives, and evidence dissemination or interpretation that may exist in the medical arena. Although some of the issues with IDET are particularly problematic, its story is emblematic of problems present throughout interventional spine care. The widespread clinical application of new techniques before the establishment of a sound physiologic rationale for their use, an appropriate safety profile, and evidence of efficacy in a clinically valid group of patients may be detrimental to patients, providers, and the financial stability of our health system.

The IDET story is not unique in interventional pain. There are several other spine interventions introduced into clinical practice with limited data whose effectiveness has subsequently been called into question by rigorous RCTs. Vertebroplasty is the most recent example. Vertebroplasty is a widely used spine intervention now under substantial scrutiny after the publication of 2 large RCTs that show no additional benefit to the procedure over sham or placebo intervention.[77,78]

Surgical Interventions

Given the epidemiology of LBP within the United States and the extraordinary health care costs associated with its treatment,[79,80] it is not surprising to find that rates of lumbar spine surgery, like those for spinal injections, are increasing dramatically.[48,49] The rates of spinal fusion, in particular, have been increasing rapidly. The Agency for Healthcare Research and Quality's Healthcare Cost and Usefulness Project reported up to a 40% increase in spinal fusions in the 7-year period from 1998 to 2004,[8] and Deyo and colleagues[81] recently reported that the rate of complex fusion procedures being performed for lumbar spinal stenosis increased 15-fold from 2002 to 2007. Data on discectomies and other spine surgeries also reflect an increase over time, although not to the same degree as for spinal fusions.[49] It is possible that discectomies and other less invasive spine procedures may be underreported in current data because many are being performed in outpatient settings and are thus not captured in analyses of the inpatient databases typically used to estimate spine surgery rates.[49] The advancing rates for lumbar fusion surgeries are troublesome because these procedures generally have less well-defined indications and less well-documented success rates than some of the procedures mentioned previously such as microdiscectomy. In addition, fusion procedures are associated with increased costs, complications, and reoperation rates when compared with less complex surgical approaches. As with ESIs, there is no clear answer in the medical literature as to why the rates of lumbar fusion are escalating in such a disproportionate manner to other surgical approaches to the spine, but some of this is likely related to the availability of numerous new technologies and approaches to attaining fusion, many of which, like IDET, have entered the clinical arena without substantial data on clinical superiority over existing techniques.

Physical Therapy and Exercise Programs

The use of physical therapy and other specific exercise programs for back pain has also been controversial. Although there is strong evidence to suggest that staying active and engaging in physical activity can reduce disability associated with back pain,[82] there are conflicting data regarding the clinical effectiveness as well as the cost-effectiveness of physical therapy in chronic LBP.[83] One recent study suggested that adherence to an early physical therapy program in people with acute LBP was associated with lower subsequent health care costs.[84] Another study using the Medicare claims database determined that early physical therapy after a first visit to a doctor for LBP is associated with decreased subsequent health care use (emergency department visits, ESIs, surgery).[85] However, a recent systematic review of the cost-usefulness of physical therapy found that only 54% of the studies showed a net benefit in terms of cost, whereas the remainder found no benefit to physical therapy.[83]

Several difficulties are associated with studying the efficacy of physical therapy and exercise programs for LBP, including the variability in treatment protocols and patient characteristics within and between studies. Defining clinical subgroups for study has also been challenging, and there is no widely accepted method of distinguishing between many individuals with LBP in any meaningful way for research purposes. Numerous studies on exercise and LBP apply multifaceted treatment programs to what are likely widely heterogeneous groups of patients, frequently showing unimpressive results. Given the complexities associated with this topic, these studies are also frequently methodologically challenged and underpowered. Although positive benefits of physical therapy interventions for LBP have been reported, one systematic review found that only one-third of studies on this topic reporting positive outcomes showed clinically significant changes in addition to statistically significant changes.[86] In general, it has been difficult to determine if any one physical therapy protocol is more effective than others, and there is still controversy about the overall usefulness of physical therapy treatments for LBP.

There are scant data on the changes in use of physical therapy. A large cross-sectional survey study in 2006 reported that use of physical therapy to treat LBP is common, with 30% of people with LBP reporting being seen by a physical therapist, with an average of 21 visits per person per year.[87] In this sample population, use of passive modalities such as transcutaneous electrical nerve stimulation units, corsets, traction, electrostimulation, and ultrasound, all of which have limited data on efficacy, were more common than better-studied structured rehabilitation or exercise-based programs.[87] Limited data suggest that the use of physical therapy is increasing, but at a slower rate than other available treatments.[5] This is a topic that will likely come under increasing scrutiny as the drive toward evidence-based medicine and cost-effectiveness analysis continues.

Opioid Use

The safety and efficacy of opioids for treatment of nonmalignant pain, particularly chronic spinal pain, is another controversial topic. Some clinicians advocate the use of opioids in this setting as a pain relief strategy,[88] whereas others strongly oppose their use. Opioid use among persons with chronic LBP is common. Survey data from the late 1990s on more than 20,000 individuals revealed that about 12% of those with back pain had received prescriptions for opioids.[80] Data from the Medicaid system in the United States showed that overall opiate use increased by 309% from 1992 to 2002.[89]

Concerns regarding opioid use for chronic LBP arise from issues related to the potential for abuse, a possible lack of effectiveness, and the high rates of concurrent mental illness in those with chronic LBP. A recent systematic review of opioid use in the setting of chronic pain suggested a lifetime prevalence of substance abuse of 36% to 56% among those using prescription opiates, with up to 24% of patients inappropriately taking their opioid medications.[90] In addition, a meta-analysis of the available study data showed a nonsignificant difference in pain relief comparing those taking opioids and those not taking opioids.[90] The quality of the available studies is suboptimal and there are few data on the long-term efficacy of opioids for chronic pain. Despite the limitations of the data on the direct clinical benefit of opiates for LBP, a large survey has shown that patients who were prescribed opioids at their last office visit for back pain were more satisfied with their care and less likely to seek care from additional providers than those not prescribed opioids.[91]

Further complicating the picture of opiate use are recent data indicating that people taking opioids for back pain were more likely to have underlying depression, anxiety, and other comorbid medical conditions.[92] These findings suggest that there may be factors associated with opioid use that are unrelated to the severity or specific cause of back pain but more related to broader physical and mental health issues. Given the strong relationship between chronic LBP and psychosocial factors such as depression, anxiety, and somatization,[93-98] effective treatment of this problem often necessitates a multimodal approach that encompasses the full scope of comorbidities associated with chronic spinal pain. The concept that addressing the psychological state of the individual with LBP is an important component of care is supported by a large literature base on operative and nonoperative therapies.[99,100]

Reliance on the use of opiates to manage chronic LBP raises many of the same issues seen in the previous discussions on interventional spine care. There is increasing concern that the shift in training of providers has led to an increasing number of interventionalists who perform only interventional procedures without addressing underlying mental health issues or other psychosocial factors associated with chronic back pain that may influence outcomes and health care use. Successful administration of opioid medications in those with spinal pain may depend on using these medications in a comprehensive framework that addresses the biopsychosocial nature of the problem.

DISCUSSION

Individuals with LBP are receiving an increasing number of interventional treatments for pain without any available evidence to support a substantial overall improvement in functional status. This situation presents a challenging dilemma for health care providers. There is a vast and ever-expanding array of potential treatment options for LBP, many of which have some evidence of efficacy in select patients but none of which has offered long-term benefit for most patients with LBP. There are many difficulties with patient selection, and it is often unclear which patients respond to which treatments. Nonetheless, it seems that patient demand for services to address LBP is increasing, and there may be shifts in societal belief systems that create unrealistic expectations of improvement from focused interventions. The conflict between the level of patient demand and the level of evidence for various care options for LBP often leaves physicians obligated to provide treatment recommendations based on an insufficient database. Entering this care environment is an increasing supply of physicians trained in the delivery of interventional spine care, and several economic factors seem to provide incentives for them to perform these procedures with greater frequency. The result is a system that increasingly emphasizes the performance of narrowly focused and insufficiently studied procedures to address what are likely complex biopsychosocial pain problems.

The outcome of this is not good from the perspective of the individual or the society as a whole. Given the increasing health care costs associated with interventions for LBP, and the subsequent scrutiny of third-party payers, we are facing an extremely important crossroads in the care of people with chronic LBP. If we are going to identify the optimal treatment modalities for patients with LBP and show the value in our care, we must invest in high-quality outcomes research and clinical trials to determine which treatments are effective for which subsets of patients. It is imperative that we carefully examine each patient individually and determine a rational, evidence-based approach to treat their pain.

There is a need for high-quality RCTs comparing the efficacy and effectiveness of many of the interventions commonly used to treat spinal pain, including ESIs. However, there are several significant barriers to performing research of this type. There are few physicians performing these interventions with research training and interest; funding for this research is often limited; there is no consensus as to the appropriate methodology; and recruitment of patients into placebo-controlled studies for pain is difficult. There has also been significant discussion and debate about the various outcome tools used in spine research, particularly in trials of treatments for pain. What are the most important outcome measures to assess and how do we define success? Are self-reported pain, satisfaction with treatment, function, and global assessment of improvement adequate outcome measures? How do you interpret studies that document improvement in some measures of success, but not others (ie, improvement in pain scores, but no differences in opioid use, subsequent surgery rates, or return to work)? From a societal perspective, are return to work and health care use more important than self-reported pain relief or patient satisfaction? Recent recommendations from the IMMPACT (Initiative on Methods, Measurement, and Pain

Assessment in Clinical Trials) group include the use of a composite outcome measure that includes at least 2 individual outcome measures encompassing self-reported pain, physical function, emotional well-being, and global assessment of improvement in clinical trials of pain interventions.[101] Many of the available studies report improvements in only one outcome measure and fail to meet the recommended criteria for a successful outcome.

Future study designs will also have to identify and address the most important predictors of success for each of the available treatments. There are subsets of patients who benefit from many of the available treatments, but there are no consistent ways to predict the success of any given treatment of LBP. The evidence suggests that the outcomes for people with nonspecific LBP are better predicted by psychosocial factors such as current job satisfaction, fear avoidance beliefs/behaviors, and gender than they are by biomedical factors.[102] The type of provider seen, insurance coverage, age, and ethnicity also may contribute to a patient's perceived improvement in pain as well as satisfaction with care.[91] Although these psychosocial yellow flags are important predictors of the development of chronic pain,[98] it is less clear how they may be used to predict response to individual interventions for people with chronic back pain. However, they are clearly indicators of the complexity of the situation.

When considering the role of interventional care for chronic LBP, it is important to take a step back and make sure that we are addressing the associated medical and psychosocial factors that are likely contributing to the ongoing pain and disability. Factors such as sleep disturbance, fear avoidance, catastrophizing, obesity,[103] depression, anxiety, and socioeconomic issues need to be addressed in any treatment plan for chronic LBP, or the intervention is doomed to fail. Perhaps it is time to revisit old concepts with respect to the treatment of chronic LBP: interdisciplinary, comprehensive programs that encourage physical activation despite pain, improving coping strategies and self-efficacy, addressing underlying mental health issues, and fostering lifestyle behavior modification.[100,104–106] As Deyo and colleagues[3] have recently stated, "chronic back pain may benefit from sustained commitment from health care providers, involvement of patients as partners in their care, education in self-care strategies, coordination of care, and involvement of community resources to promote exercise, provide social support and facilitate a return to work." The conflicting evidence regarding the effectiveness of a myriad of treatments for LBP is likely reflective of the multifactorial and complex nature of the problem. In most circumstances, it seems that LBP, particularly in the chronic state, cannot be successfully treated with individual interventions of any kind.

REFERENCES

1. Deyo RA, Weinstein JN. Low back pain. N Engl J Med 2001;344(5):363–70.
2. Anderson G. The epidemiology of spinal disorders. In: Frymoyer JW, editor. The adult spine: principles and practice. 2nd edition. Philadelphia: Lippincott-Raven; 1997.
3. Deyo RA, Mirza SK, Turner JA, et al. Overtreating chronic back pain: time to back off? J Am Board Fam Med 2009;22(1):02–8.
4. Martin BI, Deyo RA, Mirza SK, et al. Expenditures and health status among adults with back and neck problems. JAMA 2008;299(6):656–64.
5. Weiner DK, Kim YS, Bonino P, et al. Low back pain in older adults: are we utilizing healthcare resources wisely? Pain Med 2006;7(2):143–50.

6. Paulozzi LJ, Budnitz DS, Xi Y. Increasing deaths from opioid analgesics in the United States. Pharmacoepidemiol Drug Saf 2006;15(9):618–27.

7. Paulozzi LJ, Ryan GW. Opioid analgesics and rates of fatal drug poisoning in the United States. Am J Prev Med 2006;31(6):506–11.

8. Katz S, editor. The burden of musculoskeletal diseases in the United States. Rosemont (IL): Bone and Joint Decade, American Academy of Orthopaedic Surgeons; 2008.

9. Deyo RA, Mirza SK, Martin BI. Back pain prevalence and visit rates: estimates from U.S. national surveys, 2002. Spine 2006;31(23):2724–7.

10. Freburger JK, Holmes GM, Agans RP, et al. The rising prevalence of chronic low back pain. Arch Intern Med 2009;169(3):251–8.

11. Weinstein JN, Lurie JD, Tosteson TD, et al. Surgical vs nonoperative treatment for lumbar disk herniation: the Spine Patient Outcomes Research Trial (SPORT) observational cohort. JAMA 2006;296(20):2451–9.

12. Weinstein JN, Lurie JD, Tosteson TD, et al. Surgical compared with nonoperative treatment for lumbar degenerative spondylolisthesis. four-year results in the Spine Patient Outcomes Research Trial (SPORT) randomized and observational cohorts. J Bone Joint Surg Am 2009;91(6):1295–304.

13. Watters WC 3rd, Bono CM, Gilbert TJ, et al. An evidence-based clinical guideline for the diagnosis and treatment of degenerative lumbar spondylolisthesis. Spine J 2009;9(7):609–14.

14. Martin CR, Gruszczynski AT, Braunsfurth HA, et al. The surgical management of degenerative lumbar spondylolisthesis: a systematic review. Spine (Phila Pa 1976) 2007;32(16):1791–8.

15. Weinstein JN, Lurie JD, Tosteson TD, et al. Surgical versus nonsurgical treatment for lumbar degenerative spondylolisthesis. N Engl J Med 2007;356(22): 2257–70.

16. Atlas SJ, Keller RB, Wu YA, et al. Long-term outcomes of surgical and nonsurgical management of sciatica secondary to a lumbar disc herniation: 10 year results from the Maine lumbar spine study. Spine (Phila Pa 1976) 2005;30(8): 927–35.

17. Chou R, Baisden J, Carragee EJ, et al. Surgery for low back pain: a review of the evidence for an American Pain Society Clinical Practice Guideline. Spine (Phila Pa 1976) 2009;34(10):1094–109.

18. Deyo RA. Back surgery–who needs it? N Engl J Med 2007;356(22):2239–43.

19. Birkmeyer NJ, Weinstein JN. Medical versus surgical treatment for low back pain: evidence and clinical practice. Eff Clin Pract 1999;2(5):218–27.

20. Mirza SK, Deyo RA. Systematic review of randomized trials comparing lumbar fusion surgery to nonoperative care for treatment of chronic back pain. Spine (Phila Pa 1976) 2007;32(7):816–23.

21. Wang MC, Chan L, Maiman DJ, et al. Complications and mortality associated with cervical spine surgery for degenerative disease in the United States. Spine (Phila Pa 1976) 2007;32(3):342–7.

22. Lievre JA, Block-Michel H. L'injection transsacree. [Etude clinique and radiologigue]. Bull Soc Med Paris 1957;73:1110–8 [in French].

23. Carrette S, Leclaire R, Marcoux S, et al. Epidural corticosteroid injections for sciatica due to herniated nucleus pulposus. N Engl J Med 1997;336:1634–40.

24. Nelemans PJ, deBie RA, deVet HC, et al. Injection therapy for subacute and chronic benign low back pain. Spine 2001;26(5):501–15.

25. Fukusaki M, Kobayashi I, Hara T, et al. Symptoms of spinal stenosis do not improve after epidural steroid injection. Clin J Pain 1998;14(2):148–51.

26. Butterman GR. Treatment of lumbar disc herniation: epidural steroid injection compared with discectomy. A prospective, randomized study. J Bone Joint Surg Am 2004;86(4):670–9.
27. Riew KD, Yin Y, Gilula L, et al. The effect of nerve-root injections on the need for operative treatment of lumbar radicular pain. J Bone Joint Surg Am 2000;82(11): 1589–93.
28. Weinstein SM, Herring SA. Lumbar epidural steroid injections. Spine J 2003;3(3 Suppl):37S–44S.
29. Rivest C, Katz JN, Ferrante FM, et al. Effects of epidural steroid injection on pain due to lumbar spinal stenosis or herniated disks: a prospective study. Arthritis Care Res 1998;11(4):291–7.
30. Valat JP, Giraudeau B, Rozenberg S. Epidural corticosteroid injections for sciatica: a randomized, double blind, controlled clinical trial. Ann Rheum Dis 2003;62(7):639–43.
31. Delport EG, Cucuzzella AR, Marley JK, et al. Treatment of lumbar spinal stenosis with epidural steroid injections: a retrospective outcome study. Arch Phys Med Rehabil 2004;85(3):479–84.
32. Vad VB, Chat A. Transforaminal epidural steroid injections in lumbosacral radiculopathy: a prospective randomized study. Spine 2002;27(1):11–5.
33. Arden NK, Price C, Reading I, et al. A multicentre randomized controlled trial of epidural corticosteroid injections for sciatica: the WEST study. Rheumatology (Oxford) 2005;44(11):1399–406.
34. Botwin KP, Gruber RD, Bouchlas CG, et al. Fluoroscopically guided lumbar transforaminal epidural steroid injections in degenerative lumbar stenosis: an outcome study. Am J Phys Med Rehabil 2002;81(12):898–905.
35. Rydevik BL, Cohen DB, Kostuik JP. Spine epidural steroids for patients with lumbar spinal stenosis. Spine 1997;22(19):2313–7.
36. Banaszkiwicz PA, Kader D, Wardlaw D. The role of caudal epidural injections in the management of low back pain. Bull Hosp Jt Dis 2003;61(3–4):127–31.
37. Cluff R, Mehio AK, Cohen SP, et al. The technical aspects of epidural steroid injections: a national survey. Anesth Analg 2003;95(2):403–8.
38. Riew KD, Park JB, Cho YS, et al. Nerve root blocks in the treatment of lumbar radicular pain. A minimum five-year follow-up. J Bone Joint Surg Am 2006; 88(8):1722–5.
39. Cuckler JM, Bernini PA, Wiesel SW, et al. The use of epidural steroids in the treatment of lumbar radicular pain. A prospective, randomized, double-blind study. J Bone Joint Surg Am 1985;67(1):63–6.
40. Price C, Arden N, Coglan L, et al. Cost-effectiveness and safety of epidural steroids in the management of sciatica. Health Technol Assess 2005;9(33): 1–58, iii.
41. Wilson-MacDonald J, Burt G, Griffin D, et al. Epidural steroid injection for nerve root compression. A randomised, controlled trial. J Bone Joint Surg Br 2005; 87(3):352–5.
42. Bush K, Hillier S. A controlled study of caudal epidural injections of triamcinalone plus procaine for the management of intractable sciatica. Spine 1991; 16:572–5.
43. Schaufele MK, Hatch L, Jones W. Interlaminar versus transforaminal epidural injections for the treatment of symptomatic lumbar intervertebral disc herniations. Pain Physician 2006;9(4):361–6.
44. DePalma MJ, Slipman CW. Evidence-informed management of chronic low back pain with epidural steroid injections. Spine J 2008;8(1):45–55.

45. Staal JB, de Bie RA, de Vet HC, et al. Injection therapy for subacute and chronic low back pain: an updated Cochrane review. Spine (Phila Pa 1976) 2009;34(1):49–59.

46. Carrino JA, Morrison WB, Parker L, et al. Spinal injection procedures: volume, distribution, and reimbursement in the U.S. Medicare populations from 1993 to 1999. Radiology 2002;225(3):723–9.

47. Friedly J, Chan L, Deyo R. Increases in lumbosacral injections in the Medicare population: 1994 to 2001. Spine 2007;32(16):1754–60.

48. Weinstein JN, Bronner KK, Morgan TS, et al. Trends and geographic variations in major surgery for degenerative diseases of the hip, knee, and spine. Health Aff (Millwood) 2004;(Suppl Web Exclusive):VAR81–9.

49. Deyo RA, Mirza SK. Trends and variations in the use of spine surgery. Clin Orthop Relat Res 2006;443:139–46.

50. Friedly J, Nishio I, Maynard C, et al. The relationship between repeated epidural steroid injections on subsequent opioid use and lumbar surgery. Arch Phys Med Rehabil 2008;89(6):1011–5.

51. Compton WM, Volkow ND. Major increases in opioid analgesic abuse in the United States: concerns and strategies. Drug Alcohol Depend 2006;81(2):103–7.

52. Vogt MT, Starz TW, Kwoh CK. Opioid usage among older adults with low back pain: comment on the article by Solomon et al. Arthritis Rheum 2006;55(3):513 [author reply: 513–4].

53. Friedly J, Chan L, Deyo R. Geographic variation in epidural steroid injection use in Medicare patients. J Bone Joint Surg Am 2008;90(8):1730–7.

54. Menachemi N, Chukmaitov A, Brown LS, et al. Quality of care in accredited and nonaccredited ambulatory surgical centers. Jt Comm J Qual Patient Saf 2008;34(9):546–51.

55. Mitchell JM. The prevalence of physician self-referral arrangements after Stark II: evidence from advanced diagnostic imaging. Health Aff (Millwood) 2007;26(3):w415–24.

56. Mitchell JM. Utilization changes following market entry by physician-owned specialty hospitals. Med Care Res Rev 2007;64(4):395–415.

57. MedPac report to congress: Medicare payment policy. 2004. Chapter 3F: p. 185–204.

58. Chukmaitov AS, Menachemi N, Brown S, et al. A comparative study of quality outcomes in freestanding ambulatory surgery centers and hospital-based outpatient departments: 1997–2004. Health Services Research 2008;43(5):1485–504

59. Manchikanti L, Boswell MV. Interventional techniques in ambulatory surgical centers: a look at the new payment system. Pain Physician 2007;10(5):627–50.

60. Centers for Medicare & Medicaid Services (CMS), HHS. Medicare program; revised payment system policies for services furnished in ambulatory surgical centers (ASCs) beginning in CY 2008. Final rule. Fed Regist 2007;72(148):42469–626.

61. Strope S, Sarma A, Ye Z, et al. Disparities in the use of ambulatory surgical centers: a cross sectional study. BMC Health Serv Res 2009;9:121.

62. Strope SA, Daignault S, Hollingsworth JM, et al. Medicare reimbursement changes for ambulatory surgery centers and remuneration to urological physician-owners. J Urol 2008;180(3):1070–4.

63. Binder DS, Nampiaparampil DE. The provocative lumbar facet joint. Curr Rev Musculoskelet Med 2009;2(1):15–24.

64. Wilde VE, Ford JJ, McMeeken JM. Indicators of lumbar zygapophyseal joint pain: survey of an expert panel with the Delphi technique. Phys Ther 2007;87(10):1348–61.

65. Kalichman L, Hunter DJ. Lumbar facet joint osteoarthritis: a review. Semin Arthritis Rheum 2007;37(2):69–80.
66. Cavanaugh JM, Lu Y, Chen C, et al. Pain generation in lumbar and cervical facet joints. J Bone Joint Surg Am 2006;88(Suppl 2):63–7.
67. Dreyfuss PH, Dreyer SJ, Vaccaro A. Lumbar zygapophysial (facet) joint injections. Spine J 2003;3(3 Suppl 1):50–9.
68. Nath S, Nath CA, Pettersson K. Percutaneous lumbar zygapophysial (Facet) joint neurotomy using radiofrequency current, in the management of chronic low back pain: a randomized double-blind trial. Spine 2008;33(12):1291–7 [discussion: 1298].
69. Bogduk N. Evidence-informed management of chronic low back pain with facet injections and radiofrequency neurotomy. Spine J 2008;8(1):56–64.
70. Slipman CW, Bhat AL, Gilchrist RV, et al. A critical review of the evidence for the use of zygapophysial injections and radiofrequency denervation in the treatment of low back pain. Spine J 2003;3(4):310–6.
71. Saal JS, Saal JA. Management of chronic discogenic low back pain with a thermal intradiscal catheter. A preliminary report. Spine (Phila Pa 1976) 2000;25(3):382–8.
72. Pauza KJ, Howell S, Dreyfuss P, et al. A randomized, placebo-controlled trial of intradiscal electrothermal therapy for the treatment of discogenic low back pain. Spine J 2004;4(1):27–35.
73. Freeman BJ, Fraser RD, Cain CM, et al. A randomized, double-blind, controlled trial: intradiscal electrothermal therapy versus placebo for the treatment of chronic discogenic low back pain. Spine (Phila Pa 1976) 2005;30(21): 2369–77 [discussion: 2378].
74. Andersson GB, Mekhail NA, Block JE. Intradiscal electrothermal therapy (IDET). Spine (Phila Pa 1976) 2006;31(12):1402 [author reply: 1402–3].
75. Appleby D, Andersson G, Totta M. Meta-analysis of the efficacy and safety of intradiscal electrothermal therapy (IDET). Pain Med 2006;7(4):308–16.
76. Manchikanti L, Boswell MV, Singh V, et al. Comprehensive evidence-based guidelines for interventional techniques in the management of chronic spinal pain. Pain Physician 2009;12(4):699–802.
77. Buchbinder R, Osborne RH, Kallmes D. Vertebroplasty appears no better than placebo for painful osteoporotic spinal fractures, and has potential to cause harm. Med J Aust 2009;191(9):476–7.
78. Kallmes DF, Comstock BA, Heagerty PJ, et al. A randomized trial of vertebroplasty for osteoporotic spinal fractures. N Engl J Med 2009;361(6): 569–79.
79. Pai S, Sundaram LJ. Low back pain: an economic assessment in the United States. Orthop Clin North Am 2004;35(1):1–6.
80. Luo X, Pietrobon R, Sun SX, et al. Estimates and patterns of direct health care expenditures among individuals with low back pain in the United States. Spine 2004;29:79–86.
81. Deyo RA, Mirza SK, Martin BI, et al. Trends, major medical complications, and charges associated with surgery for lumbar spinal stenosis in older adults. JAMA 2010;303(13):1259–65.
82. Weiner SS, Nordin M. Prevention and management of chronic back pain. Best Pract Res Clin Rheumatol 2010;24(2):267–79.
83. Roine E, Roine RP, Räsänen P, et al. Cost-effectiveness of interventions based on physical exercise in the treatment of various diseases: a systematic literature review. Int J Technol Assess Health Care 2009;25(4):427–54.

84. Fritz JM, Cleland JA, Speckman M, et al. Physical therapy for acute low back pain: associations with subsequent healthcare costs. Spine (Phila Pa 1976) 2008;33(16):1800–5.

85. Gellhorn A, Martin B, Chan L, et al. Management patterns in acute low back pain: the role of physical therapy. J Spine, in press.

86. van Tulder M, Malmivaara A, Hayden J, et al. Statistical significance versus clinical importance: trials on exercise therapy for chronic low back pain as example. Spine (Phila Pa 1976) 2007;32(16):1785–90.

87. Carey TS, Freburger JK, Holmes GM, et al. A long way to go: practice patterns and evidence in chronic low back pain care. Spine (Phila Pa 1976) 2009;34(7): 718–24.

88. Mahowald ML, Singh JA, Majeski P. Opioid use by patients in an orthopedics spine clinic. Arthritis Rheum 2005;52(1):312–21.

89. Zerzan JT, Morden NE, Soumerai S, et al. Trends and geographic variation of opiate medication use in state Medicaid fee-for-service programs, 1996 to 2002. Med Care 2006;44(11):1005–10.

90. Martell BA, O'Connor PG, Kerns RD, et al. Systematic review: opioid treatment for chronic back pain: prevalence, efficacy, and association with addiction. Ann Intern Med 2007;146(2):116–27.

91. Wallace AS, Freburger JK, Darter JD, et al. Comfortably numb? Exploring satisfaction with chronic back pain visits. Spine J 2009;9(9):721–8.

92. Rhee Y, Taitel MS, Walker DR, et al. Narcotic drug use among patients with lower back pain in employer health plans: a retrospective analysis of risk factors and health care services. Clin Ther 2007;29(Suppl):2603–12.

93. Campello MA, Weiser SR, Nordin M, et al. Work retention and nonspecific low back pain. Spine (Phila Pa 1976) 2006;31(16):1850–7.

94. Pincus T, Burton AK, Vogel S, et al. A systematic review of psychological factors as predictors of chronicity/disability in prospective cohorts of low back pain. Spine (Phila Pa 1976) 2002;27(5):E109–20.

95. Nickel R, Egle UT, Eysel P, et al. Health-related quality of life and somatization in patients with long-term low back pain: a prospective study with 109 patients. Spine (Phila Pa 1976) 2001;26(20):2271–7.

96. Bacon NM, Bacon SF, Atkinson JH, et al. Somatization symptoms in chronic low back pain patients. Psychosom Med 1994;56(2):118–27.

97. Cleland JA, Fritz JM, Brennan GP. Predictive validity of initial fear avoidance beliefs in patients with low back pain receiving physical therapy: is the FABQ a useful screening tool for identifying patients at risk for a poor recovery? Eur Spine J 2008;17(1):70–9.

98. Deyo RA, Diehl AK. Psychosocial predictors of disability in patients with low back pain. J Rheumatol 1988;15(10):1557–64.

99. Palmer KT, Calnan M, Wainwright D, et al. Disabling musculoskeletal pain and its relation to somatization: a community-based postal survey. Occup Med (Lond) 2005;55(8):612–7.

100. Newman RI, Seres JL, Yospe LP, et al. Multidisciplinary treatment of chronic pain: long-term follow-up of low-back pain patients. Pain 1978;4(3):283–92.

101. Dworkin RH, Turk DC, Wyrwich KW, et al. Interpreting the clinical importance of treatment outcomes in chronic pain clinical trials: IMMPACT recommendations. J Pain 2008;9(2):105–21.

102. Ritzwoller DP, Crounse L, Shetterly S, et al. The association of comorbidities, utilization and costs for patients identified with low back pain. BMC Musculoskelet Disord 2006;7:72.

103. Shiri R, Karppinen J, Leino-Arjas P, et al. The association between obesity and low back pain: a meta-analysis. Am J Epidemiol 2010;171(2):135–54.
104. Ahern DK, Bishop D, Follick MJ, et al. Interdisciplinary perspectives on mechanisms and management of low back pain. R I Med J 1990;73(1):21–31.
105. Beekman CE, Axtell L. Ambulation, activity level, and pain. Outcomes of a program for spinal pain. Phys Ther 1985;65(11):1649–57.
106. Branthaver B, Stein GF, Mehran A. Impact of a medical back care program on utilization of services and primary care physician satisfaction in a large, multi-specialty group practice health maintenance organization. Spine (Phila Pa 1976) 1995;20(10):1165–9.

Functional Anatomy and Pathophysiology of Axial Low Back Pain: Disc, Posterior Elements, Sacroiliac Joint, and Associated Pain Generators

Ariana J. Vora, MD[a,b,c],*, Katherine D. Doerr, MD[a,c],
Lee R. Wolfer, MD, MS[d]

KEYWORDS

- Low back pain • Tensegrity • Ligament • Fascia • Anatomy
- Disc • Zygapophysial joint

Despite thorough clinical examinations and advances in diagnostic technology, the precise pain generator is difficult to identify in many patients with axial low back pain. The literature reveals significant limitations to the measures used to implicate a particular anatomic structure as an axial low back pain generator. The intervertebral disc, zygapophysial joint, and sacroiliac joint are believed to be common pain generators in axial low back pain, with prevalences reported as 5% to 39%,[1] 15% to 40%,[2] and 6% to 13%,[3] respectively. Infection, malignancy, fracture, and inflammatory arthropathy are rare causes of low back pain. Recent research shows that a symptomatic hip joint commonly refers pain to the buttock.[4] Most physical examination and imaging findings lack sensitivity and specificity. Degenerative changes of the lumbar spine visualized on magnetic resonance imaging (MRI) do not reliably predict low back pain.[5] At present,

[a] Department of Physical Medicine and Rehabilitation, Harvard Medical School, 55 Fruit Street, Boston, MA 02144, USA
[b] Massachusetts General Hospital Physical Medicine and Rehabilitation, 5 Longfellow Place, Suite 201, Boston, MA 02144, USA
[c] Spaulding Rehabilitation Hospital, 125 Nashua Street, Boston, MA 02144, USA
[d] Spinal Diagnostics and Treatment Center, 901 Campus Drive, Suite 312, Daly City, CA 94015, USA
* Corresponding author. Department of Physical Medicine and Rehabilitation, Harvard Medical School, Massachusetts General Hospital, 5 Longfellow Place, Suite 201, Boston, MA 02144.
E-mail address: arianavora@gmail.com

Phys Med Rehabil Clin N Am 21 (2010) 679–709
doi:10.1016/j.pmr.2010.07.005
1047-9651/10/$ – see front matter © 2010 Elsevier Inc. All rights reserved.

our most precise estimates of prevalence of various pain generators are based on strict diagnostic criteria such as the dual block paradigm used for diagnosis of posterior element or sacroiliac pain. Provocation discography remains a controversial test.

Therapeutically, the individual presenting with acute or subacute axial low back pain is commonly offered a range of interventions including physical therapy, medication, functional restoration, acupuncture, chiropractic, epidural injections, or facet injections. Most individuals with low back pain have a favorable natural history and recover within a few weeks to months. In cases of severe or chronic pain, increasingly sophisticated treatment strategies have been developed based on a continually evolving understanding of lumbosacral anatomy and pathophysiology. Advanced imaging studies are often obtained to corroborate clinical findings and inform a variety of fluoroscopically guided diagnostic and therapeutic injections directed at the nerve roots, zygapophysial joints, or sacroiliac joints. Patients with severe, intractable axial low back pain often undergo provocative discography and may proceed to intradiscal injections, minimally invasive percutaneous decompression, or spinal fusion. When clinical findings and imaging identify a putative pain generator, a single, expertly performed invasive procedure and/or surgery may improve symptoms; however, relief is often partial or short lived.

The modest diagnostic and therapeutic success with low back pain may in part be the result of attempts to localize and target only one structure. Most medical and health professionals are still taught anatomy in a piecemeal fashion, studying one structure at a time rather than appreciating the spine as an integrated, interdependent, and dynamic biologic structure, suggesting that perhaps the focus on a single target may blind the physician to the big picture: the functional and pathophysiologic context of axial low back pain. The lumbosacral discs, posterior elements, and sacroiliac joint do not act in isolation; they function interdependently within a complex network of ligaments, muscles, nerves, and fascia via direct blending of tissue types. The low back is not a passive structure; it is dynamic and responsive to the environment via its specific connective tissue properties, biomechanical capacity, and sophisticated neurologic enneagrams. Diagnostic and therapeutic success in treating low back pain may ultimately lie in identifying dysfunction within this integrated network of structures rather than in searching for a single pain generator.

In addition to the visible physical connections among the discs, posterior elements of the spine, truncal muscles, and extremities, an increasing body of literature establishes that, at a cellular and biomechanical level, no anatomic structure acts in isolation. For example, multiple experimental studies in rat models have shown that, when a muscle's extracellular matrix is subjected to mechanical force, the force is transmitted to the extracellular matrix of adjacent muscles,[6,7] antagonist muscles,[8] and to surrounding bony structures.[9] Additional human studies have shown that force generation in a single human finger is coupled by force production in adjacent fingers,[10] and that truncal muscles act synergistically during voluntary body sway.[11]

Kinematically, the human spine's capability for combined flexion, extension, twisting, and bearing weight from any direction is not consistent with its classic description as a pillar or column.[12] The theory of biotensegrity (proposed by Stephen Levin[12]), grounded in cellular studies of surface tension and cytoskeletal structures, proposes support of the vertebral bodies by a highly organized continuous tension network consisting of muscles, ligaments, and fascia. In this system, the bones act as compression rods and the soft tissues as the tension elements. By this concept, a mechanical load encountered anywhere in the body is distributed through a continuous network of fascia, ligaments, and muscles suspending the entire skeleton, including the lumbar spine and sacrum. The membrane of a cell is another example of a structure with both elastic and rigid properties. The term biotensegrity was derived from the term tensegrity, or tensional integrity, first coined by Buckminster Fuller. This term was originally applied to artistic and architectural structures reflecting a balance between tension (cables) and compression (steel rods) elements. The original artistic inspiration is credited to Kenneth Snelson (**Figs. 1** and **2**) for his classic Needle Tower which resembles a spine.

This article discusses lumbosacral anatomy and functional biomechanics and explores how these structures can malfunction in the setting of axial low back pain. Key anatomic structures and the functional interdependence of the elements at both the macroscopic and microscopic levels are discussed in detail. Lumbosacral anatomy and function are examined from a biotensegrity perspective.

INTERVERTEBRAL DISC
Disc Anatomy and Histology

The intervertebral disc is composed of a central nucleus pulposus surrounded by a tough annulus fibrosus (**Fig. 3**). Within the annulus fibrosus, fibroblast cells continuously synthesize type I and II collagen into obliquely and perpendicularly oriented lamellar fibers, forming an overlapping pattern of near-complete circumferential rings.[13] Lamellae are interconnected through a network of smaller fibers consisting of fibrillin, elastin, and aggrecan.[14,15] The nucleus pulposus is composed of an extracellular matrix of type II collagen, proteoglycans, and noncollagenous proteins synthesized by chondrocytes to form a gelatinous inner core. The proteoglycans contain core proteins linked to chains of glycosaminoglycans and chains of hyaluronic acid. This

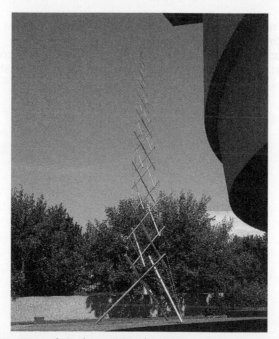

Fig. 1. Needle Tower, Kenneth Snelson, 1968, aluminum and stainless steel. (*From* Hirshhorn Museum and Sculpture Garden, Smithsonian Institution, Gift of Joseph H. Hirshhorn, 1974. Photography by Lee Stalsworth; with permission.)

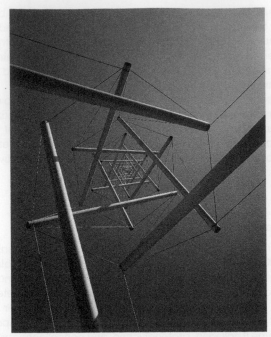

Fig. 2. Suspension system; Needle Tower, Kenneth Snelson, 1968, aluminum and stainless steel. (*From* Hirshhorn Museum and Sculpture Garden, Smithsonian Institution, Gift of Joseph H. Hirshhorn, 1974. Photography by Lee Stalsworth; with permission.)

matrix gives the nucleus pulposus its hydrostatic properties to allow for compression and bracing by the annulus fibrosus.[16]

In a healthy disc, the extracellular matrix undergoes a balance of continual synthesis and degradation. Synthesis is primarily activated by fibroblast growth factor,

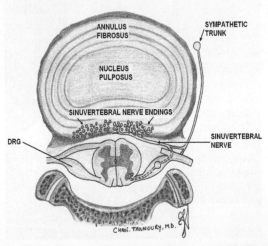

Fig. 3. Intervertebral disc in a cross section. (*From* Zhang Y, An TS, Tannourey C, et al. Biologic treatment for degenerative disc disease: implications for the field of physical medicine and rehabilitation. Am J Phys Med Rehabil 2008;87(9):697.)

transforming growth factor, and insulinlike growth factor, which inhibit the matrix metalloproteinases and allow for increased production of the matrix.[17] Macrophages in the matrix secrete interleukin (IL)-1, interferon, and tumor necrosis factor (TNF)-α.[18] These cytokines stimulate chondrocytes to secrete matrix metalloproteinases and facilitate degradation of the matrix. TNF-α in particular has been found to activate cell migration, increase vascular permeability, and reduce matrix synthesis in the nucleus pulposus.[19] In a comparative study of cytokine expression, Lee and colleagues[20] detected increased TNF-α and IL-8 in herniated disc tissue, and increased vascular endothelial growth factor and nerve growth factor in degenerated discs.

Pioneering anatomic studies of disc tissue revealed the inner annulus fibrosus and the nucleus pulposus to be avascular. Terminal vessels to the vertebral body endplates supply only the outer rings of the annulus fibrosus. Nutrition is believed to reach these areas via diffusion through the inner annulus fibers and extracellular matrix. In an early study of 4 cadavers (wherein history of low back pain was not reported), Bogduk and colleagues[21] observed innervation of lumbar intervertebral discs by sinuvertebral nerve fibers on the outer posterior aspect of the annulus fibrosus. He hypothesized dual innervation from a sympathetic branch from the gray ramus communicans and a somatic branch from the ventral ramus.[22] Subsequent immunohistochemistry studies indicate that the sympathetic pathway comprises most of the nerve fibers. Further anatomic studies revealed an extensive network of nerve fibers located on the disc surface and relatively few nerve endings, mainly unmyelinated and unencapsulated, within the annulus fibrosus itself.[23] Nerve extension deep to the outer annulus is not seen in healthy discs.

Disc Biomechanics

Acting as a buttress and buffer between consecutive vertebral bodies, the intervertebral disc maintains structural integrity throughout a variety of movements. The annulus fibrosus provides both tensile and compression stiffness through its configuration of lamellar rings, and the semifluid nucleus pulposus can change its shape without losing volume. The nucleus pulposus transmits radial pressure on the vertebral endplates in response to a compressive load, which in turn is balanced by opposing tension within the annulus.[24]

During forward sliding of vertebral bodies or application of shear force, the annulus resists slide via anteriorly and posteriorly oriented lamellar fibers. During flexion and extension, the corresponding anterior or posterior annulus compresses and stretches, resisting tension and pressure via deformation of the nucleus pulposus.[25] Rotation causes circumferential movement of adjacent vertebral bodies, requiring that half of the lamellae separate and the other half approximate. Because only half of the fibers resist rotation, the annulus fibrosus may be more susceptible to rotational injury compared with compression injuries.[26]

Disc Pathology

Disc degeneration is a state of histochemical dysfunction and gross structural changes of the annulus fibrosus and nucleus pulposus. Pain can be caused by obvious disc herniations and/or pathologic disc degeneration (vs normal aging). Disc herniation was first described by Dandy[27] in 1929 and later by Mixter and Barr[28] in 1934. Using oil-contrast myelography, Dandy[27] described "loose cartilage simulating a tumor of the spinal cord." During the herniated disc era, most axial and radicular low back pain was attributed to herniated discs; however, discography has shown that degenerated discs, particularly those with annular tears, were a significant cause of back pain.[29,30] In 1980, Crock[31] hypothesized that, following mechanical trauma, vertebral discs produce chemical substances that irritate the disc and nerve root, causing pain. Numerous subsequent studies have shown an imbalance between synthesis and degradation, resulting in histochemical changes in the extracellular matrix.[32] As catabolic activity of matrix metalloproteinases, IL-1, and TNF-α increases, anabolic activity of insulinlike growth factor-1, transforming growth factor-β, and bone morphogenetic factors decreases.[33] Consequently, the concentration of cells and matrix in the annulus fibrosus decreases.[34] In addition, the proportion of collagen fiber types in the nucleus pulposus changes from type II to type I as the nucleus pulposus becomes desiccated and fibrotic.[35,36] Declining nutrition, cell senescence, and the accumulation of degraded matrix products seem to contribute to this process.

Unlike healthy discs, degenerated discs develop pathologic innervation with extension of nerve fibers to the inner annulus and nucleus pulposus. Coppes and colleagues[37] found that 8 of 10 degenerated disc specimens contained nerves within the inner annulus. Through nerve antibody testing in pathologic discs of patients with low back pain, Peng and colleagues[38] detected both innervation and vascularization from the outer annulus fibrosus into the inner nucleus pulposus. Freemont and colleagues[39] also detected nerve fibers in the inner annulus and nucleus pulposus tissue in degenerated discs of patients with low back pain, and found that these nerve fibers expressed substance P, a marker commonly associated with pain generation. Further studies have identified calcitonin gene–related peptide, also associated with pain generation, within the inner annulus and nucleus pulposus.[40]

Mechanical factors have been implicated in disc degeneration. Disc degeneration occurs more commonly in the lower lumbar discs, discs immediately above a transitional vertebra, and discs adjacent to lumbar fusion. Several hypotheses involving mechanical changes at these levels are suggested. In vitro studies show that physiologic loading induces collagen formation, but excessive loading induces gene expression of matrix metalloproteinases, resulting in decreased gene expression of nearly all anabolic proteins.[41] In cadaveric studies, acute torsion injuries are associated with tears in the posterior annulus similar to compression injury, whereas degenerative changes may cause tears in the inner annulus with extension into the periphery.[42,43]

However, these studies have not been replicated in vivo. Animal studies of the association of compression with disc degeneration often have conflicting results,[44] and human studies show that the intervertebral disc is able to withstand a wide range of compression forces during various activities of living.[25] This finding is corroborated by an MRI study comparing elite equestrians with nonriding volunteers. Although the equestrian group had a higher rate of low back pain, there was no difference in disc degenerative findings between equestrians and age-matched controls.[45] In a study of long-term effects of physical loading and exercise on back-related symptoms, elite weight lifters and soccer players showed greater degeneration throughout the lumbar spine compared with competitive runners and historically matched controls. Although imaging showed more degenerative findings, back pain was less common among athletes versus controls.[46]

Biomechanical studies indicate that the vertebral endplate is more vulnerable to excessive compressive load than the intervertebral disc. Endplates can fracture in response to a sudden, large compressive load, or repeated large compressive loads.[25,47] Endplate fractures are believed to increase interlaminar shear stress on the posterior annulus, resulting in depressurization such that the nucleus pulposus is unable to brace the annulus. The inner annulus then buckles anteriorly and the outer annulus buckles posteriorly, increasing the shear stress from compressive loads and thereby facilitating annular tears.[26]

Conditions that reduce blood supply to the lumbar spine are associated with ischemic degenerative changes to the disc. Atheromatous lesions in the abdominal aorta and congenital hypoplasia of the lumbar arteries have been associated with disc degeneration.[48,49] In addition, arteriolar constriction secondary to smoking has been associated with an increased incidence of disc herniation.[50] When a vertebral fracture occurs, the resulting callus formation can occlude blood vessels providing nutrition to the disc, impairing maintenance of the matrix.

Although once attributed only to age-related changes, recent research has redefined the process of disc degeneration such that it can no longer be attributed to a singular process. Hadjipavlou and colleagues[44] observe that "degeneration of the intervertebral disc can be defined as an age-dependent, cell-mediated molecular degradation process under genetic influence that is accelerated primarily by nutritional and mechanical factors, and secondly by toxic and metabolic factors."

Clinical Correlates: Localization of Discogenic Pain Generators

Clinically, pain related to disc degeneration is currently distinguished from other sources of axial low back pain by first ruling out other pain generators (negative sacroiliac and facet joint blocks) and then proceeding to provocation discography. Provocation discography involves insertion of a small needle into the disc using fluoroscopic guidance, followed by pressure-, rate-, and volume-monitored instillation of contrast into the disc. The contrast provides hydraulic distension of the disc to determine whether it is chemically and/or mechanically sensitive.[51] As a diagnostic test, provocative discography is controversial. In one study, Carragee and colleagues[52] reported an unacceptably high (40%) false-positive rate for provocative discography in patients with chronic low back pain. Significant questions were raised about whether psychological comorbidity confounded provocative discography. In patients with somatization disorder, he reported a false-positive rate of 75%.[53] However, a recent meta-analysis of false-positive rates for discography by Wolfer and colleagues[54] showed a false-positive rate of less than 10% when the International Spine Interventional Society guidelines were followed.

Despite continuing controversy among stakeholders, discography remains the most reliable available test of the intervertebral disc as a pain generator. Schwarzer and colleagues[55] used pain reproducible on provocation discography to assess the prevalence of disc disruption in 92 patients. Each patient was also required to have evidence of internal disc disruption on computed tomography (CT) and no reproduction of pain on testing of an additional disc. In this study, the prevalence of discogenic low back pain was calculated at 39%.[56] When discogenic low back pain is suspected, clinical assessment includes identifying the location of pain and its relation to movements of the lumbar spine. There is wide variation in the sensitivity and specificity of the association between symptom location and positive discography. Identification of a directional preference, such as standing flexion, standing extension, supine flexion, prone extension, and rotation, is associated with positive provocation during discography, but two studies have indicated that these directional preferences are more specific than sensitive, and are not reliable.[57]

In summary, the lumbar intervertebral disc contains a strong outer annulus fibrosus and a semifluid inner nucleus pulposus. Through the unique histochemistry of these two elements, the disc is designed to provide significant spinal support during a variety of movements, including forward slide, rotation, flexion, and extension. Numerous studies indicate that a significant subset of axial low back pain localizes to the intervertebral disc. However, disc degeneration is a complex biomechanical and histologic process that does not necessarily cause symptoms. The process by which some discs generate pain and others do not remains an area of active investigation.

ZYGAPOPHYSIAL JOINTS
Zygapophysial Joint Anatomy and Histology

Each lumbar spinal segment contains 2 posterolateral zygapophysial joints, often referred to colloquially as facet joints. Each zygapophysial joint consists of paired right and left inferior articular facets of one vertebra articulating with the paired superior articular facets of the vertebra below. The articular facets vary in shape and orientation to the sagittal plane. Superior articular facets may be flat or curved, containing either a C or J shape, and orientation may vary from 0 to 90 degrees based on level, with lower vertebrae oriented further from the sagittal plane. Zygapophysial joints have classic synovial joint features including hyaline cartilage, synovial membrane, and a joint capsule. The capsule is composed of 1 mm thick collagenous tissue located around the dorsal, superior, and inferior margins of the joint transversely connecting each articular process. The capsule contains 1 to 1.5 mL of fluid and consists of 2 layers: an outer layer of dense, parallel collagen fibers and an inner layer of irregular elastic fibers.[58] Similarly to traditional synovial joints, a synovial lining lies deep to the fibrous capsule. Capsule fibers blend posteriorly with the multifidus muscle and anteriorly with the ligamentum flavum, which is continuous with the joint capsule.

The zygapophysial joint is innervated by 2 medial branches from consecutive vertebral levels. Each medial branch courses over the respective transverse process 1 level above its origination. The medial branch also innervates the multifidus muscle, the interspinous ligament, and the periosteum of the neural arch.[21,59] One in 9 people may have variant innervation of the joint.[60] Additional proposed innervation sources include the dorsal root ganglion and the paravertebral sympathetic ganglion (**Fig. 4**).[61]

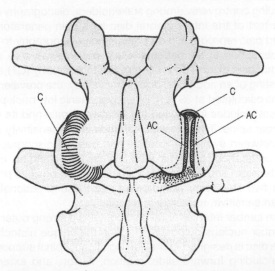

Fig. 4. Zygapophysial joint. (*From* Bogduk N. The zygapophysial joints. In: Bogduk N, editor. Clinical anatomy of the lumbar spine. 4th edition. London: Elsevier; 2005. p. 30.)

Zygapophysial Joint Biomechanics

Through its orientation and shape, the zygapophysial joint stabilizes the spine by limiting motion. The orientation of the joint determines its pattern of resistance. At the lower lumbar levels, zygapophysial joints contain greater surface area and are oriented more obliquely to provide more resistance to shear load and forward displacement; at higher lumbar levels, their sagittal orientation offers no resistance to forward displacement but strongly resists rotation.[62] The shape of the joint provides additional resistance; C-shaped facets have increased surface area posteriorly and provide greater resistance to forward dislocation than J-shaped facets. Within the capsule, transverse orientation of fibers provides maximum resistance to flexion.[63] With age, the zygapophysial joints weaken and change orientation from coronal to sagittal, providing less resistance against forward displacement.[64,65]

Zygapophysial Joint Pathology

In 1911, Goldthwaite[66] first suggested an association between facet joint variation and low back pain. In 1927, Putti[67] dissected 75 cadavers and noted that degenerative changes in the facet joints were associated with sciatica. In 1933, Ghormley[68] coined the term facet syndrome after finding similar symptoms in specimens subjected to sudden rotational strain. Although interest in the zygapophysial joint waned with increasing interest in the intervertebral disc, this joint has acquired significant attention in the last few decades.

Zygapophysial pathology is believed to occur through intimately linked direct and indirect processes. In the direct process, repetitive mechanical strain leads to osteoarthritic changes within the joint, including subchondral sclerosis and cartilage degeneration. This in turn leads to the indirect process, including zygapophysial hypertrophy and cystic formation of the synovial membrane.[69] This cystic formation occurs most commonly at the L4 to L5 level.[70]

On review of autopsy studies describing zygapophysial joints, Uhrenholt and colleagues[71] observed subchondral sclerosis, cartilage fibrillation and splitting, and thinning of the articular surface in degenerated joints. In samples taken from a series of patients undergoing lumbar spinal fusion, histologic changes similar to chondromalacia patellae and osteoarthritis of large joints were visualized, including cartilage necrosis and exposure of subchondral bone.[72] Similar changes were visualized in patients who underwent repetitive strain patterns. In response to repetitive strain, these joints can fill with fluid, distend, and cause pain likely related to capsular stretch. Capsular stretch is also associated with reflex spasm of the erector spinae and multifidus muscles.[73–75]

Facet tropism is defined as asymmetry between the right and left facet orientation and has also previously been implicated as a pain generator. Loss of coronal orientation is seen with age in 20% to 40% of the population.[64,76] This change in orientation was strongly associated with osteoarthritis in a study of 111 patients by Fujiwara and colleagues.[65] A more recent study involving 188 patients in the Framingham Heart Study showed that sagittal orientation of the joint was only associated with osteoarthritis at the L4 to L5 level, but neither study reflected an association between facet tropism and zygapophysial osteoarthritis.[77]

Because the zygapophysial joint is richly innervated, these degenerative changes could result in pain. Recent findings of substance P and calcitonin gene–related peptide within the capsule suggest its capacity to serve as a pain generator.[78,79] Phospholipase A2 has also been implicated as an inflammatory mediator within the zygapophysial joint, increasing inflammation and edema and causing prolonged nociceptive excitation.[80]

Clinical Correlates: Localization of Zygapophysial Joint Pain Generators

The prevalence of zygapophysial joint pain is hypothesized to range between 15% and 40%. Diagnosis of lumbar back pain secondary to zygapophysial joint degenerative changes is often challenging. Most clinicians rely on several history-related characteristics of the pain, including unilateral pain worse with extension, and pain slightly lateral to the midline. Clinicians may then confirm possible causes using imaging consistent with facet degeneration. However, currently there is no evidence to suggest that any specific history, physical examination findings, or imaging findings will predict response to a medial branch block.[81]

Revel and colleagues[82,83] created 7 diagnostic criteria for identifying zygapophysial joint pain: age more than 65 years; pain relieved by recumbent position; no exacerbation with cough, flexion, or extension; no pain with rising from flexion; and the extension-rotation test. He reported that 92% of patients having 5 of 7 criteria responded to a medial branch block.[82,83] However, in a subsequent study, these results were not replicated; and the 7 criteria exhibited specificity near 90% and a sensitivity of only 17%.[84]

In a series of 192 patients who reported positive response to a medial branch block, Cohen and colleagues[85] studied multiple factors believed to predict this outcome, including duration of pain, MRI abnormalities, and levels treated. The only factor associated with a successful medial branch block was paraspinal tenderness.[85] A prospective statistical study showed no correlation between radiographic evidence of zygapophysial joint degeneration and response to a medial branch block.[86] More recently, MRI with sagittal short-tau inversion recovery (STIR) seems promising. In a study of serial STIR imaging of axial low back pain in patients with visible zygapophysial joint edema, patients who noted change in their pain score were also noted to have changes in the intensity of edema at the zygapophysial joint.[87]

In summary, the zygapophysial joint connects the superior articular facet of each consecutive vertebra with the inferior articular facet of the vertebra above. These true synovial joints are particularly active in resisting flexion and forward slide of the vertebrae. With age and trauma, these joints can exhibit pathologic changes similar to those in seen large joint osteoarthritis. Pain generation in the zygapophysial joint may result from osteoarthritic changes and altered orientation of the joint in space. The current state of the art for diagnosis of zygapophysial joint pain uses fluoroscopically guided comparative medial branch blocks.

THE SACROILIAC JOINT/LIGAMENT COMPLEX
Sacroiliac Anatomy

The sacroiliac joint connects the spine and the pelvis through a diarthrodial joint between 2 bony surfaces: the sacrum and ilium. The sacrum is wedged between 2 iliac bones to form the posterior wall of the pelvis. The space between the concave sacrum and convex ilium is approximately 1 to 2 mm wide,[88] and the joint maintains a C shape with convexity directed anteriorly and inferiorly. The joint surfaces are lined with 1 mm of hyaline cartilage at the iliac end and 6 mm at the sacral end. The superior portion of the joint has the histologic qualities of a symphysis and is attached to a dense network of surrounding stabilizing ligaments, whereas the inferior portion of the joint has the histologic characteristics of a synovial joint.[89]

Several strong ligaments maintain the integrity, shape, and position of the sacroiliac joint. The dense interosseous fibers constitute the thickest connections between the sacrum and the ilium. The anterior and posterior sacroiliac ligaments strengthen this connection on their respective aspects of the sacrum and ilium (**Fig. 5**).[90] The

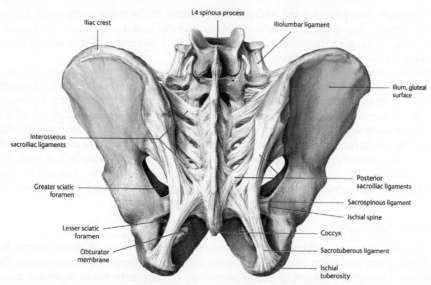

Fig. 5. Sacroiliac joint. (*From* Vleeming A, Stoeckart R. The role of the pelvic girdle in coupling the spine and legs: a clinical-anatomic perspective on pelvic stability. In: Vleeming A, Mooney V, Stoeckart R, editors. Movement, stability and lumbopelvic pain: integration of research and therapy. London: Elsevier; 2007. p. 115; with permission.)

ligaments and the joint are so closely connected that the anterior sacroiliac ligament is a continuation of the anterior capsule.[91] The sacrotuberous ligament attaches at the sacroiliac joint capsule, the coccygeal vertebrae, and the ischial tuberosity. Sacrotuberous fibers also blend with the biceps femoris tendon distally,[92] and the deep multifidus and piriformis proximally.[93] Caudal traction on the long head of the biceps femoris increases tension in the sacrotuberous ligament. The sacrospinous ligament attaches at the sacroiliac joint capsule, the lower sacral and coccygeal vertebrae, and the ischial spine.[94]

The innervation of the sacroiliac joint is under debate. Mechanoreceptors and nerve fascicles have been observed in the sacroiliac joint with gold chloride staining.[95] Further histologic studies verify the presence of innervation to the joint capsule and the ligaments. Nerve fascicles containing myelinated fibers, unmyelinated fibers, paciniform mechanoreceptors, and nonpaciniform mechanoreceptors have been identified, suggesting that both pain and proprioception are transmitted through the sacroiliac joint.[96] However, the source of these nerves is controversial. Based on cadaveric studies, Fortin proposes that the joint receives exclusive innervations from the sacral S1 to S4 dorsal rami.[97] Electrical and mechanical stimulation studies suggest that the innervation arises predominantly via the L4 to S1 nerve root, with secondary contribution from the superior gluteal nerve.[98]

Sacroiliac Biomechanics

The sacroiliac joint transmits vertical forces through the spine, the pelvis, and the extremities.[99] Its C shape, with interlocking lever arms at S2 and numerous ridges and depressions, is believed to increase stability. During activity, this joint allows 2 to 3 degrees of rotation[100] and 0.5 to 1.6 mm of translation.[75] The axis of motion crosses the pelvis obliquely. During hip flexion, the ipsilateral ilium moves posteriorly and caudally, compressing the sacrum and pivoting at the pubic symphysis. During hip extension, the ipsilateral ilium moves anteriorly and away from the sacrum. This oblique plane of movement is consistent with 3 dimensional movement of the pelvis required during ambulation.[101]

The thick interosseous sacroiliac ligament intimately connects the sacrum and ilium and is believed to secure the bony interlocking mechanism.[102] In addition to strengthening the interosseous ligament, the anterior and posterior sacroiliac ligaments prevent forward rocking (nutation) and backward rocking (counternutation) of the pelvis, respectively.[103] The sacrospinous and sacrotuberous ligaments prevent rotation of the caudal end of the sacrum. Although the sacroiliac ligament attaches to multifidus fibers directly and to additional muscles via the sacrotuberous ligament, the joint's movement is minimal.[104] Rotational axis studies by Lavignolle and colleagues[105] suggest that the sacroiliac joint's primary function is absorption of mechanical force from the lower limbs across the pelvic girdle.

Sacroiliac Pathology

Mechanical changes, inflammation, trauma, and degeneration all occur within the sacroiliac joint, and each can be associated with pain generation. Anatomically, the joint can undergo significant changes secondary to osteoarthritis or repetitive strain patterns, including capsular or synovial disruption, chondromalacia, and cartilage destruction. In a study by Chou and colleagues,[106] the most likely cause of sacroiliac joint pain confirmed by injection was trauma in 44% of patients, idiopathic in 35% of patients, and repeated stress in 21% of patients.

The extra-articular ligaments and muscles may contribute to sacroiliac joint pathology through hypomobility or hypermobility, abnormal joint mechanics, soft tissue injury, and inflammation.[107] Sacroiliac ligaments also seem to be significant pain generators. In a comparative study, Murakami and colleagues[108] found that 36% of patients receiving intraarticular injections alone experienced relief of low back pain, in contrast to 92% of patients receiving extra-articular injections.

Biomechanical and muscle length discrepancies may predispose a patient to sacroiliac pain secondary to altered gait patterns and repetitive stress on the joint. Fortin and Falco[109] hypothesized that an imbalanced unilateral load changes the balance of the C-shaped joint and increases sacral rotation when 1 ilia is fixed and the other is rotationally loaded. They identified biomechanical dysfunction of the sacroiliac joint in athletes who participate in unidirectional repetitive activities, including forward displacement and rotation. Pregnancy also predisposes to sacroiliac pain through weight gain, lordotic posturing, and hormone-induced ligamentous laxity.

Clinical Correlates: Localization of Sacroiliac Pain Generators

Overall, clinical tests for sacroiliac pain have shown much better sensitivity and specificity than those for disc pain or facet pain. Clinical tests used to assess for sacroiliac pain generators include the Faber test, distraction/compression, focal joint tenderness, the Gillett femoral shear test, and the modified Gaenslen test. Young and colleagues[110] found that the likelihood of low back pain arising from the sacroiliac joint was significantly higher if 3 or more of these tests are positive and if the pain is unilateral below L5 without lumbar pain. However, in a study of 12 physical examination findings individually and in combination, Dreyfuss and colleagues[111] found that none could predict intraarticular sacroiliac joint pain as determined by a single positive block with more than 90% pain relief. A recent systematic review validated the thigh thrust test and sacroiliac compression test as diagnostic indicators of sacroiliac joint pain, finding that, if 3 of 5 provocation tests including compression, distraction, thigh thrust, Gaenslen test, and Patrick sign were positive, the specificity reached 100% and the sensitivity was 77% to 87%.[112] Several small studies have shown a positive correlation between successful sacroiliac joint block and clinical localization of primary pain to the Fortin point, which lies within 2 cm of the posterior superior iliac crest.[113]

In the last decade, a newer functional physical examination test, called the active straight leg raise (ASLR), has been used to assess pelvic load transfer in patients with sacroiliac or posterior pelvic girdle pain.[114] Lying supine, with legs extended, the patient is asked to raise the heel approximately 30 cm off the table. A positive test is described if the patient subjectively reports one leg to be heavier than the other. The ASLR test reveals that sacroiliac joint pain can cause global dysfunction of lumbopelvic motor control patterns and respiration in low load conditions. O'Sullivan and colleagues[114] found that subjects with sacroiliac joint pain combined with positive ASLR test had increased pelvic floor descent, decreased diaphragmatic excursion, and increased minute ventilation. With manual compression of the ilia (similar to using a sacroiliac belt), participants with sacroiliac pain exhibited neuromuscular patterns normalized to those of matched controls.

Imaging is of limited diagnostic value, with CT sensitivity of 57% and specificity of 69% in predicting positive response to intraarticular sacroiliac injection.[115] Specificity of bone scans has been calculated to be as high as 90%, but with only 46% sensitivity in predicting positive response to intraarticular sacroiliac block. Imaging is most useful when there is suspicion for a fracture, infection, or malignant or rheumatologic cause of sacroiliac joint pain.

In summary, the sacroiliac joint binds the spine to the pelvis and plays a critical role in force transmission to the extremities. Given its unique position, this joint and its supportive ligaments and muscles provide minimal amounts of rotation and translation on an oblique axis to allow a variety of pelvic movements during stance and ambulation. The sacroiliac joint is also believed to be intimately involved in core stability, including pelvic floor function. Increased success of periarticular, compared with intraarticular, injections indicates that sacroiliac joint pain is not confined to the joint capsule alone but also can arise from with well-innervated contiguous ligaments and muscle fibers.

LIGAMENTS OF THE LUMBOSACRAL SPINE
Ligamentum Flavum

The ligamentum flavum lies just superficial to the vertebral canal and connects consecutive vertebral laminae. Medially, the ligamentum flavum attaches to the interspinous ligament. Laterally, it attaches to the zygapophysial joint capsule.[116] Unlike other ligaments of the lumbosacral spine, its histology is 80% elastic fibers and 20% collagenous fibers.[117] Its uniquely rich composition of elastic fibers is believed to prevent buckling of the vertebral column during flexion/extension movements.

When disc herniation occurs, the ligamentum flavum can buckle inferiorly. Although the structure itself has little innervation, buckling of the ligamentum flavum has been implicated as a contributor to nerve root compression in disc herniation.[118] With advancing age, the elastic fibers are increasingly replaced by collagenous fibers and high-molecular-weight proteoglycans, and calcium deposition occurs within ligamentous fibers. Calcification and thickening of the ligamentum flavum is commonly seen in spinal stenosis, and ligamentum flavum hypertrophy has been implicated in the pathogenesis of disc degeneration.[119] Ossification of the ligamentum flavum was found in 100% of samples in a cadaveric study of spinal stenosis.[120] A recent

MRI study evaluating 162 patients with low back pain showed a high correlation between increasing age and ligamentum flavum hypertrophy; these changes began at the L4 to L5 level in the fourth decade of life.[121]

Longitudinal Ligaments

The anterior longitudinal ligament covers the anterior aspect of the entire vertebral column. It attaches to the anterior aspects of the lumbar vertebral bodies and annuli fibrosi, and to the psoas muscle fibers laterally.[93] It receives innervation from branches of the gray rami.[61] Biomechanically, it resists separation of the anterior intervertebral discs during spinal extension. The posterior longitudinal ligament similarly extends from occiput to sacrum. It attaches to the outer layer of the annuli fibrosi, with shorter fibers connecting consecutive annulus fibers. Narrowing around the bases of each pedicle, it has a serrated appearance. Innervated by the sinuvertebral nerves, its biomechanical function is to resist separation of the posterior intervertebral discs during spinal flexion.

Interspinous and Supraspinous Ligaments

The interspinous ligament connects consecutive spinous processes. Innervated by the dorsal rami, it is fan shaped, with the middle fibers lying parallel to the spinous processes.[122] Anteriorly, it is continuous with the ligamentum flavum. Posteriorly, it blends with the supraspinous ligament, which is continuous with the thoracolumbar fascia (Fig. 6). Although these fibers provide resistance at end range of lumbar flexion,[123] they do not resist forward bending movements,[124] nor do they provide significant extensor mechanical assistance. In addition to opposing separation between consecutive vertebral spinous processes, Willard[125] proposes that the interspinous ligament serves as an anchor transmitting anterior-posterior forces from the extremities to the spine via contiguous thoracolumbar fascia and vertebral bodies. He describes the interspinous ligament as part of an interspinous-supraspinous-thoracolumbar (IST) complex, which secures the thoracolumbar fascia and multifidus sheath to the facet capsules and is considered to be the central support for the lumbosacral spine (Fig. 7).

Iliolumbar Ligament

The iliolumbar ligament is also a fan-shaped structure providing a strong attachment between the L5 transverse processes and the ilium. It receives innervation from the dorsal rami and the L4 to L5 spinal nerve ventral rami. Although this ligament is classically depicted as 5 distinct bands of fibers (Fig. 8), the exact morphology of the iliolumbar ligament is a subject of controversy because of anatomic variations and the density of connective tissue in the region. A magnetic resonance study of 15 adults showed only two bands extending from the L5 transverse process to form an anterior fan, inserting along the anterior iliac tuberosity, and a posterior cone distribution of fibers, inserting from the anterior margin of the iliac crest to the apex of the iliac crest.[126] A larger cadaveric study corroborated these findings, although some of the specimens in that study did not have visibly distinct separation between anterior attachments and bands.[127] Some studies document proximal iliolumbar ligament fibers attaching to both L4 and L5 transverse processes, and others suggest distal fibers extending to the sacroiliac joint capsule.[128] Three-dimensional volume data and computer-reformatted magnetic resonance images may provide a more accurate anatomic representation of the iliolumbar ligament than routine MRI.[129]

Biomechanically, the iliolumbar ligament restrains lumbosacral movement including side bending,[130] flexion, and extension.[131] Cadaveric studies indicate that this is likely

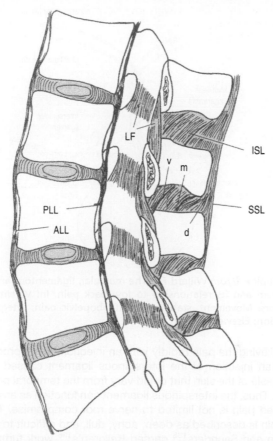

Fig. 6. Sagittal view of lumbar spine ligaments. (*From* Bodguk N. The ligaments of the lumbar spine. In: Bogduk N, editor. Clinical anatomy of the lumbar spine and sacrum. London: Elsevier; 2005. p. 41.)

to be an important function in the normal spine and in the setting of L5 spondylolysis.[132] The iliolumbar ligament is also believed to stabilize the sacroiliac joint in the sagittal plane.[133] Sims and Moorman[134] hypothesize that as annular fibers become less effective in absorbing mechanical forces in the setting of disc degeneration, the iliolumbar ligament may take on additional stress and become subject to tears. A recent cadaveric study indicated that the iliolumbar ligament is primarily innervated by Pacinian and Ruffini mechanoreceptors, and also contains plentiful free nerve endings.[135] This suggests that although its primary role is proprioceptive, the iliolumbar ligament has the capacity to contribute to low back pain.[135]

Clinical Correlates: Ligamentous Pain Generators

The early research on the interspinous ligament introduced important clinical correlates and a more sophisticated understanding of deep somatic pain generators beyond the disc, facet, and sacroiliac joint. The interspinous ligament can be a source of referred pain to the spine, trunk, abdomen, and upper/lower limbs, as first described by Kellgren[136] in 1939 using injections of 0.3 mL or less of 6% saline. In 1958, Whitty[137] confirmed Kellgren's[136] work by first using hypertonic saline to create

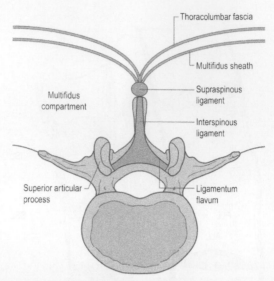

Fig. 7. The IST complex. (*From* Willard FH. The muscular, ligamentous and neural structure of the lumbosacrum and its relationship to low back pain. In: Vleeming A, Mooney V, Stoeckart R, editors. Movement, stability and lumbopelvic pain: integration of research and therapy. London: Elsevier; 2007. p. 11.)

pain and then relieving the pain rapidly with an injection of 2% procaine. Kellgren[136] also noted that an injection of the interspinous ligament caused palpable muscle spasm; hyperalgesia of the skin that could vary from the temporal profile and location of the deep pain. Thus, the interspinous ligament can function as an independent pain generator; referred pain is not limited to nerve root compromise. The quality of the deep somatic pain is described as deep, achy, dull, and difficult to localize.

In 1944, Inman and Saunders[138] carried Kellgren's[136] work further, using varying noxious methods to stimulate multiple, deep somatic tissues, including the interspinous ligament. They ranked the sensitivity of deep somatic tissues (periosteum>ligament>joint capsule>tendon>fascia>muscle).[138] From this and subsequent works

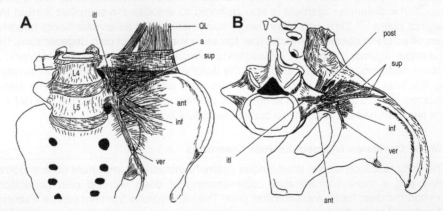

Fig. 8. The iliolumbar ligament. (*From* Bogduk N. The ligaments of the lumbar spine. In: Bogduk N, editor. Clinical anatomy of the lumbar spine and sacrum. London: Elsevier; 2005. p. 41.)

arose the concept of sclerotomal pain or deep somatic referred pain. Sclerotomes are described as the pain referral zones for bone, joints, and ligaments sharing spinal segmental innervations. Bogduk[139] asserts that maps of referred pain refer to segmental spinal innervations, not always to a specific structure. The overlap between pain referral maps between discs and zygapophysial joints is well established. Inman and Saunders'[138] work indicates that the same is true for these other deep somatic structures. Deep somatic referral patterns overlap with our classically taught referral patterns and deserve closer scrutiny in the diagnosis and treatment of patients with spinal pain.

Recent advanced imaging studies support the presence of deep somatic structures as pain generators in patients with low back pain. Gatehouse and colleagues[140] used ultrashort echo time (TE) MRI pulse sequences to image patients with degenerative disease of the lumbar spine compared with normals. The sequences revealed high signal in the anterior and posterior longitudinal ligaments, the cartilaginous endplate, the annulus fibrosus, the ligamentum flavum, interspinous ligaments, and insertions of ligaments. Hypertrophied ligaments and scar tissue enhanced with contrast. These findings suggest that degenerative disc disease is not confined to the disc itself, but compromises the entire functional unit of the lumbosacral spine with specific findings in the tension elements, or supportive ligaments, and the compression elements, or bony structures.

Dysfunction of the IST ligamentous complex may explain why ultrasensitive MRI sequences of patients with disc degeneration also show increased signal in all surrounding major ligaments and their attachments. When this biotensegrity system fails via microscopic or macroscopic failure of the thoracolumbar fascia, supraspinous ligament, or interspinous ligament, the ligamentum flavum may buckle toward the spinal cord. This in turn may place more stress on the bony compression elements (the vertebral bodies, sacroiliac bones, and articular processes) and, by extension, the disc, sacroiliac joint, and facet joint. This theory implies that, for example, a disc may be more prone to herniate after progressive failure of these supporting tissues.

ENTHESIS ORGAN

An enthesis is the site of tendon, ligament, joint capsule, or fascia attachment to bone. Some entheses are close to bursae and fat, as in the insertion of the patellar or Achilles tendons. Entheses serve important biomechanical functions of shock absorption and maintain a constant length despite high levels of force applied to the junction between bone and soft tissue fibers. Degenerative changes in entheses, such as partial tearing and calcification, with fibroblast proliferation and neovascularization, have been implicated in overuse injuries such as lateral epicondylosis. Benjamin and McGonagle[141] have advanced the notion of an enthesis organ composed of the enthesis, fibrocartilage, fascia, bursa, fat pad, and adjacent trabecular bone. The enthesis organ is thus the functional unit of the musculoskeletal system, present throughout the body. As noted in the ultrashort TE MRI study of patients with degenerative disc disease, numerous entheses or sites of ligamentous attachment show high signal. Because mechanical forces directed at the lumbosacral region surround the body's center of gravity, enthesopathy warrants further exploration in the setting of axial low back pain.

MUSCLES OF THE LUMBOSACRAL SPINE
Multifidus

The multifidus muscle consists of short and long fibers. The short fibers originate at the posteroinferior vertebral laminae and spinous processes of the vertebral body above and insert at the vertebral mamillary process below (**Fig. 9**A). The lowest level of this series originates at the L5 laminar fibers and inserts onto the sacrum superior to the first dorsal sacral foramen. The long fibers are 5 sets of fascicles, each originating at the most caudal aspect of its lumbar spinous processes and attaching in a fanlike projection to the mamillary processes, iliac crest, and sacrum below (**Fig. 9**B-F). Cadaveric studies show continuity of multifidus fibers with the deep laminae of the posterior thoracolumbar fascia, the long dorsal sacroiliac ligament, and the sacrotuberous ligament. The course of these fibers is slightly more oblique in women compared with men.[142]

In addition to facilitating sagittal movements of the lumbar spine, the multifidus muscle is believed to facilitate a self-bracing mechanism of the lumbosacrum via compression of the intervertebral discs, facilitation of the lumbar lordosis, and counteraction of the abdominal muscles during lumbar flexion. It may also transfer energy from the upper body to the lower extremities. Multiple electromyogram (EMG) studies have shown activation of the multifidus fibers during standing, sitting, trunk movements, lifting activities, and gait.[143,144]

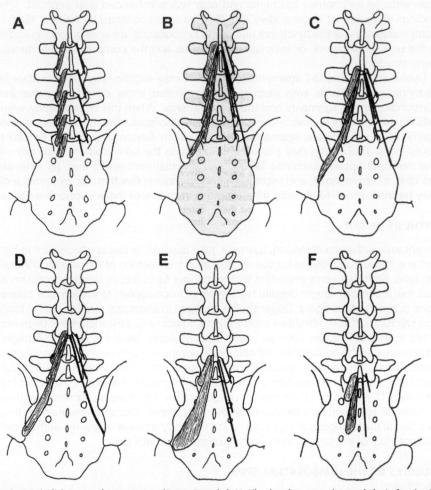

Fig. 9. Multifidus muscle anatomy. (*From* Bogduk N. The lumbar muscles and their fascia. In: Bogduk N, editor. Clinical anatomy of the lumbar spine. 4th edition. London: Elsevier; 2005. p. 102.)

There is a strong association between low back pain and lumbar multifidus atrophy.[145] In a case series of CT images, decreased bulk of the combined multifidus and erector spinae muscles was associated with zygapophysial joint hypertrophy at L4 to L5 but not low back pain; this study did not isolate the multifidus muscle.[146] A recent MR spectroscopy study showed increased multifidus mean fat content in individuals with low back pain compared with controls; the longissimus muscle was also measured and no significant association with low back pain was found.[147]

Neuromuscular changes are also seen in low back pain. A recent EMG study revealed prolonged mean motor latency of short multifidus fibers when provoked by rapid arm movement in individuals in remission from recurrent low back pain, compared with healthy controls.[148] Biopsies of the multifidus muscle in individuals with low back pain reveal a higher distribution of type II fibers and reduced diameter in both type I and type II fibers compared with healthy controls.[149] In a recent experimental pain protocol inducing unilateral low back pain via hypertonic saline injection, ultrasound visualization during arm lifts revealed reduced bilateral multifidus thickness change during automatic contraction associated with arm movement.[150]

Interspinales/Intertransversalis

The interspinales are 4 pairs of short muscles located just lateral to the interspinous ligament, connecting consecutive spinous processes. The intertransversalis muscles consist of ventral fibers that connect consecutive transverse processes, and dorsal fibers that connect the accessory process above to the transverse process below. The intertransversalis muscles connect the accessory and mamillary processes of each lumbar vertebra to the mamillary process below.[151] Although these small segmental muscles exert negligible mechanical force, their high density of spindle fibers suggests a primarily proprioceptive function.[152]

Erector Spinae

The lumbar erector spinae consist of the longissumus and iliocostalis fibers, which are divided into distinct lumbar and thoracic muscle groups. Together, the erector spinae muscle fibers form an aponeurosis that serves as an indirect connection between the lumbar vertebrae and the ilium. The lumbar division of the longissimus thoracis originates at the dorsal aspect of each lumbar transverse process and attaches to the medial aspect of the posterior superior iliac spine. The lumbar division of the iliocostalis originates from the lumbar transverse processes and attaches to the iliac crest. These lumbar erector spinae fibers are believed to counteract lumbar flexion and derotate the spine. The longissimus thoracis pars thoracis are a bundle of long, narrow fascicles originating at each transverse process and rib from T1 to T12, each level forming its own tendinous attachment at a point several levels down on the lumbar spinous processes or sacrum.[153] The iliocostalis pars thoracis originates from the T1 to T12 rib angles and inserts at the posterior superior iliac spine. Among their functions is the facilitation of thoracic side flexion.

Additional Muscles of Interest to the Lumbosacral Spine

Frequently targeted in core strengthening exercises, the transversus abdominus muscle is considered a critical muscle for the strength and stability of the lumbar spine.[154] Transversus abdominus fibers originate at the lowest 6 ribs, the thoracolumbar fascia, the anterior iliac crest, and the lateral inguinal ligament.[155] Superior fibers insert at the linea alba, and inferior fibers insert at the anterior wall of the pelvis. Its horizontally oriented fibers share an aponeurosis with the more superficial internal and external oblique fibers, both of which connect to the thoracolumbar fascia, the ribs, and the iliac crest. Electrophysiologic studies indicate anticipatory activity in these fibers before rapid upper and lower limb movements.[156] In subjects with low back pain, activation of the transversus abdominus was delayed.[157] Current rehabilitation strategies focus on motor reeducation with activation of the transversus abdominus muscle first to stabilize the spine, followed by activation of the larger, global prime mover muscles of the low back.

The psoas major originates at the anterior surface of the T12 to L5 transverse processes, the annuli fibrosi, and the vertebral bodies, and inserts at the lesser trochanter of the femur. Its primary action is hip flexion,[158] but it also exerts compression load on the lower lumbar discs.[159] The quadratus lumborum is a complex network of oblique and longitudinally directed fibers connecting the 12th rib, the L1 to L4 transverse processes, and the ilium. It is believed to serve as a posterior anchor for the 12th rib, but this has not been objectively shown. It has been shown to exert a modest amount of extensor and lateral bending action on the lumbar spine.[160] The latissimus dorsi attaches the thoracolumbar fascia, the iliac crest, the lowest 3 ribs, and the humerus. Although its principal actions are related to arm movement, it may facilitate lumbar stability via its extensive bony and fascial connections.

The gluteus maximus fibers originate at the posterior surface of the iliac crest, the thoracolumbar fascia, the lateral sacrum, and the coccygeal vertebrae; they insert onto the iliotibial band and the lateral femur. Electrophysiologic studies confirm its classically described action as a trunk extensor.[161] Recent biomechanical studies suggest that it may limit pelvic torsion and thereby contribute to self-bracing of the pelvis.[162] Contraction of the gluteus maximus fibers is believed to compress the sacroiliac joint. Electrophysiologic studies show a close relationship between the gluteus maximus and the sacroiliac joint; compression force affects the onset of gluteus maximus contraction and has only inconsistent effect on erector spinae and semitendinosis contraction.[163] The piriformis muscle attaches the sacrum, the sacrotuberous ligament, and the greater trochanter of the femur. It therefore facilitates external rotation of the hip joint and exerts tensile force between the sacrum and the ilium. Numerous anatomists throughout history have described anomalous passage of the sciatic nerve through or above piriformis fibers. "Piriformis syndrome" refers to low back, buttock or posterior thigh pain, with occasional descriptions of foot drop, and is attributed to entrapment of the sciatic nerve by the piriformis muscle. A recent meta-analysis of over 6,000 cadavers showed 16.9 percent prevalence of sciatic nerve passage through the piriformis muscle.[164] Interestingly, this anomaly was not statistically any less prevalent (16.2%) in 130 patients undergoing hip replacement who lacked "piriformis" symptoms. While further studies of local inflammation, edema and muscle spasm are warranted, this large study indicates that the "piriformis syndrome" can not be attributed to common congenital variations in the passage of the sciatic nerve through the piriformis muscle.

THORACOLUMBAR FASCIA

The muscular anatomy described earlier reflects the complex overlap of muscle, tendon, and ligament fiber attachments in the lumbosacral region. Given their multiple shared attachments, none of the muscles outlined earlier can function in isolation. How are motor and proprioceptive forces coordinated to align the spine, transmit mechanical forces, and control subtle and gross movements of the lumbosacral spine? How might dysfunction of the fascia play a role in axial low back pain, as its own pain generator, or by affecting the function and proprioception of the muscles, ligaments, and biomechanical alignment? A growing body of literature is devoted to the potential role that fascia may play.

Classically, fascia is described as a multilayered, soft tissue sheath dividing muscles into organized groupings and protecting nerve and vascular structures. More recently, fascia has been described as "a connective tissue continuum throughout the body, uniting and integrating its different regions."[165] The thoracolumbar fascia envelops the lumbar spine muscles and divides them into anterior, middle, and posterior layers. The anterior layer attaches the anterior lumbar transverse processes, intertransverse ligaments, quadratus lumborum fascia, and the other layers of thoracolumbar fascia (**Fig. 10**).[166] The middle layer attaches the tips of the lumbar transverse processes and intertransverse ligaments with the aponeurosis of the transversus abdominus. The posterior layer is discussed later; all 3 layers also attach to each other.

The posterior layer of the thoracolumbar fascia has been the subject of increasing scientific attention (**Fig. 11**). Loukas and colleagues[167] studied the posterior layer of the thoracolumbar fascia in 40 cadavers and revealed inferomedially oriented fibers comprising a superficial layer with extensive attachments at the gluteus maximus, the median sacral crest, the spinous processes, the serratus posterior inferior aponeurosis, the latissimus dorsi aponeurosis, and, in 10 specimens, the trapezius aponeurosis. The deeper layer, also known as the vertebral aponeurosis, consists of inferolaterally oriented fibers forming numerous attachments to the thoracic spinous processes, rib angles, serratus posterior superior, and the deep fascia of the neck. Both the superficial and deeper layers of the posterior thoracolumbar fascia converge inferiorly to attach at the sacrotuberous ligament.

It is believed that the posterior layer of the thoracolumbar fascia transfers force between the spine and the extremities. Vleeming and colleagues[168] found that traction applied to the latissimus dorsi, gluteus maximus, erector spinae, and biceps femoris muscles of 10 cadavers caused displacement of the posterior thoracolumbar fascia, and postulated that a similarly integrated load transfer system occurs in vivo. This transfer of force may also have a stabilizing effect on the lumbar spine and sacroiliac joint. Barker and colleagues[169] showed that application of physiologic amounts of

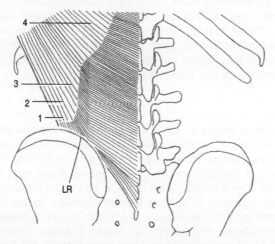

Fig. 10. Superficial thoracolumbar fascia. (*From* Bogduk N. The lumbar muscles and their fascia. In: Bogduk N, editor. Clinical anatomy of the lumbar spine. 4th edition. London: Elsevier; 2005. p. 102.)

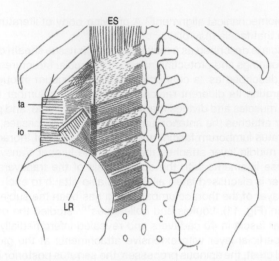

Fig. 11. Deep thoracolumbar fascia. (*From* Bogduk N. The lumbar muscles and their fascia. In: Bogduk N, editor. Clinical anatomy of the lumbar spine. 4th edition. London: Elsevier; 2005. p. 102.)

tension to the thoracolumbar fascia of 9 unembalmed cadavers reduced axial displacement during flexion and extension at most lumbar segments. Because of its multiple attachments, tension applied to the thoracolumbar fascia via muscle contraction may similarly affect spinal alignment.

The question has arisen whether the thoracolumbar fascia itself can generate pain. In a simple but novel study, thoracolumbar fascia tissue samples were obtained intraoperatively from 24 patients undergoing their first lumbar surgery following a positive discogram or facet joint block. Histologic examination revealed aneural tissue with no microscopic evidence of the ubiquitous neural end organs. The tissue showed unexpected evidence of ischemic changes[170]; this raises questions of whether an ischemic insult could be a pain generator. The diseased thoracolumbar fascia was compared with tissue changes seen in diabetic microangiopathy. These findings raise speculation about the thoracolumbar fascia as a primary pain generator, and, given its critical biomechanical role, suggest that micro- and macroscopic failure of the thoracolumbar fascia could affect the biomechanical function of the entire lumbosacral region.

DISCUSSION

Review of the anatomy shows no clear delineation of where one structure ends and another begins; hence, no anatomic structure can function in isolation. Endplate changes compromise nutrition to the intervertebral disc. By limiting motion, the lumbar ligaments and zygapophysial joints protect the annular fibers from excessive torsion and rotation forces. The sacroiliac joint capsule fibers are histologically continuous with the sacroiliac ligament. Multifidus fascicles cement to the vertebral laminae and apply support to the annulus fibrosus. In addition, fascial networks connect seemingly unrelated structures; thoracolumbar fascia attaches firmly to the spinous processes and ilium and connects these bony structures to the arms via the latissimus, and to the abdomen via the transversus abdominus. Via the erector spinae aponeurosis, the thoracic iliocostalis and longissimus muscles support the lumbar vertebral bodies without touching them. This complex interplay of structures affects spine alignment, strength, mobility, and stability.

Vleeming's study of transmission of force from the gluteus maximus to the latissimus dorsi muscles via the thoracolumbar fascia, described earlier, is in accordance with these findings.[166] DeRosa and Porterfield[171] similarly observed a myofascial network connecting seemingly unrelated muscles of the trunk and extremities. Willard[125] proposed that the interspinous ligament, supraspinous ligament, and thoracolumbar fascia act in concert as the central support system for the lumbosacral spine via a functional unit called the IST complex. Recent research, supported by histologic examination and advanced imaging findings, has introduced a new organ in the body, unique to the musculoskeletal system: the enthesis or the specific site of attachment of ligaments, tendons, and fibrocartilage.

SUMMARY

Dysfunction of an element can cause pain, and clinicians are most familiar with the disc, facet joints, and sacroiliac joint as pain generators. Objective abnormalities in multiple anatomic structures have been associated with axial low back pain; for example, cellular changes occur in the nucleus pulposus. Gross and microscopic changes are noted in the annulus fibrosus. Altered bone metabolism is seen in the zygapophysial joints. Careful consideration of functional lumbosacral anatomy reveals association of low back pain with other potential pain generators, such as interspinous ligament degeneration, multifidus atrophy, and microvascular ischemic changes in the thoracolumbar fascia. These structures are inextricably bound to the lumbosacral spine via a complex, dynamic tensegrity network.

These compelling findings raise further questions. How is intercellular communication coordinated among these structures, and how does it break down? What role do genetics, cellular nutrition, and metabolism play in the overall health of the musculoskeletal tissues? Does disc degeneration initiate a cascade of cellular reactions and degenerative changes in the posterior elements, or does it result from failure of myofascial or ligamentous structures to provide structural support to the disc? Further exploration of the dynamic, interdependent structures that affect the lumbosacral spine may facilitate more accurate diagnosis and treatment of low back pain.

REFERENCES

1. Bogduk N. The anatomical basis for spinal pain syndromes. J Manipulative Physiol Ther 1995;18(9):603–5.
2. Schwarzer AC, Wang SC, Bogduk N, et al. Prevalence and clinical features of lumbar zygapophysial joint pain a studying an Australian population with chronic low back pain. Ann Rheum Dis 1995;54(2):100–6.
3. Schwarzer AC, Aprill C, Bogduk N. The sacroiliac joint in chronic low back pain. Spine 1995;20(1):31–7.
4. Lesher JM, Dreyfuss P, Hager N, et al. Hip joint pain referral patterns: a descriptive study. Pain Med 2008;9(1):22–5.
5. Jensen MC, Brant-Zawadzki MN, Obuchowski N, et al. Magnetic resonance imaging of the lumbar spine in people without back pain. N Engl J Med 1994; 331(2):69–73.
6. Yucesoy CA, Koopman BH, Baan GC, et al. Effects of inter-and extramuscular myofascial force transmission on adjacent synergistic muscles: assessment by experiments and finite-element modeling. J Biomech 2003;36:1797–811.

7. Maas H, Baan GC, Huijing PA. Intermuscular interaction via myofascial force transmission: effects of tibialis anterior and extensor hallucis longus length on force transmission from rat extensor digitorum muscle. J Biomech 2001;34:927–40.

8. Yucesoy CA, Baan G, Huijing PA. Epimuscular myofascial force transmission occurs in the rat between the deep flexor muscles and their antagonistic muscles. J Electromyogr Kinesiol 2010;20:118–26.

9. Rijkelijkhuizen JM, Baan GC, Ruiter CJ, et al. Extramuscular myofascial force transmission for in situ rat medial gastrocnemius and plantaris muscles in progressive stages of dissection. J Exp Biol 2005;208:129–40.

10. Zatsiorsky VM, Gregory RW, Latash ML. Force and torque production in statis multifinger prehension: biomechanics and control. II. Control. Biol Cybern 2002;87(1):40–9.

11. Wang Y, Asaka T, Zatsiorsky VM, et al. Muscle synergies during voluntary body sway: combining across-trials and within-a-trial analyses. Exp Brain Res 2006; 174(4):679–93.

12. Levin SM. A suspensory system for the sacrum in pelvic biomechanics: biotensegrity. In: Vleeming A, Mooney V, Stoeckart R, editors. Movement, stability and lumbosacral pain: integration of research and therapy. 2nd edition. Edinburgh; London; NY: Churchill Livingstone/Elsevier; 2007. p. 229–31.

13. Marchand F, Ahmed AM. Investigation of the laminate structure of lumbar disc annulus fibrosus. Spine 1990;15:402–10.

14. Melrose J, Smith SM, Appleyard RC, et al. Aggrecan, versican and type VI collagen are components of annular translamellar crossbridges in the intervertebral disc. Eur Spine J 2008;17(2):314–24.

15. Yu J, Tirlapur U, Fairbank J, et al. Microfibrils, elastin fibres and collagen fibres in the human intervertebral disc and bovine tail disc. J Anat 2007;210(4):460–71.

16. Urban JP, Maroudas A. Swelling of the intervertebral disc in vitro. Connect Tissue Res 1981;9:1–10.

17. Shinmei M, Masuda K, Kikuchi T, et al. Interleukin-1, tumour necrosis factor, and interleukin-6 as mediators of cartilage destruction. Semin Arthritis Rheum 1989; 18:27–32.

18. Adams MA, Green TP. Tensile properties of the annulus fibrosus. I. The contribution of fibre-matrix interactions to tensile stiffness and strength. Eur Spine J 1993;2(4):203–6.

19. Weiler C, Nerlich AG, Bachmeier BE, et al. Expression and distribution of tumor necrosis factor alpha in human lumbar intervertebral discs: a study in surgical specimen and autopsy controls. Spine 2005;30(1):44–53.

20. Lee S, Moon CS, Sul D, et al. Comparison of growth factor and cytokine expression in patients with degenerated disc disease and herniated nucleus pulposus. Clin Biochem 2009;42(15):1504–11.

21. Bogduk N, Tynan W, Wilson AS. The nerve supply to the human lumbar intervertebral discs. J Anat 1981;132:39–56.

22. Jackson HC 2nd, Winkelmann RK, Bickel WH. Nerve endings in the human lumbar spinal column and related structures. J Bone Joint Surg Am 1966;48: 1272–81.

23. Edgar MA. The nerve supply to the lumbar intervertebral disc. J Bone Joint Surg Br 2007;89:1135–9.

24. Meakin JR, Hukins DW. Effect of removing the nucleus pulposus on the deformation of the annulus fibrosus during compression of the intervertebral disc. J Biomech 2000;33(5):575–80.

25. White AA, Panjabi MM. Clinical biomechanics of the spine. Philadelphia: Lippincott; 1978.

26. Farfan HF, Cossette JW, Robertson GH, et al. The effects of torsion on the lumbar intervertebral joints: the role of torsion in the production of disc degeneration. J Bone Joint Surg Am 1970;52:468–97.
27. Dandy W. Loose cartilage from intervertebral disc simulating tumor of the spinal cord. Arch Surg 1929;19:660.
28. Mixter WJ, Barr JS. Rupture of the intervertebral disc with involvement of the spinal canal. N Engl J Med 1934;211:210–5.
29. Yu SW, Haughton VM, Sether LA, et al. Comparison of MR and discography in detecting radial tears of the annulus: a postmortem study. AJNR Am J Neuroradiol 1989;10(5):1077–81.
30. Yu SW, Sether LA, Ho PS, et al. Tears of the annulus fibrosus: correlation between MR and pathologic findings in cadavers. AJNR Am J Neuroradiol 1988;9(2):367–70.
31. Crock HV. Internal disc disruption. A challenge to disc prolapse fifty years on. Spine 1986;11(6):650.
32. Buckwalter JA, Mow VC, Boden SD, et al. Intervertebral disk structure, composition, and mechanical function. Orthopaedic basic science - biology and biomechanics of the musculoskeletal system. Rosemont (IL): American Academy of Orthopaedic Surgeons; 2000.
33. Zhang Y, An HS, Tannoury C, et al. Biological treatment for degenerative disc disease: implications for the field of physical medicine and rehabilitation. Am J Phys Med Rehabil 2008;87:694–702.
34. Trout JJ, Buckwalter JA, Moore KC, et al. Ultrastructure of the human intervertebral disc I: changes in notochordal cells with age. Tissue Cell 1982;14:359–69.
35. Haefeli M, Kalberer F, Saegesser D, et al. The course of macroscopic degeneration in the human lumbar intervertebral disc. Spine 2006;31:1522–31.
36. Vernon-Roberts B, Pirie CJ. Degenerative changes in the intervertebral discs of the lumbar spine and their sequelae. Rheumatol Rehabil 1977;16:13–21.
37. Coppes MH, Marani E, Thomeer RT, et al. Innervation of "painful" lumbar discs. Spine 1997;22(20):2342–9.
38. Peng B, Wu W, Hou S, et al. The pathogenesis of discogenic low back pain. J Bone Joint Surg Br 2005;87(1):62–7.
39. Freemont AJ, Peacock TE, Goupille P, et al. Nerve ingrowth into diseased intervertebral disc in chronic back pain. Lancet 1997;350(9072):178–81.
40. Ozawa T, Ohtori S, Inoue G, et al. The degenerated lumbar intervertebral disc is innervated primarily by peptide-containing sensory nerve fibers in humans. Spine 2006;31(21):2418–22.
41. Neidlinger-Wilke C, Wurtz K, Urban JP, et al. Regulation of gene expression in intervertebral disc cells by low and high hydrostatic pressure. Eur Spine J 2006;15(Suppl 3):372–8.
42. Hansoon TH, Keller TS, Spengler DM. Mechanical behaviour of the human lumbar spine II: fatigue stretch during dynamic compressive loading. J Orthop Res 1987;5:479–87.
43. Vernon-Roberts B, Fazzalari NL, Mathey BA. Pathogenesis of tears of the annulus investigated by multi-level transaxial analysis of the T12-L1 disc. Spine 1997;22:2641–6.
44. Hadjipavlou AG, Tzermiadianos MN, Bogduk N, et al. The pathophysiology of disc degeneration: a critical review. J Bone Joint Surg Br 2008;90:1261–70.
45. Kraft CN, Pennekamp PH, Becker U, et al. Magnetic resonance imaging findings of the lumbar spine in elite horseback riders: correlations with back pain, body mass index, trunk/leg-length coefficient, and riding discipline. Am J Sports Med 2009;37(11):2205–13.

46. Videman T, Sarna S, Battie MC, et al. The longterm effects of physical loading and exercise lifestyles on back-related symptoms, disability and spinal pathology among men. Spine 1995;20(6):699–709.

47. Adams MA, McNally DS, Wagstaff J, et al. Abnormal stress concentrations in lumbar intervertebral discs following damage to the vertebral bodies: a cause of disc failure? Eur Spine 1993;1:214–21.

48. Kauppila LI. Can low back pain be due to lumbar-artery disease? Lancet 1995; 346:888–9.

49. Kauppila L, Pentitila A, Karhunen PJ, et al. Lumbar disc degeneration and atherosclerosis of the abdominal aorta. Spine 1994;19:932–9.

50. Benneker LM, Heini PF, Alini M, et al. Vertebral endplate marrow contact channel occlusions and intervertebral disc degeneration. Spine 2005;30:167–73.

51. Lindblom K. Diagnostic puncture of intervertebral discs in sciatica. Acta Orthop Scand 1948;17:231–9.

52. Carragee EJ, Chen Y, Tanner CM, et al. Provocative discography in patients after limited lumbar discectomy: a controlled, randomized study of pain response in symptomatic and asymptomatic subjects. Spine 2000;25: 3065–71.

53. Carragee EJ, Tanner CM, Khurana S, et al. The rates of false-positive lumbar discography in select patients without low back symptoms. Spine 2000;25: 1373–80.

54. Wolfer LR, Derby R, Lee JE, et al. Systematic review of lumbar provocation discography in asymptomatic subjects with metaanalysis of false-positive rates. Pain Physician 2008;11(4):513–38.

55. Schwarzer AC, Aprill C, Derby R, et al. The prevalence and clinical features of internal disc disruption in patients with chronic low back pain. Spine 1995;20(1): 1878–83.

56. Manchikanti L, Singh V, Rivera JJ. Effectiveness of caudal epidural injections In discogram positive and negative chronic low back pain. Pain Physician 2002; 5(1):18–29.

57. Werneke M, Hart DL, Cook D. A descriptive study of the centralization phenomenon: a prospective analysis. Spine 1999;24(7):676–83.

58. Glover JR. Arthrography of the joints of the lumbar vertebral arches. Orthop Clin North Am 1977;8:37–42.

59. Bogduk N, Wilson AS, Tynan W. The human lumbar dorsal rami. J Anat 1982; 134:383–97.

60. Kaplan M, Dreyfuss P, Halbrook B, et al. The ability of the lumbar medial branch blocks to anesthetize the zygapophysial joint: a physiologic challenge. Spine 1998;23:1847–52.

61. Bogduk N. The innervation of the lumbar spine. Spine (Phila Pa 1976) 1983;8(3): 286–93.

62. Bogduk N. The zygapophysial joints. Clinical anatomy of the lumbar spine and sacrum. 4th edition. New York: Elsevier; 2005. p. 29–37.

63. Yahia LH, Garzon S. Structure on the capsular ligaments of the facet joints. Ann Anat 1993;175:185–8.

64. Murtagh FR, Paulsen RD, Rechtine GR. The role and incidence of facet tropism in lumbar spine degenerative disc disease. J Spinal Disord 1991;4:86–9.

65. Fujiwara A, Tamai K, An HS, et al. Orientation and osteoarthritis of the lumbar facet joint. Clin Orthop Relat Res 2001;385:88–94.

66. Goldthwaite JE. The lumbrosacral articulation: an explanation of many cases of lumbago, sciatica, and paraplegia. Boston Med Surg J 1911;164:365–72.

67. Putti V. New concepts in the pathogenesis of sciatica pain. Lancet 1927;2: 53–60.
68. Ghormley RK. Low back pain with special reference to the articular facets with presentation of an operative procedure. JAMA 1933;101:1773–7.
69. Doyle AJ, Merrilees M. Synovial cysts of the lumbar facet joint in a symptomatic population: prevalence on magnetic resonance imaging. Spine 2004;29(8): 874–8.
70. Sandhu FA, Santiago P, Fessler R, et al. Minimally invasive surgical treatment of lumbar synovial cysts. Neurosurgery 2004;54(1):107–12.
71. Uhrenholt L, Grunnet-Nilsson N, Hartvigsen J. Cervical spine lesions after road traffic accidents: a systematic review. Spine 2002;27(17):1934–41.
72. Eisenstein SM, Parry CR. The lumbar facet arthrosis syndrome. Clinical presentation and articular surface changes. J Bone Joint Surg Br 1987;69(1).3–7.
73. Gray DP, Bajwa ZH, Warfield CA. Facet block and neurolysis. In: Waldman SD, editor. Interventional pain management. 2nd edition. Philadelphia: WB Saunders; 2001. p. 446–83.
74. Yang YM, Choi WS, Pickar JG. Electrophysiologic evidence for an intersegmental reflex pathway between lumbar paraspinal tissues. Spine 2002;7: E56–63.
75. Indahl A, Kaigle A, Reikeras O, et al. Electromyographic response of the porcine multifidus musculature after nerve stimulation. Spine 1995;20:2652–8.
76. Bogduk N. Age changes in the lumbar spine. Clinical anatomy of the lumbar spine and sacrum. 4th edition. London: Elsevier; 2005. p. 168–9.
77. Kalichman L, Suri P, Guermazi A, et al. Facet orientation and tropism: associations with facet joint osteoarthritis and degeneratives. Spine 2009;34(16): 579–85.
78. Giles LG, Taylor JR. Human zygapophyseal joint capsule and synovial fold innervation. Br J Rheumatol 1987;26(2):93–8.
79. Ahmed M, Bjurholm A, Creicbergs A, et al. Sensory and autonomic innervation of the facet joint in the rat lumbar spine. Spine 1993;18(14):2121–6.
80. Lee HM, Weinstein JN, Meller ST, et al. The role of steroids and their effects on phospholipase A2. An animal model of radiculopathy. Spine 2000;25(15): 2004–5.
81. Sehgal N, Shah RV, McKenzie-Brown AM, et al. Diagnostic utility of facet (zygapophysial) joint injections in chronic spinal pain: a systematic review of evidence. Pain Physician 2005;8(2):211–24.
82. Revel ME, Listrat VM, Chevalier XJ, et al. Facet joint block for low back pain: identifying predictors of a good response. Arch Phys Med Rehabil 1992; 73(9):824–8.
83. Revel M, Poiraudeau S, Auleley GR, et al. Capacity of the clinical picture to characterize low back pain relieved by facet joint anesthesia. Proposed criteria to identify patients with painful facet joints. Spine 1998;23(18):1972–6.
84. Laslett M, Oberg B, Aprill CN, et al. Zygapophysial joint blocks in chronic low back pain: a test of Revel's model as a screening test. BMC Musculoskelet Disord 2004;5:43.
85. Cohen SP, Hurley RW, Christo PJ, et al. Clinical predictors of success and failure for lumbar facet radiofrequency denervation. Clin J Pain 2007;23(1):45–52.
86. Jackson RP, Jacobs RR, Montesano PX. Facet joint injection in low-back pain: a prospective statistical study. Spine 1988;13:966–71.
87. Freidrich KM, Nemec S, Peloschek P, et al. The prevalence of lumbar facet joint edema in patients with low back pain. Skeletal Radiol 2007;26(8):755–60.

88. Bogduk N. The sacroiliac joint. In: Bogduk N, editor. Clinical anatomy of the lumbar spine and sacrum. 4th edition. New York: Churchill Livingstone; 2005. p. 173–81.

89. Puhakka KB, Melsen F, Jurik AG, et al. MR imaging of the normal sacroiliac joint with correlation to histology. Skeletal Radiol 2004;33:15–28.

90. Schunke M, Schulte E, Schumacher U. Bones, ligaments, and joints. In: Lamperti E, Ross L, editors. Thieme atlas of anatomy: general anatomy and musculoskeletal system. New York: Thieme; 2007. p. 114.

91. Loukas M, Louis RG, Hallner B, et al. Anatomical and surgical considerations of the sacrotuberous ligament and its relevance in pudendal nerve entrapment syndrome. Surg Radiol Anat 2006;28(2):163–9.

92. Vleeming A, Stoeckart R, Snijders CJ. The sacrotuberous ligament: a conceptual approach to its dynamic role in stabilizing the sacroiliac joint. Clin Biomech 1989;4:201–3.

93. Willard FH. The muscular, ligamentous, and neural structure of the lumbosacrum. In: Vleeming A, Mooney V, Stoeckart R, editors. Movement, stability and lumbopelvic pain: integration of research and therapy. Churchill Livingstone/Elsevier; 2007. p. 7–21.

94. Williams PL, editor. Gray's anatomy. 38th edition. Edinburgh (UK): Churchill Livingstone; 1995. p. 308.

95. Rosatelli AL, Agur AM, Chhaya S. Anatomy of the interosseous region of the sacroiliac joint. J Orthop Sports Phys Ther 2006;36(4):200–8.

96. Forst SJ, Wheeler MT, Fortin JD, et al. Sacroiliac joint: anatomy, physiology & clinical significance. Pain Physician 2006;9(1):61–7.

97. Fortin JD, Kissling RO, O'Connor BL, et al. Sacroiliac joint innervation and pain. Am J Orthop 1999;28:687–90.

98. Hom S, Indahl A, Solomonow M. Sensorimotor control of the spine. J Electromyogr Kinesiol 2002;12:219.

99. Dietrichs E. Anatomy of the pelvic joints- a review. Scand J Rheumatol 1991; 88(Suppl):4–6.

100. Scholten PJM, Schultz AB, Luchico CW, et al. Motions and loads within the human pelvis: a biomedical model study. J Orthop Res 1988;6:840–50.

101. Foley BS, Buschbacher RM. Sacroiliac joint pain: anatomy, biomechanics, diagnosis, and treatment. Am J Phys Med Rehabil 2006;85(12):997–1006.

102. Bogduk N. The sacroiliac joint. Clinical anatomy of the lumbar spine and sacrum. 4th edition. New York: Elsevier; 2005. p. 176.

103. Vleeming A, Pool-Goudzwaard AL, Hammudoghlu D, et al. The function of the long dorsal sacroiliac ligament: its implication for understanding low back pain. Spine 1996;21:556–62.

104. Sturesson B, Uden A, Vleeming A. A radiostereometric analysis of the movement of the sacroiliac joints during the standing hip flexion test. Spine 2000;25:214–7.

105. Lavignolle B, Vitam JM, Senegas J, et al. An approach to the functional anatomy of the sacroiliac joints in vivo. Anat Clin 1983;5:169–76.

106. Chou LH, Slipman CW, Bhagia SM, et al. Inciting events initiating injection-proven sacroiliac joint syndrome. Pain Med 2004;5:26–32.

107. Cohen SP. Sacroiliac joint pain: a comprehensive review of anatomy, diagnosis, and treatment. Anesth Analog 2005;101(5):1440–53.

108. Murakami E, Tanaka Y, Aizawa T, et al. Effect of periarticular and intraarticular lidocaine injections for sacroiliac joint pain: prospective comparative study. J Orthop Sci 2007;12(3):274–80.

109. Fortin JD, Falco F. Enigmatic causes of spine pain in athletes. Phys Med Rehabil State Art Rev 1977;11:445–64.

110. Young S, Aprill C, Laslett M. Correlation of clinical examination characteristics with three sources of chronic low back pain. Spine J 2003;3:460–5.
111. Dreyfuss P, Dreyer SJ, Cole A, et al. Sacroiliac joint pain. J Am Acad Orthop Surg 2004;12:255–65.
112. Szadek KM, van der Wurff P, van Tulder MW, et al. Diagnostic validity of criteria for sacroiliac joint pain: a systemic review. J Pain 2009;10(4):354–68.
113. Murakami E, Aizawa T, Noguchi K, et al. Diagram specific to sacroiliac joint pain site indicated by one-finger test. J Orthop Sci 2008;13(6):492–7.
114. O'Sullivan PB, Beales DJ, Beetham JA, et al. Altered motor control strategies in subjects with sacroiliac joint pain during the active straight-let raise test. Spine 2002;27(1):E1–8.
115. Elgafy H, Semaan HB, Ebraheim NA, et al. Computed tomography findings in patients with sacroiliac pain. Clin Orthop Relat Res 2001;382:112–8.
116. Bogduk N, Twomey LT. Clinical anatomy of the lumbar spine. Melbourne: Churchill Livingstone; 1991.
117. Yahia LH, Garzon S, Strykowski H, et al. Ultrastructure of the human interspinous ligament and ligamentum flavum: a preliminary study. Spine 1990;15:262–8.
118. Okuda T, Fujimoto Y, Tanaka N, et al. Morphological changes of the ligamentum flavum as a cause of nerve root compression. Eur Spine J 2005;14:277–86.
119. Yoshida M, Shima K, Taniguchi Y, et al. Hypertrophied ligamentum flavum in lumbar spinal canal stenosis. Pathogenesis and morphologic and immunohisto-chemical observation. Spine 1992;17:1353–60.
120. Shrader PK, Grob D, Rahn BA, et al. Histology of the ligamentum flavum in patients with degenerative lumbar spinal stenosis. Eur Spine J 1999;8:323–38.
121. Sakamaki T, Sairyo K, Sakai T, et al. Measurements of ligamentum flavum thickening at lumbar spine using MRI. Arch Orthop Trauma Surg 2009;129(10):1415–9.
122. Aspden RM, Bornsetin NH, Hukins DW, et al. Collagen organization in the inter-spinous ligament and its relationship to tissue function. J Anat 1987;155:141–51.
123. Hindle RJ, Pearce MJ, Cross A. Mechanical function of the human lumbar inter-spinous and supraspinous ligaments. J Biomed Eng 1990;12(4):340–4.
124. Hukins DW, Kirby MC, Sikoryn TA, et al. Comparison of structure, mechanical properties and functions of lumbar spinal ligaments. Spine 1990;15:787–95.
125. Willard FH. The muscular, ligamentous and neural structure of the lumbosacrum and its relationship to low back pain. In: Vleeming A, Mooney V, Stoeckart R, editors. Movement, stability and lumbopelvic pain. Integration of research and therapy. Edinburgh (UK): Elsevier; 2007. p. 7–11.
126. Rucco V, Basadonna P, Gasparini D. Anatomy of the iliolumbar ligament: a review of its anatomy and a magnetic resonance study. Am J Phys Med Reha-bil 1996;75(6):451–5.
127. Fujiwara A, Tmal K, Yoshida H, et al. Anatomy of the iliolumbar ligament. Clin Or-thop Relat Res 2000;380:167–72.
128. Pool-Goudzwaard AJ, Kleinrensink GJ, Snijders CJ, et al. The sacroiliac part of the iliolumbar ligament. J Anat 2001;199:457–63.
129. Hartford JM, McCullen GM, Harris R, et al. The iliolumbar ligament: three dimen-sional volume imaging and computer reformatting by magnetic resonance: a technical note. Spine 2000;25(9):1098–103.
130. Leong JC, Luk KD, Chow DH, et al. The biomechanical functions of the iliolum-bar ligament in maintaining stability of the lumbosacral junction. Spine 1987;12:669–74.
131. Yamamoto I, Panjabi MM, Oxlan TR, et al. The role of the iliolumbar ligament in the lumbosacral junction. Spine 1990;15:1138.

132. Aihara T, Takahashi K, Yamagata M, et al. Biomechanical functions of the iliolumbar ligament in L5 spondylolysis. J Orthop Sci 2000;5:238–42.

133. Pool-Goudzwaard A, Van Dijke GH, Mulder P, et al. The iliolumbar ligament: its influence on stability of the sacroiliac joint. Clin Biomech 2003;18(2):99–105.

134. Sims JA, Moorman SJ. The role of the iliolumbar ligament in low back pain. Med Hypotheses 1996;46:511–5.

135. Kiter E, Karaboyun T, Tufan AC, et al. Immunochemical demonstration of nerve endings in the iliolumbar ligament. Spine 2010;35(4):101–4.

136. Kellgren JH. On the distribution of pain arising from deep somatic structures with charts of segmental pain areas. Clin Sci 1939;4:35–46.

137. Whitty CW. Some aspects of referred pain. Proc R Soc Med 1958;51:159–60 section of neurology.

138. Inman VT, Saunders JB. Referred pain from skeletal structures. J Nerv Ment Dis 1944;99:660–7.

139. Bogduk N. The physiology of deep, somatic pain. Australasian Musculoskeletal Medicine 2002;7(1):6–15.

140. Gatehouse PD, He T, Hughes SP, et al. MR imaging of degenerative disc disease in the lumbar spine with ultrashort TE pulse sequences. MAGMA 2004;16(4):160–6.

141. Benjamin M, McGonagle D. The enthesis organ concept and its relevance to the spondyloarthropathies. Adv Exp Med Biol 2009;649:57–70.

142. Biedermann HJ, DeFoa JL, Forrest WJ. Muscle fibre directions of iliocostalis and multifidus: male-female differences. J Anat 1991;179:163–7.

143. Moseley FL, Hodges PW, Gandevia SC. External perturbation of the trunk in standing humans differentially activates components of the medial back muscles. J Physiol 2003;547:581–7.

144. Danneels LA, Vanderstraeten GG, Cambier DC, et al. A functional subdivision of hip, abdominal and back muscles during asymmetric lifting. Spine 2001;26: E114–21.

145. Freeman MD, Woodham MA, Woodham AW. The role of the lumbar multifidus in chronic low back pain: a review. PM R 2010;2(2):142–6.

146. Kalichman L, Kim D, Li L, et al. Computed tomography-evaluated features of spinal degeneration: prevalence, intercorrelation, and association with self-reported low back pain. Spine J 2010;10:200–8.

147. Mengiardi B, Schmid M, Boos N, et al. Fat content of lumbar paraspinal muscles in patients with chronic low back pain and asymptomatic volunteers; quantification with MR spectroscopy. Radiology 2006;240:786–92.

148. MacDonald D, Moseley GL, Hodges PW. Why do some patients keep hurting their back? Evidence of ongoing back muscle dysfunction during remission from recurrent back pain. Pain 2008;142:183–8.

149. Mazis N, Papachristou DJ, Zouboulis P, et al. The effect of different physical activity levels on muscle fiber size and type distribution of lumbar multifidus. A biopsy study on low back pain patient groups and healthy control subjects. Eur J Phys Rehabil Med 2009;45(4):459–67.

150. Dickx N, Cagnie B, Parlevliet, et al. The effect of unilateral muscle pain on recruitment of the lumbar multifidus during automatic contraction. An experimental pain study. Man Ther 2010;15(4):364–9.

151. Bogduk N. The lumbar mamillo-accessory ligament. Its anatomical and neurosurgical significance. Spine 1981;6:162–7.

152. Nitz AJ, Peck J. Comparison of muscle spindle concentrations in large and small muscles acting in parallel combinations. Am Surg 1986;52:273–7.

153. Middleditch A, Oliver J. Muscles of the vertebral column. In: Functional anatomy of the spine. 2nd edition. London: Elsevier; 2005. p. 87–152.
154. Akuthota V, Nadler SF. Core strengthening. Arch Phys Med Rehabil 2004;85(3 Suppl 1):S86–92.
155. Urquhart DM, Hodges PW. Clinical anatomy of the anterolateral abdominal muscles. In: Vleeming A, Mooney V, Stoeckart R, editors. Movement, stability and lumbopelvic pain. Integration of research and therapy. Edinburgh (UK): Elsevier; 2007. p. 76–7.
156. Marshall P, Murphy B. The validity and reliability of surface EMG to assess the neuromuscular response of the abdominal muscles to rapid limb movement. J Electromyogr Kinesiol 2003;13(5):477–89.
157. Hodges PW, Richardson CA. Contraction of the abdominal muscles associated with movement of the lower limb. Phys Therapy 1997;77:132–42.
158. Skyrme AD, Cehill DJ, Marsh HP, et al. Psoas major and its controversial rotational action. Clin Anat 1999;12:264–5.
159. Bogduk N, Pearcy M, Hadfield G. Anatomy and biomechanics of psoas major. Clin Biomech 1992;7:109–19.
160. Phillips SD, Mercer S, Bogduk N. Anatomy and biomechanics of quadratus lumborum. Proc Inst Mech Eng H 2008;222(2):151–9.
161. Van Wingerden JP, Vleeming A, Buyruk HM, et al. Stabilization of the sacroiliac joint in vivo: verification of muscular contribution to force closure of the pelvis. Eur Spine J 2004;13:199–205.
162. Snijders CJ, Vleeming A, Stoeckart R. Transfer of lumbosacral load to iliac bones and legs. Part I: biomechanics of self-bracing of the sacroiliac joints and its significance for treatment and exercise. Clin Biomech 1993;8:285–94.
163. Takasaki H, Iizawa T, Hall T. The influence of increasing sacroiliac joint force closure on the hip and lumbar spine extensor muscle firing pattern. Man Ther 2009;14:484–9.
164. Smoll NR. Variations of the piriformis and sciatic nerve with clinical consequence: a review. Clinical Anatomy 2010;23:8–17.
165. Benjamin M. The fascia of the limbs and back—a review. J Anat 2009;214(1): 1–18.
166. Bogduk N. The lumbar muscles and their fascia. In: Clinical anatomy of the lumbar spine and sacrum. London: Elsevier; 2005. p. 110.
167. Loukas M, Shoka MM, Thurston T, et al. Anatomy and biomechanics of the vertebral aponeurosis part of the posterior layer of the thoracolumbar fascia. Surg Radiol Anat 2008;30:125–9.
168. Vleeming A, Pool-Goudzwaard AL, Stoeckart R, et al. The posterior layer of the thoracolumbar fascia. Its function in load transfer from spine to legs. Spine 1995;20(7):753–8.
169. Barker PJ, Guggenheimer KT, Grkovic IP, et al. Effects of tensioning the lumbar fasciae on segmental flexion and extension: young investigator award winner. Spine 2006;31(4):397–405.
170. Bednar DA, Orr FW, Simon GT. Observations on the pathomorphology of the thoracolumbar fascia in chronic mechanical back pain. A microscopic study. Spine 1995;20(10):1161–4.
171. DeRosa C, Porterfield J. Anatomical linkages and muscle slings of the lumbopelvic region. In: Vleeming A, Mooney V, Stoeckart R, editors. Movement, stability and lumbopelvic pain. Integration of research and therapy. Edinburgh (UK): Elsevier; 2007. p. 47–62.

Myofascial Low Back Pain: A Review

Gerard A. Malanga, MD[a,b,c],*, Eduardo J. Cruz Colon, MD[d]

KEYWORDS

- Myofascial pain • Low back pain • Fibromyalgia
- Trigger points

Myofascial syndrome is a common nonarticular local musculoskeletal pain syndrome caused by myofascial trigger points (MTrPs) located at muscle, fascia, or tendinous insertions. Myofascial syndrome affects up to 95% of people with chronic pain disorders[1] and has also been found to be the principal cause of pain in 85% of patients attending a pain center.[1,2] As many as 9 million people in the United States suffer with myofascial pain.[3] Initially described in the 16th century by the French physician de Baillou (who named this regional pain syndrome muscular rheumatism), this condition has received several terms throughout the years including idiopathic myalgia, regional fibromyalgia, and regional soft tissue pain, among others. It was not until the 1950s that Travell and Rinzler referred to these muscle pain patterns as myofascial pain.

Myofascial pain syndrome is characterized by the presence of trigger points, which are hyperirritable tender spots in palpable tense bands of skeletal muscles. Trigger points can be either active, which are tender and spontaneously painful, or latent, which are tender but not spontaneously painful. Snapping palpation of the taut bands may produce a transient contraction of a group of muscle fibers referred as the local twitch response. Local twitch response is caused by activation of local Ia afferents and consequent reflex response of α motor neurons, which indicates the presence of muscle spindles.[4] A patient vocalization or withdrawal from palpation when exquisite tenderness is perceived is referred as the jump sign.[5] Clinically, myofascial pain syndrome can present as painful restricted range of motion, stiffness, referred pain patterns, and autonomic dysfunction.

PATHOPHYSIOLOGY

Several hypotheses proposed have been a topic of debate for the last several years. At present the most accepted theory is the Integrated Trigger Point Hypothesis

[a] Overlook Pain Center Summit, NJ 07901, USA
[b] Atlantic Health, Morristown, NJ 07960, USA
[c] Department of Physical Medicine and Rehabilitation, UMDNJ-New Jersey Medical School, 30 Bergen Street, ADMC 101, Newark, NJ 07101-1709, USA
[d] UMDNJ – Kessler Rehabilitation Institute, West Orange, NJ, USA
* Corresponding author.
E-mail address: gmalangamd@hotmail.com

Phys Med Rehabil Clin N Am 21 (2010) 711–724
doi:10.1016/j.pmr.2010.07.003
1047-9651/10/$ – see front matter © 2010 Elsevier Inc. All rights reserved.

described by Simons.[2,5–8] Simons'[8] integrated hypothesis proposes that a sequence of events including an "energy crisis" of the muscle fibers will cause sustained sarcomere contracture. Decreased levels of adenosine triphosphate caused by reduced blood flow renders the muscle fibers with insufficient energy to return calcium to the sarcoplasmic reticulum, resulting in a rigor state where these muscle fibers are unable to relax. This situation leads to increased metabolic demands, resulting in local temporary hypoxia and the release of noxious histochemicals, which may account for the pain associated with the active MTrPs.[5,6,9]

It has also been hypothesized that the reason for this sarcomere shortening is secondary to an increase in miniature endplate potentials and excessive acetylcholine release, the reason why botulinum toxin may be effective in the treatment of MTrPs.[6,7,10] Besides the mechanism of excessive release of acetylcholine leading to abnormal depolarization, other mechanisms include upregulation of nicotinic acetylcholine-receptor activity as well as genetic or acquired defects of the L-type and N-type voltage-gated Ca^{2+} channel.[7] Excessive calcium release at the sarcoplasmic reticulum through a dysfunctional Ryanidine receptor calcium channel may also cause sustained muscle contraction.[11]

Simons' theory was supported by Shah and colleagues[9] when they measured the levels of biochemical substances at active and latent MTrPs at the upper trapezius and compared them to uninvolved sites at the gastrocnemius muscle. These biochemical substances are associated with the pain, muscle soreness, and inflammation in the soft tissue sites. The selected inflammatory mediators include neuropeptides, cytokines, and catecholamines, and also noted is a decrease in pH. These chemical substances activate the different nociceptors located at muscle, fascia, and joints, and are responsible for the pain associated with the myofascial pain syndrome. Specific substances found by Shah and Gilliams[6] in their study of microdialysis sampling of the trapezius include substance P, calcitonin gene-related peptide, serotonin, norepinephrine, prostaglandins, bradykinins, tumor necrosis factor α, interleukin (IL)-6, IL-8, and IL-1β. The acidic environment secondary to ischemia and local hypoxia inhibits acetylcholinesterase, resulting in an excess of acetylcholine, and activates nociceptors that promote hyperalgesia.[12,13]

The vasodilatory effects of several of the biochemicals released contribute to increased pain at the active trigger point.[6,9] Furthermore, Partanen and colleagues[4] suggested in 2010 that postural stresses and sustained overload of the muscle will cause inflammation of the muscle spindles, resulting in activation and sensitization of intrafusal III and IV afferents.

The pain experienced by these patients may be severe only with minimal palpation, and they may appear as if they are overreacting. This pain response is felt to be secondary to hyperalgesia as a result of sensitization.[4,6] Many of the endogenous substances mentioned may cause peripheral sensitization of nociceptors, which decrease their pain threshold in the peripheral receptors and cause a normally nonpainful stimulus to elicit pain.

ETIOLOGY

There are many factors that have been proposed to result in the development and persistence of MTrP pain. These factors include anatomic abnormalities, various postural habits, vocational activities causing excessive strain on a particular muscle, tendon, or ligament, endocrine dysfunctions, psychological stressors, sleep disorders, and lack of exercise.[14–16]

Mechanical

Postural habits contribute to the development of myofascial pain by causing excessive overload on specific muscle groups, the quadratus lumborum being the most commonly involved.[5] For example, leg crossing will cause the hemipelvis to rise, approximating the iliac crest to the 12th rib, and cause shortening of the ipsilateral quadratus lumborum. A common sleeping position such as lying on one's side with the uppermost leg in adduction will also cause shortening of the quadratus lumborum, and these patients will typically complain that their pain is worse at night.[17] Anatomic considerations include leg length inequality, short arms, and a small hemipelvis. Leg length discrepancy will cause excessive lumbar lordosis and excessive stress at the quadratus lumborum. The compensatory (functional) scoliosis produced by the quadratus lumborum is a necessary lumbar curvature needed to maintain balance, leading to overloading of this muscle. Patients with short arms can be identified by evaluating if the elbows do not reach the iliac crest. When seated, these patients will tend to slump forward or lean to one side of the chair, to be able to place their elbows at the armrest, resulting in excessive strain on the quadratus lumborum and posterior cervical paraspinal muscles.[5] One can also see shoulder tilt to accommodate the spinal curvature and chronic muscle contraction to bring the spine back to midline, which will eventually lead to trigger points.[16]

Medical

Besides mechanical causes of myofascial type pain such as structural, postural, or ergonomic; others include hormonal dysfunction, enzyme deficiencies, immunologic causes, infectious diseases, and nutritional deficiencies. Plotnikof and Quigley[16,18] found that 89% of subjects with chronic musculoskeletal pain had low levels of vitamin D. Deficiency of this vitamin has been associated with musculoskeletal pain, loss of type II fibers, and proximal muscle atrophy. Vitamin B12 and iron deficiency have also been linked to chronic pain, presenting with symptoms such as muscle pain, chronic fatigue, tiredness, and poor endurance. Iron is necessary for the generation of energy through the cytochrome oxidase system, and a deficiency of accessible iron in muscle will result in "energy crisis."[16] Other vitamins such as vitamins C, B1, and B6 have also been associated with diffuse mylagia.[16,18]

Endocrine disorders include hypothyroidism and growth hormone deficiency. Special considerations have been made with hypothyroidism in view of that it promotes a hypometabolic state thought to promote trigger point formation.[16] Low levels of thyroid hormones will affect cellular metabolism, resulting in an inadequate supply of energy for muscle contraction.[16] The same principle of active muscle contraction secondary to inadequate recovery of calcium by the sarcoplasmic reticulum is also seen in McArdle disease. This genetic myophosphorylase deficiency will affect glycolytic metabolism in muscle and will lead to lack of calcium recovery.[19] Finally, infections that have been linked to myofascial pain include chronic Lyme disease, chronic mycoplasma infections, hepatitis C, and enteroviruses.

Assessment

Identification of MTrPs is almost entirely based on history and physical examination. The patient will usually present with a chronic history of localized or regional pain, with resisted range of motion of the muscles involved. It is essential to identify from the history if the muscle pain is more focal as opposed to generalized or widespread. A focal myalgia would suggest mechanical or structural factors as the cause of pain, whereas in a widespread myalgia, laboratory tests are necessary to identify metabolic, hormonal, or nutritional disorders, or fibromyalgia as the reason for the musculoskel-etal pain syndrome.[16] There are also a series of diagrams that the patient can use to identify his or her pain pattern, for a better assessment of widespread versus localized pain.

Physical examination should begin inspecting for postural imbalances, gait, pelvic symmetry, shoulder tilt, leg length discrepancies, and for compensatory functional scoliosis. Evaluating tightness at the hip flexors and hamstrings should be part of the physical examination, as tightness in these muscle groups will promote forward pelvic tilt and an increase in lumbar lordosis, which will result in excessive strain at extensor muscles.[5] Palpation is the most important component of the physical exam-ination to assess for the presence of MTrPs. It is essential to identify if the tender points on palpation produce referred pain patterns or just local tenderness, which is the main difference between trigger points and tender spots. A systematic review in 2009 by Lucas and colleagues[20] on the reliability of physical examination for the diag-nosis or trigger points demonstrated that due to a lack of studies and interobserver reliability, physical examination cannot currently be recommended as a reliable test for the diagnosis of trigger points.[2,20–22]

When evaluating patients with suspected myofascial low back pain, muscles that may have trigger points include the iliocostalis lumborum, longissimus thoracis, multi-fidus, quadratus lumborum, and gluteus medius.[23] Travell and Simons[5] suggest that the quadratus lumborum and gluteus medius are the most frequently involved. Adequate assessment of the quadratus lumborum will require that the patient be lying on his or her side with the uppermost arm abducted above the head with knees bent. Palpation of the gluteus medius should be at the upper lateral quadrant of the buttocks when the patient is lying prone. In a prospective study by Njoo and Van der Does,[22] it was determined that the clinical usefulness of trigger points is increased when local-ized tenderness and the presence of either the jump sign or patient's recognition of his pain pattern are used as criteria for the presence of trigger points in these muscles.

Also, adequate screening for stress and anxiety is important in patients with wide-spread musculoskeletal pain. Severe depression, anxiety, and fear avoidance behavior are predominantly associated with patients with low back pain and widespread musculoskeletal pain as compared with patients who are pain free. Other psychosocial factors to consider include low income, early psychological stressors, gender, job satisfaction, and history of musculoskeletal pain in family members.[23]

MYOFASCIAL PAIN VERSUS FIBROMYALGIA

Common differential diagnoses of low back pain include mechanical, sacroiliac joint, discogenic or zygapophysial joint pain; a thorough physical examination will help rule out most of these. When considering myofascial low back pain as the cause of the patient's complaint; special attention has to be made to fibromyalgia, which is also a chronic noninflammatory muscle pain syndrome. Many questions have risen over the years regarding the diagnosis of fibromyalgia, and several have doubted its existence.

Fibromyalgia is a syndrome characterized by chronic widespread muscle tender-ness as a result of widespread sensitization. Fibromyalgia may be accompanied by fatigue, sleep disturbances, mood disturbances, depression, and visceral pain syndromes.[16]

The current American College of Rheumatology (ACR) criteria include spontaneous pain present for over 3 months, pain in all 4 quadrants of the body (above and below the waist, right and left of midline) and pain on digital palpation on 11 out of 18 tender points. Without an adequate physical examination one might confuse myofascial pain syndrome with fibromyalgia. Myofascial pain syndrome is the most common condition that must be considered in the differential diagnosis of fibromyalgia and can also present as widespread myalgia. As stated in a review by Gerwin in 2005 about myofascial pain syndrome and fibromyalgia; "many cases of fibromyalgia are in fact cases of myofascial pain syndrome that have been misdiagnosed as a result of poor muscle palpation techniques that miss the presence of taut bands and referred pain." The main difference between the two is the referral of pain produced when palpating trigger points as compared with tender spots.

In previous studies more than 10 active trigger points were found in more than half of fibromyalgia patients,[24] and active trigger points were found in about 18% of examinations in the predetermined tender points of fibromyalgia.[25] A study by Ge and colleagues[26] in 2009 evaluated if the predetermined sites of examination for tender points in fibromyalgia were frequently associated with MTrPs. Thirty women diagnosed with fibromyalgia as per the ACR criteria were chosen for the study. All of the 18 predetermined tender points were manually palpated and examined with intramuscular needle electromyographic (EMG) examination, as one would expect to see spontaneous electric activity in both active and latent trigger points. The 2 sites bilaterally at the second rib were not included in the EMG examination of thin patients, to avoid any complications. In this study more than 90% of the predetermined tender point sites were either active or latent MTrPs, as evaluated by manual palpation and confirmed by needle EMG registration of spontaneous electrical activity. In conclusion, this study demonstrated that positive tender points at predetermined sites were mostly clinically active and latent trigger points at these predetermined sites, which mimicked fibromyalgia pain.[26]

A new diagnostic tool named the Symptom Intensity Scale (SIS) has been developed for the diagnosis of fibromyalgia. This tool has been used to both diagnose and establish severity of fibromyalgia, without the need to count tender points. The scale consists of 2 parts: a regional pain score, which is the number of anatomic areas out of possible 19 in which the patient feels pain, and a fatigue visual analog scale whereby the patient makes a mark somewhere along a 10-cm line to indicate how tired they are. The SIS has been shown to be an accurate measure for general health, depression, and disability. Although still not recognized by the ACR, several investigators state that it will probably replace the current diagnostic criteria and that tender spots will no longer have to be counted.[27]

DIAGNOSTIC CRITERIA FOR MYOFASCIAL PAIN SYNDROME

Travell and Simons are identified as the principal founders of the diagnostic criteria of myofascial pain. Their proposed criteria include tender spots in a taut band, predicted pain referral pattern, patient pain recognition on tender point palpation, limited range of motion, and the local twitch response. A literature review from 2007 examined the variability of criteria used to diagnose MTrP pain syndrome. The criteria most commonly used by researchers and expert clinicians include all of the previously mentioned by Travell and Simons, except the local twitch response, which has not shown to be a reliable diagnostic test.[28] When comparing the frequency of the commonly used criteria, identifying a tender spot in a taut band is used in 65% of cases, and had been suggested by Travell and Simons to be the most sensitive and specific of all the diagnostic criteria. The frequency of the criteria used include patient pain recognition 53%, predicted pain referral pattern 44%, local twitch response 44%, and limited range of motion 22%. There is still a lack of evidence demonstrating the reliability of these maneuvers. Further research is needed to test the sensitivity, specificity, and reliability of the current diagnostic criteria.[2]

Other minor criteria proposed include the jump sign, muscle weakness, autonomic responses, reduced skin resistance, pressure algometry readings, patients' being able to identify their trigger points, and alleviation of symptoms by stretch. The combination of the criteria used has been inconsistent but the combination proposed by Simons is still the most commonly used. The most recent modifications of the diagnostic criteria include tender spot in a taut band, patient pain recognition, and painful limitation to range of motion.

The local twitch response and predicted pain referral pattern are no longer considered as part of the diagnosis. Other investigators have suggested alleviation of the pain by infiltration of a local anesthetic and pressure algometry readings as part of the diagnosis, but this has not been adopted by many.[2] In a 2009 review of the reliability of physical examination for the diagnosis of MTrPs, firm digital pressure and the patient's feedback on the pain experience are considered the best indicators of the presence of trigger points. In this same review it was concluded that no study to date has reported the reliability of trigger point diagnosis according to the currently proposed criteria in symptomatic patients.[20] Ongoing microdialysis and EMG studies will continue to define and validate the current proposed criteria. There is still poor agreement among investigators as to the most appropriate diagnostic criteria; only recently have interrater reliability studies been reported.[29]

It is well known that the pressure algometer is used by manual medicine practitioners to determine the pressure pain threshold of specific muscles, joints, tendons, ligaments, and bones. The pressure algometer measures the force in pounds or kilograms required to produce pain, and has become useful to quantify pain and track recovery.[30] It is a hand-held instrument with a 1-cm^2 surface area plunger attached to a dynamic force gauge that may be used to assess sensitivity to pressure near a trigger point. Some studies have found high validity with an excellent inter- and intrarater reliability, but algometry is more commonly used in a research setting than clinical practice.[31–33] Other studies have demonstrated that the pressure algometer may have limited validity on determining pressure pain thresholds. Recently a new muscle pain detection device (MPDD) has been developed for identification of trigger points that will also distinguish between primary and referred muscle pain. This new device elicits contractions in muscles in an attempt to identify the muscle pain generator (see the next section for more details).

DIAGNOSTIC EVALUATION

There are no laboratory tests or diagnostic images that can serve as a gold standard for trigger point identification. Physical examination may also be unreliable to adequately diagnose MTrPs. New diagnostic tools such as ultrasonography (US) and magnetic resonance elastography (MRE) have shown promising results to identify and differentiate MTrPs from normal surrounding tissue. US has recently been used to identify trigger points because of its ability to characterize viscoelastic properties of myofascial tissue and identify high resistance arterial flow at trigger point sites.

A study by Sidkar and colleagues[34] evaluated 10 patients with trigger points, as per the diagnostic criteria of Travell and Simons. Active trigger points, latent and normal tissue, were labeled after being identified by physical examination. US was performed on each of the sites by blinded physicians, as well as vibration sonoelastography (VSE). VSE uses external vibration to localize areas of stiffer tissue. On US 2-dimensional (2D) gray imaging, trigger points at the upper trapezius, which were identified previously by physical examination, appeared as focal dark (hypoechoic) elliptically shaped areas with heterogeneous echotexture. The palpated sites that were labeled as normal appeared as isoechoic with homogeneous echotexture.

Examination of the active trigger points with Doppler flow waveforms revealed abnormalities within the vasculature at active trigger points and adjacent tissue. Doppler flow at the active trigger point sites revealed an increase in vascular resistance as compared with latent and normal tissue sites. This high resistance is secondary to the sustained contracture at these active trigger point sites. US VSE was able to identify areas of stiffer tissue in view of that these areas of stiffer tissue vibrated with lower amplitude as compared with surrounding normal tissue; vibration amplitudes were 27% lower on average.[34] In conclusion, US can be used to identify MTrPs, and VSE can differentiate these sites from normal surrounding tissue and quantify the relative stiffness based on vibration amplitudes.

MRE is another diagnostic tool that can be used to evaluate for MTrPs. MRE was initially developed at the Mayo Clinic and was used primarily to diagnose liver fibrosis by measuring liver stiffness.[35] As initially described by Muthupillai in 1995, it is an noninvasive MR-based contrast imaging technique that applies an oscillating motion to detect tissue vibratory displacements that have been introduced into a tissue by an external source of shear vibration. MRE basically works by measuring the wavelengths of the vibrations sent through tissues. Shear waves travel more rapidly in stiffer tissue and hence display a longer wavelength. Myofascial taut bands, which have higher stiffness as compared with surrounding muscle fibers, will result in longer wavelengths.[36,37] Although MRE is able to identify the difference in wave propagation patterns in a taut band as compared with normal myofascial tissue, the MTrP was not identified in the taut band. 2D US combined with VSE may be a better diagnostic tool than MRE because it can localize MTrPs, provides better mechanical and physical properties of trigger points and surrounding muscle tissue, and is more cost effective.[38]

The MPDD is an electrical device that elicits contractions in muscles in an attempt to identify the muscle that is thought to cause the pain. If the muscle stimulated produces pain, it is believed that this muscle is the pain generator, as compared with normal muscle, where the patient will experience an involuntary painless contraction. This device uses current produced through an aluminum head that moves through the skin and causes the muscle to contract. There are 3 possible diagnostic outcomes when using the MPDD: no pain with the stimulus, pain that disappears with repeated stimulation, or pain that persists with repeated stimulation. When the stimulus does not produce pain, the muscle contracted is not considered the pain generator. Pain that disappears with continuous stimulation is thought to be secondary to tension or spasms, and may be reversible with conservative methods. Finally, pain that persists with a repeated stimulus is caused by histologic changes, such as trigger points within the muscle that produce painful contractions.[39]

In a randomized control study in 2010 by Hunter and colleagues,[39] the effectiveness of MPDD versus manual pressure was evaluated, based on the outcome of standardized injections to muscles identified by each technique. Subjects were injected at several sites identified by a blinded physician by either manual pressure or MPDD. The sample size included 40 patients with a minimum 3-month history of back or neck pain. Painful sites were identified in half of the patients by manual pressure and half with the MPDD. There were 45 muscles identified by manual pressure that were determined to benefit from injection and 46 muscles selected for injection by MPDD. When compared with MPDD, of the 45 muscles identified with manual pressure 24% had no pain, in 42% the pain disappeared with repeated stimulus, and only 15 muscles were identified that would benefit from injection. After treatment with 2 mL of 1% lidocaine injection, the MPDD group reported statistically significant improvements from baseline in pain, mood, and disability scores at 1 week and 1 month. Although relatively new, the MPDD demonstrates promising results in identifying muscle pain generators, for better precision of injection, as compared with manual pressure palpation.

TREATMENT

Multiple modalities and approaches have been used for the treatment of MTrPs with varying degrees of success. These methods include manual therapies such as pharmacologic management, physical therapy modalities, myofascial release, injection therapies, dry needling, and alternative medicine treatments such as acupuncture. The most common and effective treatment options used in daily clinical practice as well as other alternative treatment options such as acupuncture and herbal medications are presented in this section. The most important concept overall is treating the underlying etiologic pathology responsible for trigger point activation—far more important than treating the actual trigger point(s). In many cases, the active MTrP will automatically inactivate as soon as the underlying pathology is adequately treated.[40] Important mention has to be made of several of the principles proposed by Hong concerning inactivation of trigger points. First of all, the trigger point being targeted should be confirmed as the pain generator. This targeting might be difficult because there may be many adjacent latent trigger points that will be painful on palpation. Identification of active versus chronic trigger points should also be assessed. Furthermore, the active trigger point should not be inactivated in the acute stage because it will subsequently disappear on its own once the acute lesion is adequately treated, although inactivation might be considered if the pain is severe or intolerable. When the etiologic lesion cannot be targeted locally because of severe pain from the active MTrPs, treatment of inactive distal (satellite) trigger points can be considered. This action may result in decreased sensitivity of the surrounding muscle tissue, and will later allow for treatment of the acute lesion and active trigger points. Finally, for optimal results, perpetuating factors should be avoided. The patient should be educated on proper posture, home exercises, and self-care techniques. Special considerations have to be made to underlying anatomic abnormalities that contribute to the persistence of myofascial pain, such as limb length discrepancies and compensatory functional scoliosis.

Manual therapy is one of the most common treatment options for myofascial pain. Manual therapy is often the first line of treatment before going on to other more invasive techniques such as injections or needling. Manual therapy will mostly consist of myofascial release, deep pressure massage, osteopathic manipulative treatment, and a popular technique called spray and stretch. This technique was initially described by Simons, and consists of passively stretching the targeted muscle and simultaneously applying a vaporized cooling liquid spray such as Fluori-Methane or ethyl chloride. This temporary anesthesia allows the muscle to be stretched passively toward normal length and helps inactivate the trigger point.[3,41]

Postisometric relaxation is another effective technique whereby the patient is asked to contract the involved muscle 10% to 25% of maximum, followed by relaxation and stretching.[40] Deep digital pressure (ischemic compression) is no longer recommended by Simons in the most recent edition of the trigger point manual, in view that it theoretically contributed to additional local ischemia. The best approach is by applying a "press and stretch" technique, which is believed to restore abnormally contracted sarcomeres to their normal resting length.[7]

Pharmacologic therapy, transcutaneous electrical nerve stimulation, and thermotherapy are useful only for controlling pain symptoms. Pharmacotherapy includes muscle relaxants, nonsteroidal anti-inflammatory drugs (NSAIDs), analgesics, and tricyclic antidepressants such as amitriptyline. The latter are recommended in myofascial pain characterized by sleep disturbances.[5,42] Muscle relaxants include clonazepam, whose primary mechanism of action is enhancing GABAergic inhibition, and cyclobenzaprine, which is a centrally acting serotonin receptor antagonist that suppresses muscle spasms without interfering with muscle function. Leite and colleagues[43] have demonstrated cyclobenzaprine to be slightly superior when compared with clonazepam. Topical NSAIDs have been used in pain control for acute soft tissue damage, although their effectiveness in treating myofascial pain has not been fully studied. A randomized, double-blind, placebo-controlled study demonstrated that a 1-week treatment with a diclofenac patch produced significantly greater pain reduction and earlier mobilization of the involved muscles when compared with placebo (menthol patch). However, it did not affect pain threshold on MTrPs.[44]

US, iontophoresis, phontophoresis, and high-voltage galvanic stimulation are used by many professionals, but none of these techniques are supported by scientific evidence regarding their efficacy in eliminating MTrPs.[42] Of all available treatment options for MTrPs, the best evidence exists for trigger point injection and dry needling.[41] The main goal of treatment is to inactivate the trigger point and loosen the taut band.[45] The indications for a trigger point injection is clinical localization of active trigger points in patients with chronic low back pain with myofascial pain syndrome, who have failed to respond to medications and/or a course of active physical therapy, or when a joint is mechanically locked.[46,47] When the decision is made to proceed with injection or needling, there are several precautions to keep in mind. Contraindications to trigger point injections include bleeding disorders, anticoagulation, local infection, aspirin ingestion within 3 days of injection, and acute muscle trauma.[3,5] Bleeding tendencies will result in increased capillary hemorrhage, which will contribute to postinjection soreness.[5] If possible, the patient should be placed prone or supine to decrease the risk of vasovagal depression. Other complications include local muscle necrosis if corticosteroid is the substance being injected, pneumothorax, cervical epidural abscess, and intrathecal injection. Using botulinum toxin within trigger points may result in excessive weakness, flu-like symptoms, and transient numbness of the ipsilateral limb, and has not been shown to be superior to injection with Marcaine.[48–50]

Lidocaine is a frequently used anesthetic, although there are many different types of anesthetics or injection solutions that can be used. Procaine is also a preferred anesthetic because of its short action and minimal systemic toxicity with the absence of local irritation. Procaine also has the distinction of being the least myotoxic of all injectable anesthetics.[3] Other anesthetics cited in the literature for the treatment of MTrPs include prilocaine, mepivacaine, bupivacaine, levobupivacaine, and ropivacaine. A study in 2000 suggested that ropivacaine 0.5% was better tolerated than dry needling, bupivacaine 0.5%, bupivacaine plus dexamethasone, or ropivacaine plus dexamethasone. Corticosteroids should NOT be included as part of treatment, as there is no evidence of added benefit and local muscle necrosis is a potential risk.

Needle size is frequently 25- or 27-gauge, but a needle as large as 21-gauge has been reported. Thick subcutaneous muscles such as the gluteus maximus or paraspinals will usually require a 21-gauge, 2.0-in needle.[5] Needle length may be dependent on the depth of the muscle through subcutaneous tissue, but is reported from 0.75 to 2.5 in. The 21-gauge, 2.5-in needle will be required to reach deep muscle such as the gluteus minimus and quadratus lumborum.[3] The number of trigger points injected varies, as does the volume of solution injected. Volume may depend on the pharmacologic dosing limits of the injected mixture and the total number of trigger points. Common clinical practice is to use 0.5 to 2 mL per trigger point, which may be injected in one location of maximal tenderness or an angular array of sites. The technique recommended by Hong and Hsueh was modified from Travell and Simons. This approach described holding the syringe in the dominant hand while palpating the trigger with the thumb or index finger of the opposite hand. Needle insertion was into the subcutaneous tissue adjacent to the trigger point at a 50° to 70° angle to the skin, aiming at the taut band. Multiple insertions in different locations in different directions from the subcutaneous layer were "fast in" and "fast out" to probe for latent triggers; this technique kept a straight track of needle insertion and avoids the possibility of muscle fiber damage.[51] Each thrust coincided with the injection of 0.02 to 0.05 mL of injectate to a total of 0.5 to 1 mL in each trigger point. Compression of the point for 2 minutes allowed hemostasis, which was followed by stretching of the muscle. Some studies have emphasized that stretching the muscle after the injection will increase efficacy of treatment. Travell and Simons recommended full active range of motion of the muscles injected so that they could reach their fully shortened and lengthened position.

Hameroff and colleagues[52] compared injection of bupivacaine 0.5%, etidacaine 1%, and saline into triggers in the neck and low back. Anesthetic improved pain and activities of daily living at 1 week better than saline, but there was no difference in the type of anesthetic. Malanga and Wolff[53] compared mepivacaine 0.5% with saline in acute low back pain, and found no significant difference in pain resolution at 2 weeks. One quality trial by Garvey and colleagues[54] showed no difference between dry needling, injection of lidocaine, lidocaine plus steroid, or vapocoolant spray with acupressure in the short term. A double-blind controlled study by Hong and Simons[55] compared lidocaine injection versus dry needling for MTrP treatment. These investigators noted that lidocaine injection and dry needling were equally successful in treating MTrPs. 0.5% lidocaine was preferred over dry needling because it reduced the intensity and duration of postinjection soreness. It was also concluded that the best response to injection and immediate relief was found when the "local twitch response" was provoked by impaling the active point; little treatment effect was noted if no local twitch response during needling or lidocaine injection was elicited. Relief after injection or needling lasted for a short period of time and then returned gradually. Persistence or recurrence of pain might have been secondary to underlying pathologic lesions that had not been addressed, such as intervertebral disk lesions.[51,55]

A randomized controlled study similar to that done by Hong in 1994[51] was carried out by Ay and colleagues[45] in 2009. These investigators compared the efficacy of anesthetic injection and dry needling methods for myofascial pain syndrome, and significant improvement in pain relief was obtained with both. With dry needling, additional pain was not significant and was found to be as effective as local anesthetics in the inactivation of trigger points. Both of these injection methods were effective by causing local mechanical disruption; this leads to relaxation of taut bands, decreased pain, increased local blood flow, and improved range of motion, and causes fibrotic scar formation on trigger points.

In highly resistant trigger points botulinum toxin can be used, but its high cost does not support its use. Other investigators recommend the use of botulinum toxin in patients with chronic myofascial pain resistant to physical therapy including dry needling and oral pharmacotherapy over at least 1 month.[56] Advantages include presynaptic block of acetylcholine release from motor nerve endings, which will promote prolonged muscle relaxation for 3 to 4 months' duration.[57,58] Some studies have demonstrated the analgesic and antinociceptive effects of botulinum toxin in animal pain models.[59] Despite the theoretical advantages of botulinum toxin, a randomized, double-blind, placebo-controlled study by Ferrante and colleagues[60] did not demonstrate significant differences compared with placebo with respect to pain scores, pain thresholds with pressure algometry, or use of rescue medication. There is still concern regarding excessive muscle weakness. For example, weakening neck flexors without simultaneously weakening neck extensors can lead to postural abnormalities and increase pain.[60]

There are several alternative treatment options for myofascial pain syndrome such as acupuncture, chiropractic manipulation, and herbal medications. A recent review of the published evidence for the treatment of myofascial pain demonstrated acceptable evidentiary support by common chiropractic techniques for the treatment of myofascial pain.[61] Acupuncture's analgesic effects may be mediated by pain perception block by gate control theory whereby a pain input may be inhibited by another sensory input such as needling, elevating opioid peptides in the central nervous system, and noxious inhibitory control. Dry needling itself causes this same effect.[62] A controlled randomized trial demonstrated significant differences between the effects of trigger point acupuncture and sham acupuncture on pain and function in patients suffering from chronic low back pain.[63] Another new approach to treating trigger points is through the use of herbal medications. Some of the natural medicines that may be used include lavender, rosemary, passionflower, lemon balm, and marijuana, all of which contain the compound linalool. This compound inhibits end plate activity by reducing acetylcholine release and by modifying nicotinic acetylcholine receptors.[64]

SUMMARY

Myofascial pain is a common process resulting from a variety of causes. The diagnosis is usually made clinically, although there are recent advances in imaging that will allow for better research and may have future clinical benefits. The underlying cause (often related to muscular imbalances) should be assessed by a comprehensive physical examination and should be treated by the practitioner using a comprehensive rehabilitation program. Additional treatment options include pharmacologic, needling with or without anesthetic agents or nerve stimulation, and alternative medicine treatments such as massage and herbal medicines. Repeated trigger point injections should be avoided and corticosteroids should not be injected into trigger points. Ongoing research will continue to expand our knowledge concerning the treatment and management of myofascial pain, and provide new views concerning etiology and diagnosis.

REFERENCES

1. Fishbain DA, Goldberg M, Megher BR, et al. Male and female chronic pain patients categorized by DSM-III psychiatric diagnostic criteria. Pain 1986;26: 181–97.
2. Tough EA, White AR, Richards S, et al. Variability of criteria used to diagnose myofascial trigger point pain syndrome—evidence from a review of the literature. Clin J Pain 2007;23:278–86.
3. Alvarez DJ, Rockwell PG. Trigger points: diagnosis and management. Am Fam Physician 2002;6:653–60.

4. Partanen JV, Ojala TA, Arokoski JP. Myofascial syndrome and pain: a neurophysiological approach. Pathophysiology 2010;17:19–28.
5. Travell JG, Simons DG. Travell & Simons' myofascial pain and dysfunction: the trigger point manual. Pennsylvania: Williams & Wilkins; 1999.
6. Shah JP, Gilliams EA. Uncovering the biochemical milieu of myofascial trigger points using in vivo microdialysis: an application of muscle pain concepts to myofascial pain syndrome. J Bodyw Mov Ther 2008;12:371–84.
7. McPartland JM. Travell trigger points—molecular and osteopathic perspectives. J Am Osteopath Assoc 2004;104:244–9.
8. Simons DG. New views of myofascial trigger points: etiology and diagnosis. Arch Phys Med Rehabil 2008;89:157–9.
9. Shah JP, Danoff JV, Desai MJ, et al. Biochemicals associated with pain and inflammation are elevated in sites near to and remote from active myofascial trigger points. Arch Phys Med Rehabil 2008;89:16–23.
10. Hsieh RL, Lee WC. Are the effects of botulinum toxin injection on myofascial trigger points placebo effects or needling effects? Arch Phys Med Rehabil 2008;89:792–3.
11. Gerwin RD. The taut band and other mysteries of the trigger point: an examination of the mechanisms relevant to the development and maintenance of the trigger point. Journal of Musculoskeletal Pain 2008;16:115–21.
12. Hong CZ, Simons DG. Pathophysiologic and electrophysiologic mechanisms of myofascial trigger points. Arch Phys Med Rehabil 1998;79:863–72.
13. Kuan TS, Hong CZ, Chen JT, et al. The spinal cord connections of the myofascial trigger spots. Eur J Pain 2007;11:624–34.
14. Vedolin GM, Lobato VV, Conti PC, et al. The impact of stress and anxiety on the pressure pain threshold of myofascial pain patients. J Oral Rehabil 2009;36:313–21.
15. Chien JJ, Bajwa ZH. What is mechanical back pain and how best to treat it? Curr Pain Headache Rep 2008;12:406–11.
16. Gerwin RD. A review of myofascial pain and fibromyalgia—factors that promote their persistence. Acupunct Med 2005;23:121–34.
17. Edwards J. The importance of postural habits in perpetuating myofascial trigger point pain. Acupunct Med 2005;23:77–82.
18. Plotnikoff GA, Quigley JM. Prevalence of severe hypovitaminosis D in patients with persistent, nonspecific musculoskeletal pain. Mayo Clin Proc 2003;78:1463–70.
19. Mense S, Simons DG, Russell IJ. Muscle pain. Understanding its nature, diagnosis and treatment. Baltimore (MD): Lippincott Williams and Wilkins; 2001.
20. Lucas N, Macaskill P, Irwig L, et al. Reliability of physical examination for diagnosis of myofascial trigger points: a systematic review of the literature. Clin J Pain 2009;25:80–9.
21. Myburgh C, Larsen AH, Hartvigsen J. A systematic, critical review of manual palpation for identifying myofascial trigger points: evidence and clinical significance. Arch Phys Med Rehabil 2008;89:1169–76.
22. Njoo KH, Van der Does E. The occurrence and inter-rater reliability of myofascial trigger points in the quadratus lumborum and gluteus medius: a prospective study in non-specific low back pain patients and controls in general practice. Pain 1994;58:317–23.
23. Friedrich M, Hahne J, Wepner F. A controlled examination of medical and psychosocial factors associated with low back pain in combination with widespread musculoskeletal pain. Phys Ther 2009;89:786–803.
24. Bengtsson A, Henriksson KG, Jorfeldt L, et al. Primary fibromyalgia. A clinical and laboratory study of 55 patients. Scand J Rheumatol 1986;15:340–7.

25. Wolfe F, Simons DG, Fricton J, et al. The fibromyalgia and myofascial pain syndromes: a preliminary study of tender points and trigger points in persons with fibromyalgia, myofascial pain syndrome and no disease. J Rheumatol 1992;19:944–51.
26. Ge HY, Wang Y, Danneskiold-Samsøe B, et al. The predetermined sites of examination for tender points in fibromyalgia syndrome are frequently associated with myofascial trigger points. J Pain 2010;11(7):644–51.
27. Wilke WS. New developments in the diagnosis of fibromyalgia syndrome: say goodbye to tender points? Cleve Clin J Med 2009;76:345–52.
28. Gerwin RD, Shannon S, Hong CZ, et al. Interrater reliability in myofascial trigger point examination. Pain 1997;69:65–73.
29. Simons D. Myofascial pain management: update of myofascial pain from trigger points 2010. Available at: http://www.pain-education.com/myofascial-pain-from-trigger-points.html. Accessed April, 2010.
30. Bonci DC. Algometry validates chiropractic. Dynamic Chiropractic 1994;15:12.
31. Kinser AM, Sands WA, Stone MH. Reliability and validity of a pressure algometer. J Strength Cond Res 2009;23:312–4.
32. Delaney GA, McKee AC. Inter- and intra-rater reliability of the pressure threshold meter in measurement of myofascial trigger point sensitivity. Am J Phys Med Rehabil 1993;72:136–9.
33. Sciotti VM, Mittak VL, DiMarco L, et al. Clinical precision of myofascial trigger point location in the trapezius muscle. Pain 2001;93:259–66.
34. Sikdar S, Shah JP, Gilliams E, et al. Assessment of myofascial trigger points: a new application of ultrasound and vibration sonoelastography. Conf Proc IEEE Eng Med Biol Soc 2008;2008:5585–8.
35. Magnetic resonance elastography: an overview. Available at: http://www.mayoclinic.org/magnetic-resonance-elastography/. Accessed April, 2010.
36. Chen Q, Bensamoun S, Basford JR, et al. Identification and quantification of myofascial taut bands with magnetic resonance elastography. Arch Phys Med Rehabil 2007;88:1658–61.
37. Chen Q, Basford J, An KN. Ability of magnetic resonance imaging to asses taut bands. Clin Biomech 2008;23:623–9.
38. Sikdar S, Shah JP, Gebreab T, et al. Novel applications of ultrasound technology to visualize and characterize myofascial trigger points and surrounding soft tissue. Arch Phys Med Rehabil 2009;90(11):1829–38.
39. Hunter C, Dubois M, Zou S, et al. A new muscle pain detection device to diagnose muscles as a source of back and/or neck pain. Pain Med 2010;11:35–43.
40. Hong CZ. Treatment of myofascial pain syndrome. Curr Pain Headache Rep 2006;10:345–9.
41. Han SC, Harrison P. Myofascial pain syndrome and trigger-point management. Reg Anesth 1997;22:89–101.
42. Vázquez-Delgado E, Cascos-Romero J, Gay-Escoda C. Myofascial pain associated to trigger points: a literature review. Part 2: differential diagnosis and treatment. Med Oral Patol Oral Cir Bucal 2010;15(4):e639–43.
43. Leite FM, Atallah AN, El Dib R, et al. Cyclobenzaprine for the treatment of myofascial pain in adults. Cochrane Database Syst Rev 2009;8:CD006830.
44. Hsieh LF, Hong CZ, Chern SH, et al. Efficacy and side effects of diclofenac patch in treatment of patients with myofascial pain syndrome of the upper trapezius. J Pain Symptom Manage 2010;39:116–25.
45. Ay S, Evcik D, Tur BS. Comparison of injection methods in myofascial pain syndrome: a randomized controlled trial. Clin Rheumatol 2010;29:19–23.

46. American Medical Association. Article for trigger point injections—coding guidelines for LCD L19485. Centers for Medicare Services. Available at: http://www.Empiremedicare.com/newjpolicy/policy/119485_final.htm. Accessed March 16, 2007.
47. Fischer AA. New approaches in treatment of myofascial pain. Phys Med Rehabil Clin N Am 1997;8:153–69.
48. Wheeler AH, Goolkasian P, Gretz SS. Botulin toxin A for the treatment of chronic neck pain. Pain 2001;94:255–60.
49. Wheeler AH, Goolkasian P, Gretz SS. A randomized, double-blind, prospective pilot study of botulinum toxin injection for refractory, unilateral, cervicothoracic, paraspinal, myofascial pain syndrome. Spine 1998;23:1662–6.
50. Shafer N. Pneumothorax following "trigger point" injection. JAMA 1970;213:1193.
51. Hong CZ. Lidocaine injection versus Dry needling to myofascial trigger points. The importance of the local twitch response. Am J Phys Med Rehabil 1994;73: 256–63.
52. Hameroff SR, Crago BR, Blitt CD, et al. Comparison of bupivacaine, etidocaine, and saline for trigger-point therapy. Anesth Analg 1981;60:752–5.
53. Malanga G, Wolff E. Evidence-informed management of chronic low back pain with trigger point injections. Spine J 2008;8:243–52.
54. Garvey TA, Marks MR, Wiesel SW. A prospective, randomized, double-blind evaluation of trigger-point injection therapy for low-back pain. Spine 1989;14:962–4.
55. Hong CZ, Simons DG. Response to treatment for pectoralis minor myofascial pain syndrome after whiplash. Journal of Musculoskeletal Pain 1992;1:89–132.
56. Reilich P, Fheodoroff K, Kern U, et al. Consensus statement: botulinum toxin in myofascial [corrected] pain. J Neurol 2004;251:136–8.
57. Borodic GE, Acquadro M, Johnson EA. Botulin toxin therapy for pain and inflammatory disorders: mechanisms and therapeutic effects. Expert Opin Investig Drugs 2001;10:1531–44.
58. Göbel H, Heinze A, Reichel G, et al. Efficacy and safety of a single botulinum type A toxin complex treatment (Dysport) for the relief of upper back myofascial pain syndrome: results from a randomized double-blind placebo-controlled multicentre study. Pain 2006;125:82–8.
59. Cui M, Khanijou S, Rubino J, et al. Subcutaneous administration of botulinum toxin A reduces formalin-induced pain. Pain 2004;107:25–33.
60. Ferrante FM, Bearn L, Rothrock R, et al. Evidence against trigger point injection technique for the treatment of cervicothoracic myofascial pain with botulinum toxin type A. Anesthesiology 2005;103:377–83.
61. Vernon H, Schneider M. Chiropractic management of myofascial trigger points and myofascial pain syndrome: a systematic review of the literature. J Manipulative Physiol Ther 2009;32:14–24.
62. Furlan AD, van Tulder M, Cherkin D, et al. Acupuncture and dry-needling for low back pain: an updated systematic review within the framework of the Cochrane Collaboration. Spine 2005;30:944–63.
63. Itoh K, Katsumi Y, Hirota S, et al. Effects of trigger point acupuncture on chronic low back pain in elderly patients—a sham-controlled randomised trial. Acupunct Med 2006;24:5–12.
64. Re L, Barocci S, Sonnino S, et al. Linalool modifies the nicotinic receptor-ion channel kinetics at the mouse neuromuscular junction. Pharmacol Res 2000;42: 177–82.

Imaging the Back Pain Patient

Timothy Maus, MD

KEYWORDS

• Back pain • Magnetic resonance imaging
• Computed tomography • Spine imaging

Imaging is a single, though integral, part of the evaluation of the patient with back pain. The comprehensive evaluation must include historical data, the physical examination, and may extend to electrophysiologic tests, imaging, and response to minimally invasive interventions. Imaging can only be appropriately interpreted in the context of the totality of the evaluation; it does not stand alone. To an imaging professional, the ability of modern imaging technology to record an exquisite and accurate representation of patient anatomy and pathology is often believed to have inherent worth. To the clinician and patient, the consumers of imaging, technologically sophisticated imaging only provides value where it advances the diagnosis, excludes sinister disease, or identifies opportunities for evidence-based therapeutic intervention.

Back pain is ubiquitous in Western societies. It is the most common and expensive cause of work disability in the United States.[1] The use of sophisticated imaging in the evaluation of back pain is increasing. Lumbar spine magnetic resonance imaging (MRI), as measured by Medicare use statistics, increased by 307% in the 12-year interval from 1994 to 2005.[2] Despite the greater intensity of evaluation, there is no evidence that patient outcomes have improved. Rather, much of spine imaging is often unreasoned and adds no value to the patient's evaluation. There are very large regional variations in the intensity of spine imaging across United States; from one-third to two-thirds of spine computed tomography (CT) and MRI studies are judged to be inappropriate when measured against established guidelines.[2] It is hoped that this review of the imaging literature will provide a more rational basis for the use of imaging in patients with back or leg pain.

When considering the use of sophisticated imaging technologies in the patient with back or leg pain, it must be remembered that this occurs in the context of overwhelmingly benign disease, in terms of both the underlying pathophysiology and the clinical course. Back pain is most commonly clinically benign and self-limiting, and will benefit neither from imaging evaluation nor invasive therapies. Von Korff and colleagues[3] studied patients with a recent history of low back pain; at 6 months from onset, 76% of patients either had no pain (21%) or mild pain and disability, and 14% had

---

Department of Radiology, Mayo Clinic, 200 First Street SW, Rochester, MN 55905, USA
E-mail address: Maus.Timothy@mayo.edu

Phys Med Rehabil Clin N Am 21 (2010) 725–766
doi:10.1016/j.pmr.2010.07.004
1047-9651/10/$ – see front matter © 2010 Elsevier Inc. All rights reserved.

significant disability with moderate to severe limitation of function. Another study noted that whereas 70% of patients with acute low back pain have persistent pain at 4 weeks from onset, at 12 weeks only 35% experience persistent discomfort and at 1 year only 10% have persistent pain.[4] In an Australian study consisting of 2 populations, 49% to 67% had recovered from low back pain at 3 months following onset, and at 12 months 56% to 71% had recovered. There was a relapse rate of 7% to 27% within 1 year.[5] Although these recent studies illustrate that the clinical prognosis of low back pain is not as positive as had been thought a generation ago, the vast majority of patients will indeed recover. Many of these patients have musculoskeletal strains or sprains, or suffer from nonspecific degenerative phenomena that may elude a clear diagnosis in up to 85% of patients.[1]

In terms of underlying pathophysiology, back or leg pain is overwhelmingly caused by benign disease. A differential diagnosis of low back pain with the associated prevalence of underlying pathologic processes has been compiled by Jarvik and Deyo[1] and is presented in **Table 1**. Their analysis suggests that 95% of low back pain is due to benign processes. In patients presenting to a primary care setting with low back pain, only 0.7% will suffer from undiagnosed metastatic neoplasm. Spine infection, including pyogenic and granulomatous discitis, epidural abscess, or viral processes, will be present in only 0.01% of subjects. Noninfectious inflammatory spondyloarthropathies, such as ankylosing spondylitis, will account for 0.3% of presentations. Osteoporotic compression fractures are the most common systemic pathologic process to present as back pain, accounting for 4% of patients.[1]

Table 1
Differential diagnosis of low back pain

Mechanical Low Back or Leg Pain (97%)	Nonmechanical Spine Conditions (1%)	Visceral Disease (2%)
Lumbar strain or sprain (70%)	Neoplasia (0.7%)	Pelvic organ involvement
Degenerative process of disc and facets (usually related to age) (10%)	Multiple myeloma	Prostatitis
	Metastatic carcinoma	Endometriosis
	Lymphoma and leukemia	Chronic pelvic inflammatory disease
	Spinal cord tumors	Renal involvement
Herniated disc (4%)	Retroperitoneal tumors	Nephrolithiasis
Spinal stenosis (3%)	Primary vertebral tumors	Pyelonephritis
Osteoporotic compression fracture (4%)	Infection (0.01%)	Perinephric abscess
	Osteomyelitis	Aortic aneurysm
Spondylolisthesis (2%)	Septic discitis	Gastrointestinal involvement
Traumatic fractures (<1%)	Paraspinous abscess	Pancreatitis
Congenital disease (<1%)	Epidural abscess	Cholecystitis
Severe kyphosis	Shingles	Penetrating ulcer
Severe scoliosis	Inflammatory arthritis (often HLA-B27 associated) (0.3%)	
Transitional vertebrae		
Spondylolysis	Ankylosing spondylitis	
Internal disc disruption or discogenic back pain	Psoriatic spondylitis	
Presumed instability	Reiter syndrome	
	Inflammatory bowel disease	
	Scheuermann disease (osteochondrosis)	
	Paget disease	

From Jarvik JG, Deyo RA. Diagnostic evaluation of low back pain with emphasis on imaging. Ann Intern Med 2002;137(7):587; with permission.

The primary role of imaging is to identify the approximately 5% of patients with back pain who have undiagnosed systemic disease as the cause of their pain. A related imaging goal is to characterize and assist in therapy planning in the very small percentage of patients who have neural compressive disease resulting in radiculopathy or radicular pain syndromes that fail conservative therapy and require surgical or minimally invasive intervention. Imaging identification of degenerative disease in the patient with back pain is, as this article elaborates, seldom helpful and is at best of secondary concern.

EARLY IMAGING

This review first addresses the utility of imaging in a patient who presents acutely with back or leg pain. It is well established that there is no role for imaging in this patient population in the absence of information that would suggest underlying systemic disease or signs of neurologic impairment which may require intervention; this applies to both radiographs and advanced imaging. A study by Scavone and colleagues[6] evaluated spine radiographs in patients who present with acute low back pain; 75% of the studies provided no useful information. A United Kingdom study randomized patients who had experienced back pain for 6 weeks to further clinically guided care or lumbar radiographs.[7] At 9 months' follow-up there were no significant differences in clinical outcomes. Gilbert and colleagues[8] randomized patients between advanced imaging (CT or MRI) at presentation with back pain versus imaging only when a clear clinical indication developed. Early advanced imaging had no significant effect on patient outcomes. Chou and colleagues[9] recently performed a meta-analysis of all randomized controlled trials comparing immediate imaging (radiographs, CT, MRI) with clinically directed care in acute patients with back pain. In the pooled data from the 6 qualifying trials, analysis showed no significant differences in pain or function in imaged versus nonimaged patients in either the short term (3 months) or long-term (6–12 months). Chou and colleagues concluded "lumbar imaging for low back pain without indications of serious underlying conditions does not improve clinical outcomes."

In addition to being ineffective, early employment of imaging is costly; a cost-effectiveness analysis by Liang and Komaroff[10] showed that simply performing radiographs at the initial presentation of back pain results in a cost of $2000 (1982 dollars) to alleviate a single day of pain. Carragee and colleagues[11] elegantly demonstrated the lack of utility of imaging in the acute setting in a 5-year prospective observational study. A large cohort of asymptomatic subjects deemed to be at risk for back pain resulting from labor-intensive vocations underwent lumbar spine MRI. This patient cohort was followed periodically over the next 5 years; a subset of these subjects presented to a medical care provider with acute back or leg pain during this 5-year period and a second lumbar MRI was obtained. Less than 5% of the MRI scans obtained at the time of acute presentation with back or leg pain showed clinically relevant new findings; virtually all of the "positive findings" noted on the images at the time of presentation with back/leg pain had been present on the baseline studies obtained when the patient was asymptomatic. Only direct evidence of neural compression in patients with a corresponding radicular pain syndrome was considered to be useful imaging information. Of particular note, psychosocial factors, not the morphology seen on imaging, were the best predictors of the degree of functional disability caused by back/leg pain.[11]

Based on such data, numerous professional organizations and societies have issued guidelines that recommend against imaging early in a clinical pain syndrome.

In 1994, the Agency for Health Care Policy and Research recommended against imaging patients with back pain within the first month of a pain syndrome in the absence of signs of systemic disease.[12] The American College of Radiology practice guidelines were recently restated by Bradley[13] in 2007. Imaging the patient who presents with acute low back pain is not indicated except in the presence of "red flag" features including recent significant trauma, minor trauma in a patient older than 50 years, weight loss, fever, immunosuppression, history of neoplasm, steroid use or osteoporosis, age greater than 70 years, known intravenous drug abuse, or a progressive neurologic deficit with intractable symptoms. Similarly, a joint recommendation from the American College of Physicians and the American Pain Society stated that imaging should not be obtained in patients with nonspecific low back pain.[14] Imaging should only be performed when severe or progressive neurologic deficits are present or when serious underlying systemic disease is suspected. Furthermore, patients with signs or symptoms of radiculopathy or spinal stenosis should be imaged only if they are candidates for surgical or minimally invasive intervention (eg, epidural steroid injection). These recommendations further reinforce the primary role of imaging as a means of detecting underlying systemic disease, most commonly neoplasm, infection, or unsuspected traumatic injury.

RISK/BENEFIT ANALYSIS

In a patient who has failed conservative therapy or who has "red flag" features that suggest underlying systemic disease, the clinician may decide to begin imaging. Such a decision must be a rational balance of risk and benefit. Certainly there are benefits to be derived from imaging. Foremost, imaging may suggest, and assist in, the diagnosis of, previously unsuspected systemic disease. In the patient with a radicular pain syndrome or radiculopathy that has not responded to conservative therapy, Imaging may supply invaluable information that allows planning of minimally invasive or surgical procedures. Negative imaging should also have value, in providing reassurance that there is no sinister disease present and in stopping further workup in appropriate circumstances. Finally, in patients with chronic pain syndromes, imaging may assist in the identification of the structural cause of such pain. Only when a specific pain generator is identified can a specific plan of therapeutic intervention, whether it be conservative or invasive, be developed.

Risk, the inevitable counterweight to benefit, is often not considered in the decision to undertake imaging. Imaging does carry risks; these include the labeling effect, radiation exposure, cost, and the provocation of intervention.

The labeling effect refers to the inevitable presence of degenerative findings on any imaging study; the subject now becomes a patient carrying a diagnosis of degenerative spine disease. The word "degenerative" carries only negative connotations. This negativity is illustrated in a study performed by Modic and colleagues,[15] in which patients who presented with back pain underwent MRI but were randomized to either disclosure of the MRI findings to the patient and physician, or withholding such information. Among the findings in this study, patients who received the MRI findings of benign degenerative phenomena actually had a diminished sense of well-being when compared with subjects from whom the MRI report was withheld. This speaks to the critical need for physicians to communicate to the patient the lack of significance of the vast majority of degenerative findings identified on imaging. Unless appropriately educated to the contrary, patients may perceive this as representing the start of an inevitable downward spiral of spine degeneration, which may lead to fear avoidance behaviors with diminished activity, deconditioning, and depression.

A recent Cochrane database review established the effectiveness of active patient education, particularly in the setting of acute low back pain.[16] The irrelevance of degenerative findings on imaging studies, and the importance of maintaining functional strength and high activity levels, must be reinforced at every patient encounter.

Radiation exposure from radiographs, CT, and nuclear medicine studies carries a cumulative risk of neoplasm induction. This risk becomes particularly problematic when serial studies are performed. The biologically effective absorbed radiation dose is measured by the Sievert (Sv); in North America, the average annual natural background exposure is approximately 3 mSv.[17] A frontal and lateral chest radiograph is often considered the common currency of radiation exposure, incurring a dose of approximately 0.1 mSv. A 3-view lumbar spine radiographic series is then worth approximately 15 chest radiographs, or 1.5 mSv. A dose of 6 mSv is typical for a lumbar spine CT scan, a value of 60 chest radiographs. Similarly, a technetium bone scan has a dose of 6.3 mSv. In this context, an abdomen and pelvis CT study will incur 14 mSv on average.[17] All radiation exposure accumulates over the patient's lifetime and contributes to a risk of radiation induced cancer. Imaging studies that use radiation must be employed with careful consideration of the risk and anticipated benefits.

Imaging is costly. In the United States the medical imaging community incurs more than $100 billion of societal cost per year. The 2009 Medicare reimbursements for lumbar spine imaging include radiographs: $41; noncontrast CT: $264; myelogram: $506; noncontrast MRI: $439; whole body positron emission tomography (PET)/CT: $1183; bone scan with single-photon emission CT (SPECT): $261.[18] Nominal fees are typically 3 to 5 times the Medicare reimbursements. It is easy to appreciate how quickly imaging costs can accrue.

A less frequently considered risk of imaging is the provocation of intervention. Jarvik and colleagues[19] documented that obtaining advanced imaging (MRI) early in a patient's spine pain syndrome leads to increased surgical interventions despite equivalent pain and disability profiles, when compared with nonimaged patients. Likewise, Lurie and colleagues[20] examined the dramatic regional variation (12-fold) in the rate of surgical intervention for central canal stenosis. These investigators noted that the rate of surgical intervention correlated directly with the intensity of CT and MRI use. When advanced imaging shows an "abnormality" potentially responsible for a patient's pain, the temptation is to correct that imaging finding. Such a situation occurs despite the well-established lack of specificity of many of the spine imaging "abnormalities," which are discussed shortly. It is critical to treat the patient, not the image.

SPECIFICITY, SENSITIVITY, AND RELIABILITY

Having considered risk and benefit, it is also imperative to know the reliability of imaging findings, as well as shortcomings in sensitivity and specificity that plague all spine imaging. **Table 2**, compiled by Jarvik and Deyo,[1] describes the estimated accuracy of several imaging techniques for various lumbar spine conditions. Although the primary role of imaging is the detection of underlying systemic disease, the low prevalence of systemic disease as a cause of back pain implies most imaging studies will primarily describe degenerative phenomena. Degenerative changes are ubiquitous on imaging studies, seldom causal of an individual patient's pain syndrome, and often inappropriately considered as pain generators, precipitating unnecessary interventions.

The observation that there is a high prevalence of asymptomatic degenerative changes in the spine is not new. Hult[21] studied adults in 1954 and showed that by

Table 2
Estimated accuracy of imaging techniques for lumbar spine conditions[a]

Technique	Sensitivity	Specificity	Positive Likelihood Ratio	Negative Likelihood Ratio
Plain Radiography				
Cancer	0.6	0.95–0.995	12–120	0.40–0.42
Infection	8.82	0.57	1.9	0.32
Ankylosing spondylitis	0.26–0.45	1	ND	0.55–0.74
Computed Tomography				
Herniated disc	0.62–0.9	0.7–0.87	2.1–6.9	0.44–0.54
Stenosis	0.9	0.8–0.95	4.5–22	0.10–0.12
Magnetic Resonance Imaging				
Cancer	0.83–0.93	0.90–0.97	8.3–31	0.07–0.19
Infection	0.96	0.92	12	0.04
Ankylosing spondylitis	0.56	0.43–0.97		
Herniated disc	0.6–1.0	0.72–1.0	1.1–33	0–0.93
Stenosis	0.9		3.2–ND	0.10–0.14
Radionuclide Scanning				
Cancer				
Planar imaging	0.74–0.98	0.64–0.83	3.9	0.32
SPECT	0.87–0.93	0.91–0.93	9.7	0.14
Infection	0.9	0.78	4.1	0.13
Ankylosing spondylitis	0.26	1	ND	0.74

Abbreviations: ND, not defined; SPECT, single-photon emission computed tomography.
[a] Estimated ranges are derived from multiple studies described in the text.
From Jarvik JG, Deyo RA. Diagnostic evaluation of low back pain with emphasis on imaging. Ann Intern Med 2002;137(7):588; with permission.

age 50 years, 87% will have radiographic evidence of disc degeneration (narrowing of the disc space, marginal sclerosis with osteophytes, vacuum phenomena). In a second study including a cohort of asymptomatic workers, Hult[22] noted radiographic evidence of disc disease in 56% of those aged 40 to 44 years, which rose to 95% in subjects 50 to 59 years old. With the evolution of more sophisticated spine imaging techniques, this lack of specificity of degenerative findings has not improved. Hitselberger and Witten[23] studied plain myelography of asymptomatic volunteers and noted that 24% showed abnormalities that would have been considered significant in a clinical context of back or leg pain. A study of lumbar spine CT in asymptomatic volunteers by Wiesel and colleagues[24] showed that in patients older than 40 years, 50% had "significant" abnormalities. Similarly, Boden and colleagues[25] evaluated MRI of the lumbar spine in asymptomatic volunteers; in patients older than 60 years, 57% had abnormalities that would have been considered significant in an appropriate clinical setting. Jarvik and colleagues[26] studied a large patient population with MRI. This study noted that only extrusions, moderate to severe central canal stenosis, and direct visualization of neural compression were likely to be significant and would separate patients with pain from asymptomatic volunteers. Disc protrusions, zygapophysial joint (z-joint) arthropathy, and antero- or retrolisthesis were virtually always asymptomatic findings. Imaging studies of asymptomatic volunteers are compiled in **Table 3**.

Table 3
Imaging abnormalities in asymptomatic subjects

Test	Study[Ref], Year	Patients (N)	Age Range (Mean)	Disc Herniation	Disc Bulge	Disc Degeneration	Central Canal Stenosis	Annular Fissure
Radiograph	Hult,[22] 1954	1200	40–44 55–59			56% 95%		
Radiograph	Hellstrom et al,[27] 1990	143	14–25			20%		
Myelogram	Hitselberger and Witten,[23] 1968	300	[51]	31%				
CT	Wiesel et al,[24] 1984	51	[40]	20%			3.40%	
MRI	Weinreb et al,[28] 1989	86	[28]	9%	44%			
MRI	Boden et al,[25] 1990	53	<60 ≥60	22% 36%	54% 79%	46% 93%	1% 21%	
MRI	Jensen et al,[29] 1994	98	[42]	28%	52%		7%	
MRI	Boos et al,[30] 1995	46	[36]	76%	51%	85%		
MRI	Stadnik et al,[31] 1998	36	[42]	33%	81%	56%		56%
MRI	Weishaupt et al,[32] 1998	60	[35]	60%	28%	72%		20%
MRI	Jarvik et al,[26] 2001	148	[54]	38%	64%	91%	10%	38%

Adapted from Jarvik JG, Deyo RA. Diagnostic evaluation of low back pain with emphasis on imaging. Ann Intern Med 2002;137(7):591; with permission.

More recent studies have addressed the prevalence of degenerative imaging findings in younger populations, primarily in Scandinavian countries; these are MRI population-based studies without regard to symptomatology. Kjaer and colleagues,[33] studying children age 13 years, found a 21% prevalence of disc degeneration. In a study of adolescents, Salminen and colleagues[34] found a 31% prevalence of disc degeneration in 15-year-olds, which rose to 42% in 18-year-olds. Takatalo and colleagues[35] evaluated 558 young adults aged 20 to 22 years. Using the 5-point Pfirrmann classification of disc degeneration, they noted disc degeneration of grade 3 or higher in 47% of these young adults. There was a higher prevalence in males (54%) than in females (42%). Multilevel degeneration was identified in 17%.

The lack of specificity of degenerative imaging findings is clear. Population-based studies show a prevalence of imaging degenerative findings greatly in excess of the symptomatic disease prevalence. Studies of asymptomatic cohorts show a high prevalence of asymptomatic degenerative imaging findings. In general, one-third to two-thirds of asymptomatic subjects will exhibit degenerative findings on all imaging studies; the prevalence of asymptomatic degenerative findings increases with increasing age. Disc bulges, protrusions, facet arthropathy, and antero- or retrolisthesis are common, usually asymptomatic, and their prevalence increases with increasing age. Disc extrusions, severe central canal stenosis, and direct evidence of neural compression are more likely to be truly symptomatic imaging findings. In the individual patient, only the clear concordance of a clinical pain syndrome and imaging can suggest causation. Even in this setting, anesthetic or provocative tests may be needed to allow rational decision making, particularly where interventions of significant risk and cost are contemplated.

On the flip side of the specificity coin, spine imaging also has a basic sensitivity flaw. The literature documents well that neuroclaudicatory pain is exacerbated by extension positioning and axial loading. Schmid and colleagues[36] demonstrated that the cross-sectional area of the lumbar central spinal canal, its lateral recesses, and neural foramina all diminish when going from neutral to extension positioning and with the assumption of axial load (standing vs recumbent). Danielson and Willen[37,38] looked at cohorts of asymptomatic volunteers and patients with neuroclaudicatory pain syndromes. These investigators noted that axial loading and extension would reduce the cross-sectional dimension of the dural sac in 50% of asymptomatic patients, but in 76% to 80% of patients who had neuroclaudicatory pain. The vast majority of advanced imaging (CT, MRI) is performed with the subject in a supine, psoas relaxed position with the legs slightly elevated, which is done for patient comfort and to minimize motion during the course of the study. This loss of normal lumbar lordosis as well as lack of axial load diminishes sensitivity to the detection of dynamic neural compressive lesions. There is significant enthusiasm in the literature for more physiologic imaging, sometimes referred to as P/K (Positional/Kinetic) or upright MRI. Existing scanners that allow weight-bearing and dynamic studies are of low field strength, 0.6 T. The lower magnetic field results in a lower signal to noise ratio and ultimately lower imaging quality. Patients also find it problematic to hold a position in which their pain is exacerbated, with resultant motion artifact. Loading devices that apply a compressive load and extension positioning in the lumbar region can be used on conventional high-field MRI scanners or CT; this is certainly much more economically palatable. Studies by Danielson and Willen[37,38] suggest that loading the patient to 50% of the body weight for 5 minutes with subsequent imaging is a reasonable reproduction of upright imaging. Such devices do not allow more complex motions such as rotation or side bending.

The reliability of MRI in detecting and describing degenerative phenomena in the lumbar spine has been best and most comprehensively studied using the data from the Spine Patient Outcomes Research Trial (SPORT). Lurie and colleagues[39] studied the reliability of MRI in the detection and categorization of disc herniations, the degree of thecal sac compromise, and the grading of nerve root impingement. Interreader reliability was substantial for disc morphology (herniation), moderate for the degree of thecal sac compression, and moderate for grading nerve route impingement. Nondisc contour degenerative findings were subsequently studied by Carrino and colleagues[40]; they noted good interobserver agreement in rating the degree of disc degeneration. There was moderate interobserver agreement in the rating of spondylolisthesis, Modic endplate changes, z-joint arthropathy, and annular high-intensity zones (HIZ).

IMAGING MODALITIES

Having weighed the risks and benefits of imaging, and acknowledged its shortcomings in specificity and sensitivity, the clinician may proceed with imaging, which should begin with radiographs. This procedure will typically occur in the setting of clinical "red flags," pain unresponsive to conservative care, or progressive neurologic deficit. Weight-bearing radiographs provide essential information on vertebral enumeration and coronal and sagittal alignment, which cannot be obtained with more advanced modalities. Vertebral enumeration should not be trivialized. Up to 12% of the general population will have anomalies of segmentation (transitional segments) at the lumbosacral junction.[41] Radiographs will establish vertebral numbering for subsequent advanced imaging and intervention; this will diminish the likelihood of wrong-level interventions at a later date. Radiographs also serve as a low-sensitivity screening tool for evidence of neoplasm, fracture, or infection. Degenerative findings, including disc space narrowing, z-joint arthropathy, and minor degrees of antero- or retrolisthesis are likely insignificant and unrelated to an individual patient's pain syndrome. Single frontal and lateral standing images of the lumbar spine are adequate. Oblique views double the gonadal radiation dose and should not be obtained routinely.[42] Flexion-extension or side bending views should only be obtained in an operative planning setting.

When radiographs are not explanatory of an unremitting pain syndrome or suggest underlying systemic disease, advanced imaging (CT, MRI, nuclear medicine) is obtained. CT has undergone a revolution in the last decade with the advancement of multidetector technology. A dataset for the lumbar spine can now be obtained in a few seconds, eliminating motion artifact and dramatically improving patient tolerance. This dataset can then be reconstructed in any plane without loss of spatial resolution or additional radiation exposure.

CT provides superior imaging of cortical and trabecular bone when compared with MRI. For this reason, CT may be necessary to characterize primary bone tumors of the spine. CT also provides reasonable contrast resolution and can identify root compressive lesions such as disc herniations in the vast majority of cases. CT cannot identify intrathecal pathology and is less sensitive than MRI in the detection of early inflammatory or infectious processes, neoplasm, or paraspinal soft tissue lesions. Radiation dose must always be considered when employing CT. One by-product of the rapid recent technological advance of CT is that the literature contains no comparative studies between MRI and the current generation of multidetector CT scanners in the detection and characterization of disc herniations.

MRI has been the dominant spine imaging modality for the past 2 decades, despite relatively little technological advancement in that time span. MRI has superior contrast resolution and thus the ability to distinguish between soft tissue types, allowing it to detect intrathecal pathology and identify subtle root compressive lesions. MRI has superior sensitivity in the detection of neoplasm and infection. With the use of gadolinium contrast, or heavily T2-weighted imaging sequences (short-tau inversion recovery [STIR] or fast spin echo T2 sequences with fat saturation), MRI can detect inflammatory change. It has greater specificity than CT in characterizing the chronicity of fractures. With gadolinium enhancement, MRI can distinguish between recurrent disc herniation and scarring in the postoperative patient. MRI does not evaluate cortical bone well.

Patient acceptance remains problematic, with high cost, prolonged imaging times, and up to 10% examination failures due to claustrophobia. Open magnets have improved patient acceptance, but at the cost of image quality. A small percentage of patients are MRI incompatible due to pacemakers, spinal cord stimulators, or other implanted devices.

CT myelography retains a problem-solving role in the lumbar spine; it will substitute for MRI in the incompatible patient. CT myelography has superior spatial resolution when compared with MRI, but lacks its soft tissue contrast resolution. With the addition of intrathecal contrast material, it can provide exquisite demonstration of root compressive lesions and central canal, lateral recess, and foraminal compromise. CT myelography is minimally invasive, expensive, operator dependent to a degree, and also requires current CT technology to be maximally useful.

Nuclear medicine studies are growing in importance in spine imaging. Technetium bone scans detect accelerated bone metabolic activity. With the addition of SPECT capability, significant additional spatial resolution is possible. Such imaging is useful in assessing the burden of metastatic disease and also in the evaluation of patients with clinically suspected spondylolysis. When MRI is not technically feasible, technetium bone scanning can be used to characterize the chronicity of vertebral fractures in selecting patients for bone augmentation. Bone scans can identify noninfectious inflammatory disease in the facet and sacroiliac joints, aiding in the identification of pain generators and targeting these structures for injection. The technetium bone scan in combination with gallium scan offers sensitivity equal to MRI in the detection of spondylodiscitis. However, they do provide less anatomic information and MRI may ultimately be necessary to characterize the degree of central canal compromise that may influence surgical decision making. PET or PET/CT scans have an increasing role in assessing the burden of metastatic disease and in selecting lesions for percutaneous biopsy.

IMAGING OF DEGENERATIVE PHENOMENA

Although the primary role of imaging in the patient with back/leg pain is the detection of systemic disease, or characterization of neural compressive disease requiring intervention, the low prevalence of these processes dictates that most spine imaging will inevitably be used to evaluate degenerative disease. This section initially discusses imaging of degenerative processes, followed by imaging findings in systemic disease that may present as back or leg pain. Disc degeneration is a multifactorial process with genetic, inflammatory, traumatic, and nutritional components. It is beyond the scope of this article to deal with disc degeneration in depth, and this is covered in the article by Wolfer elsewhere in this issue.

Disc degeneration is manifest on plain radiographs as loss of disc space height, nitrogen gas within the disc space (vacuum sign), and marginal osteophytes. In the normal adult, disc space height increases as one proceeds caudally from L1 through L4; the L5 or lumbosacral disc is variable in height and may normally be less than that of L4. On CT images, particularly sagittal reconstructions, findings of disc degeneration are identical to those seen on radiographs, although detected with greater sensitivity. On T2-weighted MRI images, the normal nuclear compartment of the disc is hyperintense, bounded by the hypointense annulus. The intranuclear cleft, a horizontal hypointense band crossing the center of the nucleus, is a normal finding in the mature disc. In early disc degeneration the intranuclear cleft is lost, and the junction between the hyperintense nucleus and the low signal annulus becomes indistinct (**Fig. 1A–D**). This diminished nuclear signal reflects loss of proteoglycans and alteration in their hydration state; it is not simply dehydration.[43] There may be subsequent loss of disc space height. Failure of the fibrous annulus results in fissuring, which may be detected as a focal zone of elevated T2 signal (HIZ) or gadolinium enhancement within the outer annulus. The outer third of the annulus is known to be innervated, with afferent supply via the sinuvertebral nerve. As fissures penetrate the annulus to the epidural space, granulation tissue will invade the disc, with ingrowth of unmyelinated C-type nociceptors into the inner annulus or nuclear compartment. Exposure to the nuclear biochemical environment is postulated to sensitize these nociceptors, such that they fire at very low levels of mechanical stress, including those experienced in activities of daily living; this is thought to be the genesis of the sitting and standing intolerance of discogenic pain. Potential imaging markers of discogenic pain are now discussed. Discography as a diagnostic test is discussed in the article by Alison Stout elsewhere; its utility remains controversial.

Endplate Changes

The functional unity of the disc and the cartilaginous endplate is apparent in signal changes within the endplate and adjacent subchondral marrow that accompany disc degeneration. Endplate marrow changes were originally classified by Modic and colleagues[44] in 1988 (**Fig. 2A–F**). Type I change represents ingrowth of vascularized granulation tissue into sub-endplate marrow; it exhibits hypointense T1 and hyperintensity T2 signal on MRI and may enhance with gadolinium. Type II change exhibits elevated T1 and T2 signal and reflects fatty infiltration of sub-endplate marrow. Type III change is hypointense on T1 and T2; it correlates with bony sclerosis. Type I change is thought to represent an active inflammatory state, with type II being more quiescent, and type III postinflammatory. Ohtori and colleagues[45] noted elevated levels of protein gene product (PGP) 9.5 immunoreactive nerve fibers and tumor necrosis factor (TNF) immunoreactive cells in the cartilaginous endplates of patients with Modic changes. The immunoreactive nerve ingrowth was seen exclusively in patients with discogenic low back pain. TNF immunoreactive cells were more common in type I endplate changes.

Modic endplate changes do carry an association with low back pain, particularly type I change. Toyone and colleagues[46] found 73% of patients with type I change had low back pain as opposed to 11% with type II change. Likewise, Albert and Manniche[47] reported low back pain in 60% of patients with Modic changes but in only 20% for those without Modic change. Type I change was more strongly associated with low back pain than type II change. Several investigators (Braithwaite and colleagues,[48] Ito and colleagues,[49] Weishaupt and colleagues,[50] Lei and colleagues,[51] O'Neill and colleagues,[52] and Kang and colleagues[53]) have correlated the response to provocation discography with type I and type II endplate changes. These studies consistently

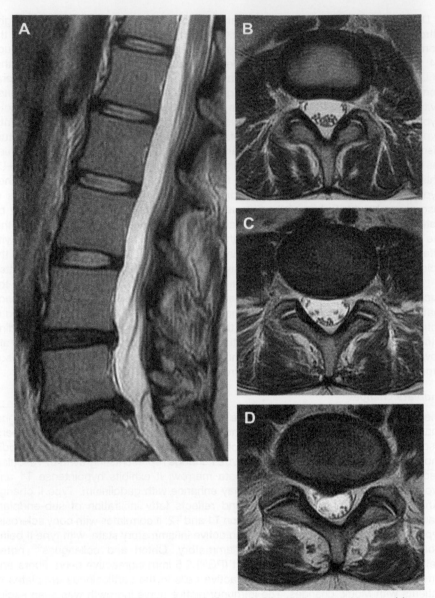

Fig. 1. Disc degeneration. (A) Mid-sagittal T2-weighted MRI image in 25-year-old woman with axial back pain. Note normal bright nuclear signal in the L3 disc, with well-defined transition to dark peripheral annulus. L1 and L2 discs contain a horizontal dark band, the intranuclear cleft, a sign of a normal mature disc. (B) Axial T2-weighted image through L3 disc. Nucleus is bright and annulus is dark with a well-defined interface. Note posterior margin of the disc is convex anteriorly—this is the normal state for L1-L4 discs. (C) Axial T2-weighted image through L4 disc. On the sagittal image (A), the L4 disc is dark, indicating loss of proteoglycans and alteration of their hydration state. On the axial Image (C), there is a broad-based protrusion present; note the posterior disc is abnormally convex dorsally. (D) Axial T2-weighted image through the L5 disc. Disc is degenerated with a small focal extrusion eccentric to the right; it contacts and minimally deforms the thecal sac, and has migrated caudally on the sagittal image (A).

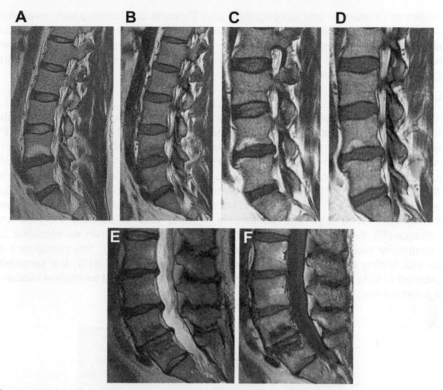

Fig. 2. Endplate (Modic) changes. (*A*) Sagittal T2-weighted MRI image shows hyperintense signal in marrow adjacent to L4 inferior endplate in a 44-year-old man with axial pain. Note loss of T2 signal in L4 and L5 discs. (*B*) Matched sagittal T1-weighted MRI in same patient shows hypointense T1 signal adjacent to L4 inferior endplate; this is Type I marrow change, vascularized granulation tissue. (*C*) Sagittal T2-weighted MRI in a 46-year-old man with radicular pain. Note increased T2 signal about anterior aspect of L4 disc; there is also T2 signal loss at the L4 and L5 levels. (*D*) Matched sagittal T1-weighted MRI in the same patient demonstrates increased T1 signal about L4 disc; this is Type II marrow change, fatty infiltration. (*E*) Sagittal T2-weighted MRI in a patient exhibiting Type III marrow change at the L4 interspace. Note marked loss of disc space height and low T2 signal. (*F*) Matched T1 sagittal image in the same patient as (*E*) demonstrates the low T1 signal about the L4 disc in Type III endplate change.

show a very high specificity (87%–98%) but a relatively low sensitivity (14%–48%) for type I and/or type II endplate change as a predictor of discogenic pain as defined by provocation discography. These studies either did not discriminate between type I and type II changes, or when differential data were available, did not show a great advantage for type I change as a predictor of discogenic pain.

Modic type I change may also be associated with segmental instability. In the study of Toyone and colleagues,[46] 70% of patients with type I change were found to have segmental hypermobility (>3 mm translation on flexion-extension films). Hypermobility was seen in only 16% of those with type II change. Similarly, in post fusion patients, the studies of Butterman and colleagues[54] and Lang and colleagues[55] showed persistent type I change in patients ultimately shown to have pseudoarthroses. Patients with solid fusions tend to have type II change or resolution of all Modic changes. The studies of Chataigner and colleagues[56] and Esposito and colleagues[57] evaluated Modic change as a predictor of fusion outcome. Patients with type I change at the operative level on preprocedure imaging tended to have much better outcomes than patients operated on with isolated disc degeneration or disc degeneration plus type II endplate change.

Annular Fissure (HIZ)

In 1992, Aprill and Bogduk[58] described the HIZ, a focus of bright T2 signal within the posterior annulus, as an MRI marker of a painful degenerated disc (**Fig. 3**A–E). Pathologically, this represents an annular fissure; it will typically enhance with gadolinium, indicating the presence of vascularized granulation tissue. Using exact pain reproduction at provocation discography as diagnostic of discogenic pain, the presence of an HIZ had a specificity of 89% and a sensitivity of 82%. In other consecutive series (Carragee and colleagues,[59] Ricketson and colleagues,[60] Smith and colleagues,[61] Ito and colleagues,[49] Weishaupt and colleagues,[50] Kang and colleagues,[53] O'Neil and colleagues[52]), the high specificity of the HIZ for discogenic pain as identified by discography has been consistently demonstrated (84%–93%). The prevalence of the HIZ finding (per disc) in these series ranged from 9% to 30%; the sensitivity spanned 11% to 57%. The HIZ is a highly specific but somewhat insensitive indicator of a painful disc.

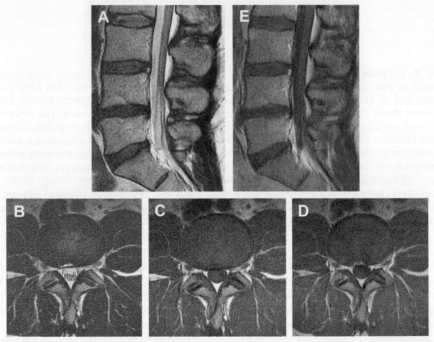

Fig. 3. High-intensity zone (HIZ). (*A*) Sagittal T2-weighted image in a 44-year-old man with axial pain shows HIZ within posterior annulus of L3 disc. Note also disc degeneration at L4 and L5. (*B*) Axial T2-weighted image at L3 demonstrates the HIZ within the bulging L3 posterior annulus. (*C*) Axial T1-weighted image at L3 shows only the mild contour abnormality (bulge). (*D*) Post-gadolinium axial T1-weighted image reveals enhancement with in the HIZ consistent with vascularized granulation tissue. (*E*) Sagittal post-gadolinium T1 image also demonstrates the enhancement in the posterior annulus of L3.

T2 Signal Abnormality

The degree of T2 signal loss has been used as an imaging marker of the painful disc. There have been several classification schemes of disc degeneration. The 5-class Pfirrmann scale is perhaps most recognized; it uses mid-sagittal T2-weighted images.[62] Grade 1: homogeneous bright T2 nuclear signal; Grade 2: inhomogeneous bright T2 nuclear signal, preservation of disc height and nuclear-annular boundary; Grade 3: inhomogeneous intermediate gray nuclear signal, nuclear-annular boundary indistinct, disc height normal or slightly decreased; Grade 4: inhomogeneous dark gray signal, nuclear-annular boundary lost, normal to moderately reduced disc height; Grade 5: inhomogeneous dark signal, no nuclear-annular boundary, disc space collapse. Series published by Ito and colleagues,[49] Weishaupt and colleagues,[50] Lei and colleagues,[51] O'Neill and colleagues,[52] and Kang and colleagues[53] have correlated T2 signal loss with provocation discography. Sensitivities for T2 signal loss as a predictor of discogenic pain at discography ranged from 90% to 98%, with a broad range of specificities, 39% to 77%. Ito and colleagues[49] and O'Neill and colleagues[52] provided data on more severely degenerated discs only, which yielded specificities of 89% and 96%, respectively, but sensitivities of 25% and 15%. Painful discs at discography overwhelmingly show abnormal T2 signal, and more severely degenerated discs are more likely to be painful.

Loss of Disc Height

The studies of Ito and colleagues[49] and O'Neill and colleagues[52] include data on disc space height. Moderate or severe loss of disc space height resulted in sensitivities of 87% and 73% with specificities of 69% and 81% in the respective studies, for a positive discogram. With the criteria as severe loss of disc space height, the specificity for discography confirmed discogenic pain rose to 97% and 98%, but the sensitivity fell to 30% and 18%, respectively. In a patient with suspected discogenic pain undergoing provocation discography, severe loss of disc space height is a strong predictor of a positive discogram.

Analysis of Multiple Variables

Kang and colleagues[53] and O'Neill and colleagues[52] evaluated combinations of imaging findings in the quest for the noninvasive diagnosis of discogenic pain. Combining imaging findings into 4 classes, Kang and colleagues concluded that the presence of a disc herniation with an HIZ was of most value, resulting in a sensitivity of 46%, specificity of 98%, and positive predictive value of 87% as a predictor of positive discography. O'Neill and colleagues[52] conducted a true multivariate analysis using receiver operator characteristic curves. Overall, they concluded that disc signal abnormality is as accurate as any other MRI parameter or combination of parameters. When disc signal is normal, discography will very likely be negative; when there is severe loss of disc signal, discography will very likely be positive. When disc signal loss is intermediate, other parameters may be helpful. Moderate disc signal loss and disc bulge had the best combination of sensitivity (80%) and specificity (79%). Adding findings of loss of disc space height or the presence of HIZ increased specificity at the cost of sensitivity.

HERNIATION NOMENCLATURE

When the disc-endplate complex undergoes degeneration with annular failure, disc herniation may occur. Discussion of disc herniations requires a brief commentary on nomenclature. Description of disc herniation has historically been chaotic, with no common terminology among various medical and surgical specialties. This was resolved by a combined task force of the North American Spine Society, American Society of Spine Radiology, American Society of Neuroradiology, American Association of Neurological Surgeons, and American Academy of Orthopedic Surgeons, whose imaging lexicon recommendations were published in 2001, allowing us to communicate better across specialties and regions.[63]

Normal aging changes are described by the term spondylosis deformans, characterized by loss of T2 signal within the disc, loss of disc space height, but the absence of radial annular tears, disc herniation, or posterior osteophytes. Intervertebral osteochondrosis is the terminology used to represent pathologic degeneration (**Fig. 4**A, B).

Herniation is the broad term describing displacement of disc material beyond its normal intervertebral disc space. If the extent of the herniation is greater than 50% of the circumference of the disc, it may be considered a bulge. A localized herniation is defined as involving less than 50% of the disc circumference. Localized herniations may be further divided into broad-based herniations, which encompass 25% to 50% of the disc circumference, and focal herniations, which constitute less than 25% of the circumference (**Fig. 5**A, B).

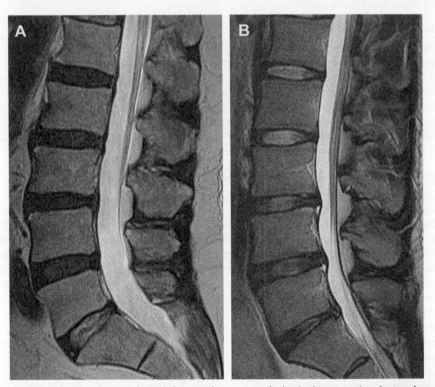

Fig. 4. Normal aging (spondylosis deformans) versus pathologic degeneration (osteochondrosis). (*A*) Spondylosis deformans: mid-sagittal T2-weighted MRI of a 62-year-old man with modest back pain. Loss of T2 signal in multiple discs is apparent, but there is preservation of disc space height, no disc contour abnormality, and a widely patent central canal. (*B*) Osteochondrosis: Mid-sagittal T2-weighted MRI of a 32-year-old man with disabling back pain. Note loss of T2 signal and disc height at L3-L5 with small disc herniations and HIZs at L3 and L4. Early central canal narrowing.

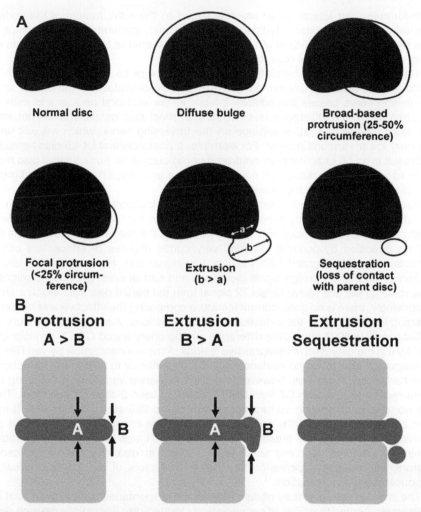

Fig. 5. Disc herniations. (*A*) Disc herniation configurations in the axial plane. (*B*) Disc herniation configurations in the sagittal plane. (*From* Benzon H, Rathmell JP, Wu CL. Raj's practical management of pain. 4th edition. Philadelphia: Elsevier/Mosby; 2008; with permission.)

The distinction between protrusion and extrusion is one of shape. In a protrusion the width of displaced disc material, in any plane, does not exceed the width of its base or the aperture through which the disc material had left its normal position. In an extrusion, the width of the displaced disc material exceeds its base or aperture in any plane. The presence of an extrusion shape suggests that there has been complete disruption of the outer annulus, and disc material has entered the epidural space. Sequestration is the term for loss of continuity of a disc fragment with the parent disc from which it arose. Displacement of disc material away from the parent disc is termed migration. In the axial plane, herniated disc material is localized into zones. It may be in the central zone, which extends from the medial margin of one facet to the contralateral facet; the subarticular zone (lateral recess), which extends from the medial margin of the facet joint to the medial margin of the pedicle; the foraminal (lateral) zone, which extends from the medial margin of the pedicle to the lateral margin of the pedicle; or extraforaminal (far lateral) zone, which is lateral to the outer margin of the pedicle. Central canal compromise is typically defined as mild, moderate, or severe, implying loss of an additional one-third of the cross-sectional area of the central canal as one progresses through these gradations.

Ninety percent of disc herniations occur at the L4 or L5 interspace levels.[64] The vector of disc displacement in most herniations is posterolateral. In the lumbar spine, the exiting nerve passes immediately inferior to the vertebral pedicle and exits the foramen above the interspace level. Therefore, most disc herniations will not affect the exiting nerve, but rather impinge on the traversing nerve, which will exit under the next lower vertebral pedicle. For example, a posterolateral L4-L5 disc herniation will result in an L5 radicular pain syndrome or radiculopathy. For a lumbar disc herniation to affect the like numbered nerve, it must be an extrusion with cephalad migration of disc material into the neural foramen.

Disc herniations are well detected by CT, CT myelography, or MRI (**Fig. 6**A–F). On CT, disc material is slightly denser (lighter gray) than the thecal sac that it deforms; epidural fat may be effaced. On CT myelography the thecal sac and root sleeves will be opacified by contrast material; very subtle degrees of effacement can be detected. On T2-weighted MRI images, low-signal disc material can be directly observed to deform the high-signal thecal sac and root sleeves. Extruded or migrated disc material will often have higher T2 signal than the parent disc from which it arose. Surprisingly, there is no good current literature comparing the effectiveness of these 3 imaging technologies in the detection of disc herniations. A study by Thornbury and colleagues[65] in 1993 found little difference among unenhanced CT, CT myelography, and MRI in the detection of compressive lesions. A more recent article by van Rijn and colleagues[66] also found no evidence that CT was inferior to MRI in the detection of disc herniation. There was, however, more interobserver variability in detecting root compressive lesions with CT than MRI. This study used 2-slice CT scanners. There are no studies comparing current generation 64- to 256-slice CT with MRI. It must also be remembered that the correlation between the imaging appearance of a disc herniation and the clinical presentation is very poor. Large herniations may produce minimal symptoms, whereas small lesions result in disabling pain. Psychosocial factors, not imaging appearance, are better predictors of the extent of disability produced by a disc hernation.[11]

The imaging natural history of disc herniations is spontaneous involution. Saal and colleagues[67] noted that 50% of conservatively treated disc herniations causing radicular pain were observed to diminish by 75% in cross-sectional area on follow-up. Maigne and colleagues[68] noted that 65% of conservatively treated herniations diminished by 75% to 100% in volume on follow-up CT, and also that the largest herniations showed the greatest percentage of resolution. This finding was further confirmed by Bush and colleagues,[69] who showed that 76% of 165 patients with extrusions or sequestrations showed complete or partial resolution on follow-up imaging. Seventy-four percent of the patients who had only annular bulges showed no change on follow-up. In this series the clinical characteristics of patients with the greatest degree of resolution were a younger population with shorter duration of symptomatology and highly positive straight leg raise at presentation. Additional literature supports the consensus that the imaging natural history of disc herniation is the overwhelming one of spontaneous resolution. Large herniations, particularly sequestrations and extrusions, are more likely to resolve. In this circumstance, the herniated material is exposed to the full fury of the immune system in the richly vascularized epidural space; this also suggests why these patients present with dramatic symptomatology. Broad bulges, confined within the annulus, are least likely to change over time.

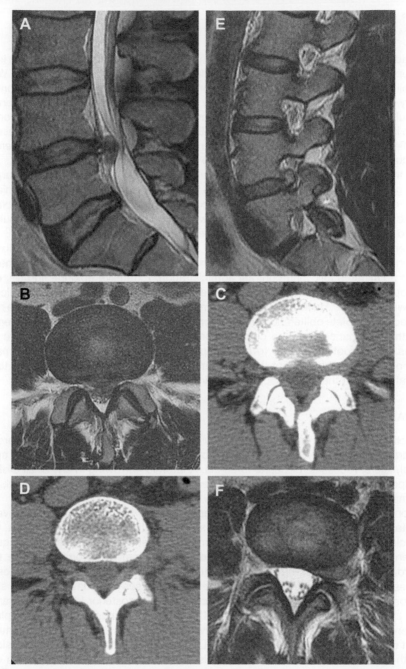

Fig. 6. Disc herniations. (*A*) Sagittal T2-weighted image in a patient with left L5 radicular pain reveals a large extrusion with cranial and caudal migration of disc material. The extrusion severely narrows the thecal sac, but the patient had no signs of cauda equina syndrome, only unilateral pain. (*B*) Axial T2-weighted image in the same patient at the L4 level. Note the compression of the thecal sac. (*C*) Axial CT image at the L4 interspace in a patient with acute left L4 radicular pain, unable to tolerate MRI. Note broad-based left-sided herniation. (*D*) CT image of the same patient cephalad to the disc reveals extruded disc material in left L4 foramen. Compare with normal fat surrounding right-sided nerve. (*E*) Sagittal T2-weighted MRI in another patient with left L4 radicular pain. L4 disc extrusion with migration of extruded material into foramen displaces the nerve superiorly. (*F*) Axial T2-weighted MRI at L4 disc level demonstrates well the foraminal extrusion.

Gadolinium contrast material is not routinely used in evaluating radicular pain in the nonoperated spine. Herniated disc material enhances minimally and slowly. When gadolinium is used, all of the material considered extruded disc on a noncontrast study is frequently shown to be a relatively small extrusion surrounded by enhancing granulation tissue. With contrast material, one occasionally may identify enhancement of an intrathecal root indicating radiculitis. Enhancement may also mark the presence of inflammatory response about an annular tear and provide the basis for a chemical radiculitis, even when there is no evidence of direct root compression.

In the postoperative spine, CT and myelography have limited utility. Postsurgical change will also confound MRI in the first 6 weeks. A diagnosis of recurrent herniation must be made with great trepidation, as expected postoperative change can exactly mimic recurrent herniation. Beyond the 6-week point, MRI with gadolinium should be up to 96% accurate in distinguishing recurrent disc material from scar.[70] This percentage is based on the differential time of enhancement: epidural fibrosis enhances very rapidly, whereas disc material shows minimal enhancement in the first 20 to 30 minutes following contrast administration. Extensive epidural fibrosis, even without recurrent herniation, is a negative prognostic sign for persistent radiculitis following surgery.[71] In its most extreme form, postoperative arachnoiditis can be manifested as complete obliteration or loculation of the subarachnoid space with extensive intrathecal enhancement and compartmentalization of the thecal sac. In more mild forms, nerve roots are seen to be clumped together on the T2-weighted images with or without enhancement. Low lumbar and sacral roots may be adherent to the lateral margin of the thecal sac, resulting in the so-called empty sac sign.

SPINAL STENOSIS

The clinical syndrome of spinal stenosis, or neurogenic claudication, must be carefully separated from the imaging observation of anatomic narrowing in the central spinal canal, lateral recesses, or neural foramina. Anatomic narrowing in any or all of these compartments may contribute to the patient's pain syndrome; all must be evaluated on imaging studies.

Considering initially the central canal, narrowing may have a congenital or developmental component in about 15% of spinal stenosis patients, most typically short, thick pedicles with a reduced anterior-posterior (AP) dimension of the canal.[64] Acquired degenerative processes that contribute to central canal compromise include facet arthropathy, central buckling of the ligamantum flavum, disc herniations, endplate osteophytes, and antero- or retrolisthesis. Systemic processes that may present as spinal stenosis may be rheumatologic (eg, ossification of the posterior longitudinal ligament [OPLL], discussed later), metabolic (epidural lipomatosis), or space occupying neoplasm.

Central canal stenosis due to degenerative processes will dominate. Compromise is most common at the L4 level, followed by L3, L5, and L1. The normal AP dimension of the thecal sac in the mid-lumbar region is 12 to 14 mm; less than 10 mm is clear anatomic evidence of stenosis, but correlation with clinical symptoms is poor.[72] The cross-sectional area of the thecal sac can be directly measured on CT or MRI; 180 ± 50 mm^2 is considered normal, 100 to 130 mm^2 may be early stenosis, while less than 100 mm^2 is a commonly quoted threshold for anatomic stenosis.[73] A more physiologically grounded parameter is the cross-sectional area at which intrathecal pressure increases; this has been measured at 77 mm^2.[74]

As with other degenerative processes, the specificity fault applies: Boden and colleagues[25] demonstrated anatomic central canal narrowing in 21% of asymptomatic subjects older than 60 years. Jarvik and colleagues[26] observed moderate to severe central canal narrowing in 7% of asymptomatic subjects younger than 45, in 11% of those 55 to 65, and in 21% of subjects older than 65 years. Dynamic lesions can also confound sensitivity: Schonstrom and colleagues[75] noted that moving from lumbar flexion to extension will reduce the area of the dural sac by 16%, while assuming axial load will also diminish cross-sectional area by 19%. The ligamentum flavum is the most important structure contributing to dynamic narrowing of the central canal with extension and axial load.[76]

Central canal narrowing can be suspected on radiographs. Short pedicles may suggest a congenitally narrow canal; the addition of disc/endplate degeneration, facet arthropathy, and antero- or retrolisthesis may conspire to produce central canal compromise. CT, CT myelography, or MRI are required to directly observe and quantify canal narrowing (**Fig. 7A–H**). In most clinical settings, central canal compromise will be rated as mild, moderate, or severe. As stenosis worsens, the dural sac can be seen to assume a trefoil, or triangular shape. On sagittal T2-weighted MRI images, serpiginous redundant roots or dilated veins can be seen in the thecal sac. On axial T2-weighted images, cerebrospinal fluid (CSF) will be effaced. When no bright CSF signal is present, only the intermediate to dark gray of crowded roots is visible, and central canal narrowing is becoming severe. One must also assess the lateral recesses and foramina; Porter and Ward[77] suggest that either multilevel central canal stenosis or central canal narrowing plus foraminal narrowing are necessary for symptoms. The study of Hamanishi and colleagues[78] also demonstrated that multiple levels of dural sac narrowing to less than 100 mm^2 strongly correlates with neuroclaudicatory pain.

In any patient with neuroclaudicatory pain, the lateral recesses and neural foramina must be evaluated as well as the central canal. As the nerve root leaves the common thecal sac, it enters the lateral recess or subarticular zone. This anatomic space is bounded anteriorly by the disc or posterior vertebral body, laterally by the medial margin of the pedicle, and posteriorly by the superior articular process and ligamentum flavum. This anterolateral extension of the central canal has a normal AP dimension of 3 to 4 mm. It is most frequently compromised by facet arthropathy, with overgrowth of the superior articular process, which encroaches on the latter recess from a posterior vector. Disc extrusions that migrate caudally may also enter the lateral recess. Lateral recess stenosis is most common at the L4-L5 interspace level.[64] Lateral recess compromise can be a subtle imaging finding on CT; it may be more evident on CT myelography or MRI (**Fig. 8A–D**).

As the exiting nerve root progresses further laterally, it enters the neural foramen. In the sagittal plane the foramen is teardrop shaped, widest in its cephalad portion; in the axial plane it extends from the medial to the lateral margins of the pedicle. The foramen is best evaluated on sagittal CT reconstructions or sagittal MRI images. On sagittal MRI images, the dorsal root ganglion can be seen in the upper portion of the foramen as a gray circle, surrounded by white fat. Additional smaller gray or black dots are veins. Compromise of the neural foramen may occur due to extruded disc material, osteophytes from the posterior margin of the vertebral body, or facet superior articular process, synovial cysts, or spondylolysis. In spondylolysis with associated spondylolisthesis, the neural foramen is narrowed in its vertical dimension by the loss of disc space height, and attains a forward-leaning, oblique configuration; direct compression or deformation of the dorsal root ganglion is often visible.

ZYGAPOPHYSIAL JOINTS

The supporting structure of the posterior column of the spine includes the paired z-joints with their associated capsules, the ligamentum flavum, the intraspinous and

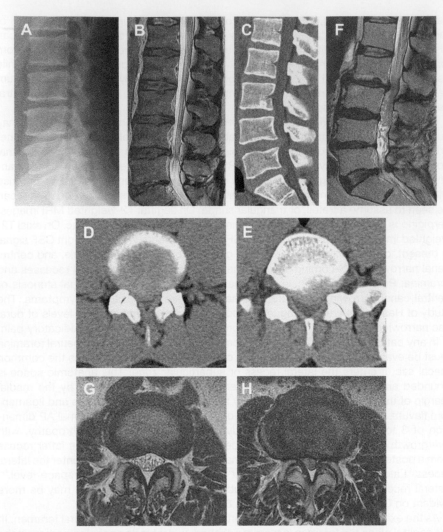

Fig. 7. Central canal stenosis. (*A*) Lateral radiograph of patient with bilateral leg pain with waking. Note short, thick pedicles, and multilevel disc space narrowing. (*B*) Sagittal T2-weighted MRI on the same patient confirms multilevel disc degeneration with small protrusion at L4; in the setting of a congenitally central canal, this causes severe central canal compromise. (*C*) Sagittal CT reconstruction in a patient with bilateral lower extremity pain. Note congenitally narrow central canal, and L4 and L5 disc herniations. (*D*) Axial CT at L4 level confirms severe central canal stenosis with tiny trefoil-shaped dural sac. (*E*) Axial CT at L5 level demonstrates large disc protrusion, but only moderate central canal compromise. (*F*) Sagittal T2-weighted MRI in another patient reveals severe central canal narrowing at L2 level with redundant nerves or dilated veins caudal to this level. (*G*) Axial T2-weighted image at L1 level shows no central canal compromise. (*H*) Axial T2-weighted image at L2 demonstrates complete effacement of CSF in this severely stenotic central canal.

supraspinous ligaments joining the spinous processes, and the intertransverse ligamentous structures. The inferior articular process of the facet joint faces anteriorly and is convex in configuration; on axial images (CT, MRI) the inferior articular process is the more posterior component of the joint. The superior articular process (SAP) has

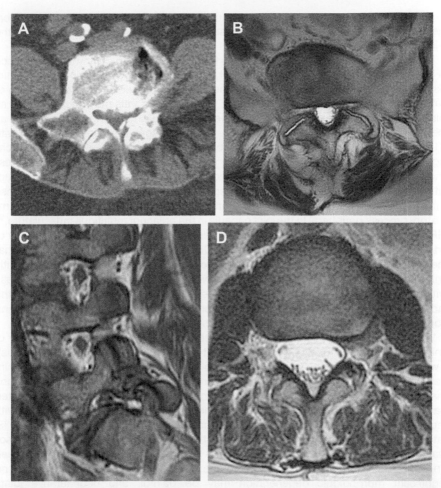

Fig. 8. Subarticular and foraminal stenosis. (*A*) Axial CT at L4 level demonstrates marked narrowing of the subarticular recesses bilaterally, due to endplate osteophytes and disc bulge. (*B*) Axial T2-weighted MRI at L5 level in a different patient illustrates bilateral subarticular recess stenosis due to facet hypertrophy. (*C*) Sagittal T1-weighted MRI in a patient with L5 spondylolysis, typical S-shaped foraminal stenosis with flattening of the dorsal root ganglion (DRG). Note normal, widely patent L3 and L4 foramina. (*D*) Axial T2-weighted MRI in a patient with "hip pain" reveals foraminal disc herniation at L3 contacting DRG.

a concave articular surface that faces posteriorly and medially; on axial images it appears as the anterior component of the joint. In an erect standing position, the lumbar z-joints bear approximately 16% of the compressive load; in a flexed sitting position they bear essentially no load.[79] In the presence of degenerative disc disease with loss of disc space height, the lumbar z-joints will bear proportionally more axial load.

The fibrous joint capsule has been demonstrated to be richly innervated by nociceptors and proprioceptive fibers.[80] In a normal state, nociceptors such as those seen in the z-joint capsule have a high threshold and would not be expected to fire unless loads are supraphysiologic. However, in the presence of pathologic joint inflammation, chemical mediators may sensitize these nociceptors, and supraphysiologic levels of stress may no longer be required to stimulate pain.[81] Such inflammatory chemical mediators (substance P, bradykinin, phospholipase A_2) have been detected in the z-joint capsule.[81,82]

There is therefore a pathoanatomic basis for z-joint pain, particularly in the presence of inflammatory mediators within the z-joint, most commonly present in osteoarthritis. Osteoarthritis of the z-joint is a common phenomenon, present in greater than 50% of patients aged 40 years or older.[79] On plain films, osteoarthritis may be manifested as joint space narrowing with associated sclerosis of the articular surfaces as well as the development of marginal osteophytes. These changes are better displayed with CT, which can also identify subchondral erosions as well as synovial cysts, outpouchings of the synovial space. MRI can directly visualize the loss of cartilage and the presence of a joint effusion. Use of fat-saturated T2-weighted images or post-gadolinium fat-saturated T1-weighted images can elegantly display the inflammatory response within the joint, synovium, adjacent subchondral bone, and the extension of the inflammatory process peripheral to the joint capsule in the adjacent multifidus musculature.[83] MRI also may show marrow edema or fatty replacement in the articular processes of arthritic joints, and in the adjacent pedicle. Cross-sectional imaging has shown that the bony changes of osteoarthritis are more pronounced in the SAP. There is frequently enlargement of the medial aspect of the SAP, which may encroach on the lateral recess with resultant neural compression. Marginal osteophytes at the posterior aspect of the facet joint are more prominent on the SAP, often covering the posterior joint margin and complicating injection access to the synovial space of the joint.

With the pathoanatomic basis of z-joint mediated pain identified, and the ability of imaging to depict the most common inflammatory condition of the joint (osteoarthritis), it would seem that imaging would play a key role in identification of patients with z-joint pain. The reality is more complex. There are no specific symptoms or physical signs that allow a clinical diagnosis of z-joint pain.[84] The diagnosis of z-joint mediated pain relies on response to controlled local anesthetic blocks. Controlled blocks with multiple anesthetic agents are critical, as there is a very high, in excess of 30%, rate of false-positive results from single anesthetic blocks.[84] Unfortunately, no association can be shown between the degree of morphologic z-joint degeneration seen on plain films or CT and the response to anesthetic blocks.[85] Z-joints that show no significant morphologic degeneration may be painful, and degenerative joints depicted by imaging are most commonly asymptomatic.

Although imaging of joint morphology has not been helpful, the detection of inflammation may be more useful. Technetium scanning with SPECT has shown a correlation between radionuclide uptake in the facet joints and response to intra-articular injections.[86] In this study there was no significant association between a positive SPECT study and morphologic changes of degeneration. Czervionke and Fenton[83] recently reported a series of patients undergoing MRI studies for back pain, and noted that fat-saturated T2-weighted images could detect z-joint synovitis that appeared to correlate with the clinical pain syndrome. STIR or fat-saturated T2-weighted sequences should be included in the MRI examination in the patient with back pain (**Fig. 9**A–E).

SYNOVIAL CYSTS

Synovial cysts are a manifestation of osteoarthritis in the facet joints. Synovial cysts arise from a traumatic or degenerative defect in the fibrous facet joint capsule with herniation of synovial membrane through the rent. There was an approximately 10% prevalence of synovial cysts in a population of patients undergoing MRI for back or leg pain studied by Doyle and Merrilees[87]; most of these cysts are posterior, extraspinal,

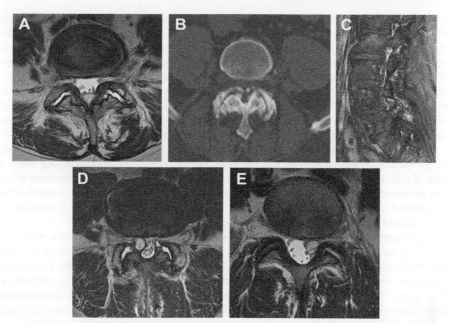

Fig. 9. Z-joint arthropathy and synovial cysts. (A) Axial T2-weighted MRI at L4 level shows bilateral z-joint effusions with subchondral degenerative cysts on the left. (B) Axial CT in another patient, also at L4, shows severe changes of osteoarthritis with joint narrowing, subchondral cysts, and osteophytes—these morphologic changes alone do not predict pain. (C) Sagittal T1-weighted, fat-saturated enhanced MRI in the same patient as (B) shows enhancement about the L4 z-joint; this finding is predictive of pain. (D and E) Axial T2-weighted MRI images in different patients demonstrating synovial cysts arising from arthritic z-joints.

and not clinically significant. A smaller proportion (2.3% prevalence) were intraspinal cysts and may act as root compressive lesions. Synovial cysts are a disease of the elderly, with an average age at presentation of 61 to 66 years in 3 large series.[88–90] Sixty to seventy percent of cysts are seen at the L4-L5 interspace level, and are often seen in association with segmental instability and associated disc degeneration.[88] Synovial cysts may be identified on CT, CT myelography, or MRI; they have widely varying histology and subsequently a very heterogeneous appearance on imaging. There is often hemorrhage within the cysts with some degree of fibrosis or calcification in the cyst wall. Synovial cysts may undergo spontaneous regression. A radicular pain syndrome caused by a synovial cyst may be treated in a minimally invasive fashion with aspiration and intra-articular instillation of steroid into the cyst or joint bearing the cyst, with a transforaminal epidural steroid injection performed at the same setting to treat the radicular pain. Such a strategy was successful in avoiding surgical intervention in 50% of patients in a series by Sabers and colleagues.[91] Other nonoperative therapies have included aspiration, fenestration, or rupture of cysts under CT or fluoroscopic guidance. Surgical excision of synovial cysts is typically a highly successful procedure, but may require partial facet resection or laminectomy.[90]

DEGENERATIVE SPONDYLOLISTHESIS

Spondylolisthesis refers to the abnormal anterior or posterior displacement of one vertebral body relative to another. Displacement due to defects in the pars interarticulari (spondylolytic spondylolisthesis) is discussed later. Degenerative anterolisthesis is the anterior displacement of a vertebral body relative to the body immediately caudal to it. The cause of degenerative anterolisthesis is primarily facet joint degeneration, often in sagittally oriented facets, with associated disc degeneration. The prevalence of degenerative anterolisthesis is up to 14% of elderly patients.[92] Anterolisthesis is most frequent at the L4 level, and less commonly at L5, followed by L3. It is significantly more common in women than men.[92] Radiographic findings of degenerative anterolisthesis include the obvious displacement itself, joint space narrowing and sclerosis in the associated facets, and findings of disc degeneration.

Degenerative retrolisthesis describes the posterior displacement of the vertebral body relative to that below it; the primary cause is disc degeneration. As there is loss of disc space height, the oblique orientation of the facet results in the more superior vertebral body gliding posterior relative to its inferior counterpart. Degenerative retrolisthesis is most commonly seen at the L2 interspace level, less commonly at L1, followed by L3.[92] There is no significant gender difference.

Degenerative spondylolisthesis may be associated with axial low back pain. The study by Kauppila and colleagues[92] showed that patients with degenerative spondylolisthesis had a higher prevalence of daily symptoms of low back pain. There was, however, no increased disability in spondylolisthesis patients relative to controls. In this study the overall prevalence of degenerative spondylolisthesis approached 20%. Degenerative spondylolisthesis carries with it the risk of neural element compromise due to secondary central canal stenosis, lateral recess stenosis, or foraminal compromise.

BAASTRUP SYNDROME

Baastrup syndrome describes an imaging finding in which lumbar spinous processes contact in extension, with radiographically evident sclerosis and flattening of the opposing bony surfaces and pseudarthrosis formation, which may be accompanied by formation of a pseudobursa. Such a pseudobursa may have a synovial membrane,[93] and can communicate with z-joints or pars defects via the retrodural space described by Okada.[94] The pseudobursa may extend anteriorly through a midline cleft in the ligamentum flavum and present on MRI or CT as a midline posterior epidural cyst, causing neural compression.[93] It may be mistaken for a synovial cyst of z-joint origin, but is distinguished by its midline posterior location, the relative absence of facet degeneration, a cystic pseudobursa, and inflammatory change in the interspinous ligament.

More commonly, Baastrup syndrome is invoked to explain midline axial pain that is exacerbated by extension, and may be relieved by local anesthetic and/or corticosteroid injection in the interspinous ligament. The posterior element findings often occur in association with disc degeneration and segmental instability; axial pain in this setting may be multifactorial. Midline posterior element activity on technetium SPECT scans may suggest the diagnosis.[95] On MRI, the author has observed marrow edema in the spinous processes, pseudobursae, and gadolinium enhancement in the interspinous ligament, particularly on fat-saturated images.

BERTOLOTTI SYNDROME

Bertolotti syndrome describes the controversial association of transitional lumbosacral segments with mechanical back pain; it does not imply a specific mechanism of pain production. Tini and colleagues[96] found no correlation between the presence of a transitional segment and low back pain. The disc at the level of the transitional segment is often rudimentary, with little nuclear material; disc herniations seldom occur at this level.[96] Rather, stresses may be accentuated at the supra-adjacent disc level, where accelerated disc degeneration and an increased incidence of disc herniations has been reported.[97]

Axial low back pain in the presence of a transitional segment has also been attributed to abnormal or asymmetric motion at this level, with the neoarticulation of the transverse process with the sacral ala, or the contralateral facet as the specific pain generator. Jonsson and colleagues[98] reported 11 cases of mechanical pain attributed to the neoarticulation despite normal bone scans. Nine of 11 patients obtained pain relief with local anesthetic injection in the neoarticulation; a similar proportion of patients had improvement in pain with resection of the neoarticulation.

SACROILIAC, COCCYGEAL DEGENERATIVE DISEASE

Osteoarthritis of the sacroiliac joints may be seen in pathologic specimens of young adults, but is not generally appreciable radiographically until middle age. Changes of cartilage degeneration are more prominent on the iliac side of the joint. Beyond age 40 years, many patients will have detectable narrowing of the sacroiliac joint, especially in its inferior portion, which may be accompanied by subchondral sclerosis and osteophyte formation, most prominent anteriorly and inferiorly. A vacuum phenomenon may be seen. The joint may undergo fibrous ankylosis over time. Intra-articular bony ankylosis is unusual as a manifestation of osteoarthritis; it is more typical of the inflammatory spondyloarthropathies. Osteoarthritic changes are evident on plain films; CT or MRI will be more sensitive. It is unclear, however, whether detection of typical changes of osteoarthritis radiographically is useful in identifying patients with a sacroiliac pain syndrome.

The prevalence of sacroiliac pain among patients with chronic axial low back pain is thus probably between 15% and 25%.[99] There is no gold standard for the diagnosis of sacroiliac joint pain. Medical history and physical examination provocative maneuvers have not been capable of consistently identifying painful sacroiliac joints,[99] and the most commonly used gold standard (intra-articular anesthetic blocks) is known to be flawed. It is not too surprising that advanced imaging has not clarified the issue. Radionuclide bone scans have been shown to have sensitivities of only 46% and 13%, although with high specificity, in the studies of Maigne and colleagues[100] and Slipman and colleagues,[101] respectively. Elgafy and colleagues[102] showed CT imaging to have a sensitivity of 58% and a specificity of 69%. MRI-based studies have primarily focused on active inflammatory disease in the spondyloarthropathies. The primary purpose of imaging in this setting is to exclude the more sinister pathology of tumor, inflammatory spondyloarthropathy, or sacral insufficiency fracture.

The radiographic evaluation of the sacrococcygeal region in patients with coccydynia remains controversial. This largely female pain syndrome is probably multifactorial in origin with contributions by somatic and neuropathic pain. A single lateral view of the coccyx to evaluate for destructive bony lesions is a reasonable screening study. Maigne and colleagues[103] has described a dynamic radiographic study to more fully evaluate the mobility of the coccyx; this has not seen broad acceptance. In persistent pain syndromes, MRI should be the final test to exclude sinister pathology.

SYSTEMIC DISEASE PRESENTING AS BACK PAIN

The final topic to be discussed is systemic disease that presents, or has as its dominant clinical manifestation, back pain. Detection of systemic disease is the primary goal of spine imaging. Comprehensive review is not possible; this section addresses inflammatory spine disease, pyogenic and granulomatous spine infection, traumatic processes that include spondylolysis, compression fractures, and insufficiency fractures, and spine neoplasms.

Inflammatory Disease

Noninfectious inflammatory disease of the spine includes rheumatoid arthritis (RA) and the seronegative spondyloarthropathies (SpA). Ankylosing spondylitis (AS) is the SpA prototype; this group also includes psoriatic arthritis, Reiter syndrome, and spondyloarthritis of inflammatory bowel disease. These diverse entities have spine involvement in common, and may present with axial back pain. RA most commonly involves the cervical segment of the spine, particularly the atlantoaxial articulation. Lumbar manifestations are rare.

AS is the prototypical seronegative spondyloarthropathy; imaging is integral to its diagnosis. The modified New York criteria require imaging evidence of sacroiliitis for diagnosis.[104] AS has a prevalence of up to 0.1% in the general population; a very high percentage will be HLA B27 positive. Males dominate by 4:1. The disease involves synovial and cartilaginous joints and entheses (ligament and tendon insertions on bone) with a strong predilection for the axial skeleton. The most common presentation is low back pain with inflammatory features (Calin criteria, 4 out of 5 of: insidious onset, age <40, 3 months' persistence, morning stiffness, and pain improved by exercise). Radiating pain mimicking sciatica may be seen in up to 50% of patients.[104]

Imaging findings in AS include sacroiliitis, ultimately bilaterally symmetric. Sacroiliitis is the initial imaging finding in 99% of cases.[105] Early plain film findings of sacroiliitis are blurring of the subchondral cortex and small erosions, predominantly on the iliac side of the joint. As the erosions coalesce, the joint space appears widened and ill-defined; sclerotic reaction develops in the trabecular bone about both sides of the joint. Over time the joint undergoes ankylosis via direct bony bridging; the joint space is no longer visible and the sclerosis resolves. Plain films can detect these structural changes (erosions, sclerosis, ankylosis) with a sensitivity equal to MRI.[106] MRI, however, can detect inflammation in and about the sacroiliac joint in symptomatic patients with normal plain films. In patients with recent onset axial low back pain with inflammatory clinical characteristics, sacroiliac joint inflammation may be detected by MRI in one-third of patients and structural changes in one-sixth.[106] Inflammation is initially seen in the iliac side of the joint at its caudal and dorsal aspects, and in the adjacent dorsal entheses.[105] Spine lesions include osteitis, syndesmophyte formation, discovertebral lesions, and inflammation leading to ankylosis of facet and costovertebral joints.[64] Osteitis is seen as sclerosis at the anterior corners of the vertebral bodies (shiny corners sign), and inflammatory remodeling (straightening) of the normally concave anterior vertebral margin (squaring of the vertebrae).[64] Thin, gracile, vertically oriented bony struts (syndesmophytes, as opposed to more horizontally oriented osteophytes) ultimately bridge the margins of adjacent vertebrae. Inflammatory discovertebral lesions may resemble Modic-1 change with progression to a Modic-2 appearance followed by ankylosis.[104] Extensive spinal ankylosis places these patients at risk for catastrophic fracture-dislocations with modest trauma; the threshold for advanced imaging in trauma situations should be low (**Fig. 10A–F**).

Psoriatic arthritis is far less common than AS, affecting 5% to 8% of all patients with psoriasis. Approximately 10% to 25% of patients with moderate to severe skin disease will have abnormal sacroiliac joint radiographs.[64] Spondylitis is present in a roughly similar proportion, but may or may not coexist with sacroiliitis. Male and females are equally affected. The spondylitis in psoriatic arthritis is characterized by

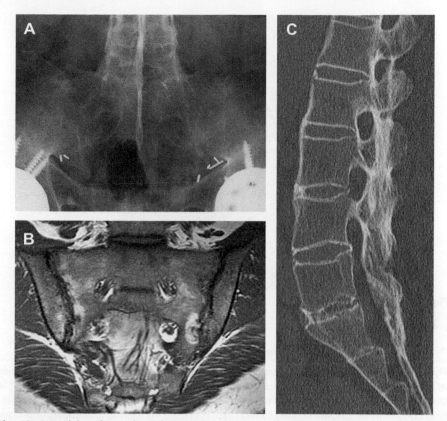

Fig. 10. Spondyloarthropathy. (*A*) Frontal radiograph of a patient with chronic ankylosing spondylitis (AS). Note fusion of sacroiliac joints, syndesmophytes bridging vertebrae, and "dagger sign" fusion of the spinous processes/interspinous ligament. (*B*) Coronal T1-weighted MRI in an AS patient showing irregular sacroiliac joints with abnormal adjacent signal, suggesting chronic inflammation. (*C*) Sagittal CT reconstruction in an AS patient clearly demonstrates syndesmophytes bridging the vertebrae as well as fusion of the z-joints. (*D*) CT scan in a patient with psoriatic arthritis shows symmetric sacroiliitis. (*E*) Enhanced, fat-saturated coronal MRI image in a patient with Reiter syndrome shows asymmetric sacroiliitis with enhancement about right sacroiliac joint only. (*F*) CT scan in a patient with Crohn's disease demonstrates symmetric sacroiliitis.

asymmetric, coarse paravertebral ossification more resembling osteophytes than syndesmophytes.[105] Reiter syndrome describes an inflammatory arthropathy, primarily in males, that may affect the spine in association with urethritis and conjunctivitis.[64] Sacroiliitis is very common, affecting up to 75% of patients with chronic disease. It is more commonly unilateral or asymmetric than in AS, but less likely to result in ankylosis. Spine involvement is infrequent.

Spondyloarthropathies may also be seen in association with ulcerative colitis, Crohn's disease, and Whipple's disease. The initial presentation of back pain may precede symptoms of gastrointestinal disease. The spondylitis and sacroiliitis seen in association with these conditions are indistinguishable from classic AS.

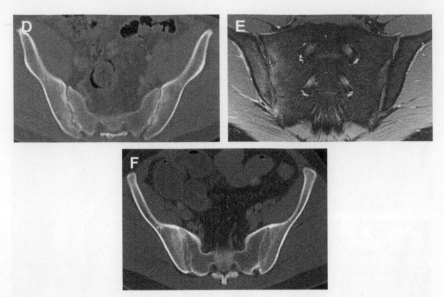

Fig. 10. (*continued*)

Pyogenic and Granulomatous Infection

Pyogenic spinal infections are usually the result of arterial seeding. In children, the disc and endplate have a rich blood supply; infection occurs initially in the disc itself.[64] In the adult the disc is avascular; an infection develops in the anterior subchondral vertebral body with secondary spread to the disc, adjacent vertebrae, and subligamentous space. Most disc space infections involve 2 adjacent lumbar vertebrae. Spread from contiguous infection or direct inoculation of the disc (surgery, discography) are much less common.

Pyogenic disc space infection involves men much more commonly than women (2–3 to 1) in the fifth to seventh decades of life.[64] Clinical symptoms may precede radiographic findings by 1 to 8 weeks. Clinical signs of elevated sedimentation rate, white blood cell count, and C-reactive protein are usually present. Plain films reveal early rarefaction of anterior subchondral bone, followed by loss of disc space height (at 1–3 weeks) with subsequent destructive changes in the vertebral endplates. Late changes include variable amounts of sclerosis, kyphotic deformity from vertebral collapse, and ankylosis. CT in pyogenic discitis shows early hypodensity in the disc, moth-eaten destruction of the vertebral endplates, inflammatory changes in paravertebral soft tissues, and epidural mass. Scattered gas formation may be seen. Extensive gas formation in the central portion of the disc is almost always a result of disc degeneration, not infection.

MRI is the preferred imaging modality for the evaluation of discitis, with a greater than 90% sensitivity and specificity in disease detection.[107,108] MRI also provides critical anatomic information. Early marrow changes are elevated T2 signal (best seen with fat saturation), diminished T1 signal, and gadolinium enhancement. There is loss of the crisp, dark cortical line of the vertebral endplate. Within the disc, the intranuclear cleft is lost and foci of elevated T2 signal develop, as well as gadolinium enhancement. The paravertebral and epidural soft tissues show diffuse enhancement (phlegmon) or frank abscess formation with zones of hypoenhancement and increased T2 signal. The imaging differential diagnosis consists of Modic type 1 degenerative change, atypical cartilaginous (Schmorl) nodes, contiguous metastatic lesions, pseudoarthroses in patients with AS, or a Charcot spine.[108]

MRI abnormalities also lag behind the clinical syndrome. Imaging may be minimally abnormal early in the disease process, and may remain quite dramatic even after a gratifying clinical response to antibiotics. In following the efficacy of antibiotic therapy, sedimentation rate, C-reactive protein, and white blood cell count will be more useful than repeated imaging, which should be reserved for patients in whom there is a clinical concern for continued infection with central canal compromise.

Nuclear medicine scans using gallium-67 citrate and technitium-99m diphosphonate are considered by some to be the primary imaging modality for suspected spondylodiscitis. Technetium and gallium scans are complementary; Hadjipavlou and colleagues[109] demonstrated 100% sensitivity, specificity, and accuracy for the combination of gallium and technetium scans when compared with surgical biopsy results; others have reported similar results. All nuclear medicine techniques, however, lack anatomic information; they are unable to define the extent of epidural or paraspinal disease or central canal compromise.

Tuberculosis (Pott disease) is the most common cause of spine infection worldwide and is increasing in frequency in the United States. Clinical symptoms are usually insidious, with 90% to 100% of patients complaining of back pain, but only 50% exhibiting constitutional symptoms or fever. Neurologic deficit is common. Radiographic imaging findings include disc space narrowing, vertebral osteolysis with collapse, and gibbus deformity. The thoracolumbar junction is the most common site of involvement.[64] The disease tends to spare the discs and posterior elements. CT will demonstrate bony destruction and paraspinal disease with greater sensitivity than radiographs, but MRI is the preferred modality for diagnosis and characterization. Early changes may be indistinguishable from pyogenic disc space infection, with marrow edema on both sides of the disc and associated paraspinal and epidural enhancement with contrast material. Epidural involvement is present in 60% to 80% of cases. Up to 50% of subjects exhibit a pattern of spondylitis without discitis.[110] The discs are completely spared, with only well-defined vertebral lesions, sometimes with paraspinal extension, which may be mistaken for metastases (**Fig. 11**A–H).

Traumatic Lesions: Spondylolysis, Compression Fractures, and Insufficiency Fractures

Isthmic spondylolysis is a fatigue fracture in an immature or deficient pars interarticularis. There is an underlying genetic predisposition, which is manifest developmentally as a diminished interfacet distance at the level of the defect[111]; this renders the pars vulnerable to impact by the inferior articular process above. In the adult United States population the prevalence is 6% to 8%, with a much higher prevalence in elite athletes who sustain supraphysiologic axial load in extension, such as divers and gymnasts.[64] Spondylolysis is most common at L5 (67%), followed by L4 (15%–20%) and L3 (1%–2%).[64] On lateral radiographs a lucent defect may be seen in the pars, as well as signs of disc degeneration and anterolisthesis. If there is clinical suspicion, a localized CT should be performed; there is no role for oblique radiographs because of their radiation dose. CT will elegantly display the morphology, allow characterization of healing potential, and evaluate the neural foramina. Beware, however, the ever present specificity flaw; there is a 5.7% prevalence of spondylolysis in an asymptomatic population.[112] Some investigators advocate combining CT with SPECT imaging to characterize and plan therapy for pars defects. Pars defects can be clearly seen on sagittal MRI, which can also detect marrow edema as a stress response before a fracture occurs.

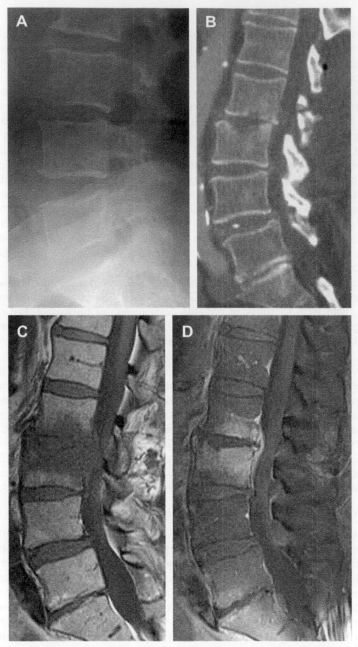

Fig. 11. Spondylodiscitis. (*A*) Lateral radiograph demonstrating early pyogenic spondylodiscitis manifesting as subtle destruction of anterior inferior aspect of L3 vertebrae. (*B*) Sagittal CT reconstruction. Sagittal T1 unenhanced (*C*), (*D*) enhanced, and (*E*) axial T1 enhanced MRI images of a patient with L2 pyogenic discitis. Note loss of disc space height, endplate destruction, low T1 signal and extensive vertebral, epidural, and paraspinal enhancement. (*F*) Sagittal T2-weighted MRI of a patient with back pain without myelopathy. Tuberculous spondylodiscitis with vertebral destruction and kyphotic deformity. (*G*) Coronal T1 enhanced MRI in the same patient demonstrates extensive paraspinal disease. (*H*) Sagittal T2-weighted MRI in another patient with tuberculous spondylodiscitis; note multiple vertebral lesions with sparing of discs.

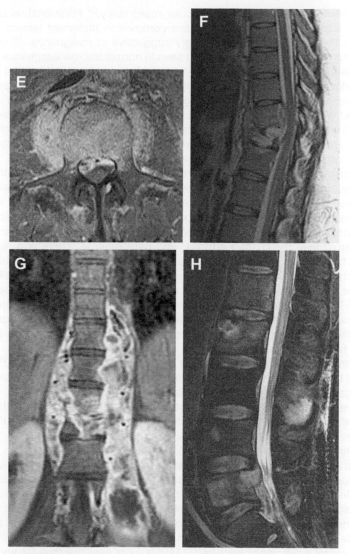

Fig. 11. (continued)

There are estimated to be in excess of 700,000 osteoporotic vertebral compression fractures in the United States per year. There is a lesser, though still substantial, number of vertebral metastatic lesions. Imaging is frequently called on to differentiate benign from malignant compression. Radiographs and CT are of little benefit in the absence of gross destruction; MRI is the preferred test for characterizing fracture etiology. Chronic benign compression fractures will exhibit marrow signal similar to that of adjacent normal vertebral bodies on T1-weighted images. Acute or early subacute fractures, however, may exhibit diminished T1 signal similar to that seen in metastatic lesions.

Malignant lesions are much more likely to exhibit hypointense T1 signal throughout the entire vertebral body. T1 signal abnormality extending into the pedicles or posterior elements is relatively specific for malignancy.[64] Paravertebral or epidural mass associated with a fracture is more common in malignant lesions. Posterior bowing of the vertebral body is strongly suggestive of malignancy.[113] Gadolinium enhancement to a level greater than that seen in normal marrow suggests a malignant lesion. Associated disc rupture or retropulsion of a bony fragment without bowing of the posterior margin of the vertebral body are features that suggest a benign lesion.[113] Discrete cystic lesions with high T2 signal within the vertebrae are also commonly associated with benign compression fractures. Myeloma remains an imaging challenge, as vertebral compression fractures in myeloma patients may exhibit a benign MRI appearance. Where clinical concern remains, image-guided biopsy of spinal lesions provides a minimally invasive means to a histologic diagnosis.[113]

Pelvic insufficiency fractures are increasingly recognized as a cause of axial and somatic referred pain experienced in the low back, pelvis, groin, and proximal lower extremities.[114] Insufficiency fractures are by definition fractures that occur in structurally inadequate bone which fails when exposed to repeated normal physiologic loads. Postmenopausal osteoporosis is the dominant risk factor, along with pelvic radiation, corticosteroid use, rheumatoid arthritis, and osteomalacia. There is a female:male ratio of 9:1; patients are typically in their sixth decade or older.[115] There is often significant morbidity associated with insufficiency fractures. Taillandier and colleagues[115] noted that 50% of their patients did not recover their former level of independence, and in 25% the insufficiency fracture precipitated institutionalization in their elderly study population. Sacral insufficiency fractures are the most common expression of this condition; pubic ramus fractures, parasymphyseal fractures, and para-acetabular fractures have also been described.

Sacral insufficiency fractures were first described by Lourie[114] in 1982. Plain radiographs of the pelvis are relatively insensitive. The most common radiographic finding is a vertical sclerotic band in the sacral ala paralleling the sacroiliac joint. CT will be more sensitive in detecting cortical disruption and the sclerotic margins of the fracture. There is often a horizontal fracture line extending through the sacral body; this may be missed on axial images and will be better seen on coronal CT images.

On technetium bone scan, the classic finding is the so-called Honda sign. Increased metabolic activity in bilateral vertical sacral ala fracture lines are bridged by a horizontal line representing a fracture through the sacral body, resulting in a representation of the letter H. In the series of Fujii and colleagues,[116] 63% of patients with sacral insufficiency fractures exhibited this sign in total, with 35% showing a variant such as 2 vertical lines without a crossbar or a single vertical and horizontal line. In this series, the Honda sign taken with its variants had 96% sensitivity and 92% positive predictive value for sacral insufficiency fracture.[116] MRI is more sensitive than CT and similar to bone scan in the early detection of insufficiency fractures. It will reveal marrow edema (low T1, high T2 signal with gadolinium enhancement) in a pattern typical of insufficiency fracture (Honda sign) before sclerosis or a fracture line can be visualized with CT.[117] Imaging in the coronal plane is preferred. Detection of increased T2 signal will be improved with fat-saturated or STIR sequences.

Spine Neoplasm

Spinal neoplasms are classified by the anatomic compartment from which they arise: extradural, intradural-extramedullary, or intramedullary. Extradural neoplasms arise from the vertebral bodies or the paravertebral soft tissues, or from within the epidural space. These neoplasms include metastatic lesions, hematologic malignancies, and primary osseous or cartilaginous tumors. Intradural-extramedullary lesions arise within the dural tube, but are extrinsic to the spinal cord itself. Lesions in this category include meningiomas, schwannomas, neurofibromas, and leptomeningeal metastatic disease. Intramedullary lesions are those which arise primarily from the spinal cord or filum terminale. Astrocytomas, ependymomas, and hemangioblastomas make up the vast majority of these lesions.

Extradural neoplasms are common. MRI provides the best combination of lesion detection, characterization, and assessment of neural compromise. Nuclear medicine techniques such as technetium bone scan and PET scanning will provide high sensitivity to lesion detection and excellent body-wide assessment of tumor burden. Nuclear medicine studies will not provide anatomic information regarding compression of neural elements. CT is less sensitive than MRI in lesion detection. Radiographs are far less sensitive; at least 50% of trabecular bone mass must be destroyed to be visible on a plain radiograph.[64]

Hemangiomas are very common benign bone tumors, characterized by high T1 and T2 signal on MRI, and a striated appearance on radiographs or CT. The vast majority are of no clinical significance; rarely aggressive hemangiomas will have a soft tissue component that invades the epidural space. Osteoid osteomas are benign but painful posterior element neoplasms of young adults. Pain is classically nocturnal and is relieved by aspirin. The lesion consists of a small nidus, less than 1.5 cm in diameter, surrounded by a larger zone of sclerotic reaction or soft tissue inflammation. The nidus is intensely enhancing on CT, MRI, or bone scan.[64]

Metastases are the most common extradural spine tumor; the spinal column is the most common site of osseous metastases. The vast majority are the result of prostate, lung, and breast primary neoplasms. Involvement of the vertebral body is most common (85%), with less frequent spread to the paravertebral tissues or epidural space. The discs, dura, and the anterior longitudinal ligament are resistant to invasion by metastatic tumor; the posterior longitudinal ligament is more readily involved, as it is penetrated by numerous venous channels. Vertebral body metastases may be blastic (bone forming), lytic (destructive), or mixed. Blastic lesions are seen as ill-defined areas of increased density on plain films or CT; on MRI blastic lesions will have low T1 and T2 signal with enhancement. Lytic metastases show destruction on plain films and CT, and low T1 and variable T2 signal with enhancement on MRI.

Myeloma is the most common malignant primary tumor of bone; it presents with bone pain in 75% of patients. Myeloma is often widespread at presentation. Its imaging appearance can range from discrete destructive lesions to diffuse loss of bone density indistinguishable from osteoporosis on plain films. CT is better able to resolve the discrete destructive lesions in trabecular or cortical bone. The MRI appearance is variable, with diminished T1 marrow signal and gadolinium enhancement in a multifocal or diffuse pattern. Compression fractures are common, and may be indistinguishable from benign osteoporotic fractures. Single focal lesions (plasmacytomas) are expansile and lytic on imaging.

Intradural-extramedullary neoplasms are situated within the dural sac, widening the subarachnoid space as they displace the cord or cauda equina. Meningiomas will typically exhibit a broad base against the dural surface and enhance uniformly. Schwannomas and neurofibromas are indistinguishable on imaging. The classic "dumb-bell" neurofibroma may issue through and widen a neural foramen. Leptomeningeal metastatic disease is most typically seen as enhancement on the surface of the cord or within the roots of the cauda equina. In some cases more discrete small masses may be seen within the cauda equina.

Intramedullary neoplasms are rare entities, but may present with pain or dysfunction that can mimic degenerative disease. Ependymomas arise from the ependymal cells lining the central canal of the cord. Ependymomas are the most common intramedullary tumor in adults; they are most frequently located in the conus medullaris and filum terminale (myxopapillary ependymoma). Because of their slow growth, they may cause bony erosion and scalloped enlargement of the central canal. MRI demonstrates an enlarged cord or filum terminale with elevated T2 signal and heterogeneous enhancement. Small cysts or hemorrhage are frequent. Astrocytomas are typically low-grade neoplasms, more commonly seen in young patients and in the cervical region. Astrocytomas typically extend over multiple vertebral segments within the cord, with poorly defined margins. The cord is enlarged with heterogeneous enhancement.. Hemangioblastomas are rare lesions characterized by enhancing nodules on the surface of the cord in the cervical and thoracic spine. About one-third of patients with hemangioblastomas will have Von Hippel Lindau syndrome.[64]

SUMMARY

Imaging has no role in the evaluation of the patient with acute back pain in the absence of signs or symptoms of underlying systemic disease or progressive neurologic deficit. The decision to undertake imaging should be a rational one, balancing risk and benefit, and should be mindful of its well-documented flaws in specificity (asymptomatic degenerative processes) and sensitivity (dynamic lesions). The primary role of imaging remains the detection of undiagnosed systemic disease. Imaging should begin with plain radiographs. Advanced imaging may be undertaken when radiographs are not explanatory and conservative therapy has failed. Degenerative processes can be well demonstrated by imaging, but they obtain significance only in the context of the patient's pain syndrome. Imaging findings of disc degeneration are ubiquitous. In patients suspected of discogenic pain, HIZs in the posterior annulus, Modic type 1 and 2 marrow changes, severe disc space narrowing, and marked T2 signal loss in the disc may predict a positive discogram; there is, however, no true gold standard for the diagnosis of discogenic pain. Disc herniations can be detected by CT, CT myelography, or MRI. The imaged morphology of disc herniations does not predict the degree of disability or the intensity of the pain syndrome. The natural history of disc herniations is resolution. Imaging the structural changes of osteoarthritis in facet or sacroiliac joints does not predict a pain syndrome or response to intra-articular interventions. Imaging the inflammatory response with bone scan or heavily T2-weighted MRI does correlate with response to intra-articular anesthetic injections. In the detection and characterization of systemic disease presenting as spine pain, MRI is the dominant and preferred imaging modality. Imaging will provide the greatest value when there is close communication between the spine clinician and the imaging professional, as all imaging is context driven.

ACKNOWLEDGMENTS

The assistance of Deb Berg in the preparation of the manuscript and figures is gratefully acknowledged.

REFERENCES

1. Jarvik JG, Deyo R. Diagnostic evaluation of low back pain with emphasis on imaging. Ann Intern Med 2002;137:586–97.
2. Deyo R, Mirza S, Turner Y. Overtreating chronic back pain: time to back off? J Am Board Fam Med 2009;22(1):62–8.
3. Von Korff M, Deyo RA, Cherkin D, et al. Back pain in primary care. Outcomes at 1 year. Spine 1993;18:855–62.

4. Van den Hoogen HJ, Koes BW, van Eijk JT, et al. On the course of low back pain in general practice: a one year follow up study. Ann Rheum Dis 1998;57: 13–9.
5. McGuirk B, King W, Govind J, et al. Safety, efficacy, and cost effectiveness of evidence-based guidelines for the management of acute low back pain in primary care. Spine 2001;26:2615–22.
6. Scavone JC, Latshaw RF, Rohrar GV. Use of lumbar spine films: statistical evaluation at a teaching hospital. JAMA 1981;246:1105–8.
7. Simmons ED, Guyer RG, Graham-Smith A, et al. Radiograph assessment for patients with low back pain. Spine J 2003;3:3S–5S.
8. Gilbert FJ, Grant AM, Gillan MG, et al. Low back pain: influence of early MR imaging or CT on treatment and outcome—multicenter randomized trial. Radiology 2004;231(2):343–51.
9. Chou R, Fu R, Carrino J, et al. Imaging strategies for low-back pain: systematic review and metanalysis. Lancet 2009;373:463–72.
10. Liang M, Komaroff AL. Roentgenograms in primary care patients with acute low back pain: a cost-effective analysis. Arch Intern Med 1982;142: 1108–12.
11. Carragee E, Alamin T, Cheng I, et al. Are first-time episodes of serious LBP associated with new MRI findings? Spine J 2006;6:624–35.
12. Agency for Health Care Policy and Research. Acute low back problems in adults: assessment and treatment. Clin Pract Guidel Quick Ref Guide Clin 1994;14:iii–iiv, 1–25.
13. Bradley W. Low back pain. AJNR Am J Neuroradiol 2007;28(5):990–2.
14. Chou R, Qaseem A, Snow B, et al. Diagnosis and treatment of low back pain: a joint clinical practice guideline from the American College of Physicians and the American Pain Society. Ann Intern Med 2007;147:478–91.
15. Modic MT, Obuchowski NA, Ross JS, et al. Acute low back pain and radiculopathy: MR imaging findings and their prognostic role and effect on outcome. Radiology 2005;237(2):597–604.
16. Engers A, Jellema P, Wensing M, et al. Individual patient education for low back pain. Cochrane Database Syst Rev 2008;1:CD004057.
17. Mettler FA, Huda W, Yoshizumi T, et al. Effective doses in radiology and diagnostic nuclear medicine: a catalog. Radiology 2008;48:254–63.
18. E-publication. Centers for Medicare & Medicaid services. 2009. Available at: http://www.cms.hhs.gov/. Accessed July 27, 2010.
19. Jarvik JG, Hollingworth W, Martin B, et al. Rapid magnetic resonance imaging vs radiographs for patients with low back pain. JAMA 2003;289:2810–8.
20. Lurie JD, Birkmeyer NJ, Weinstein JN. Rates of advanced spinal imaging and spine surgery. Spine 2003;28:616–20.
21. Hult L. The Munkfors investigation. Acta Orthop Scand Suppl 1954;16:1–76.
22. Hult L. Cervical, dorsal and lumbar spinal syndromes. Acta Orthop Scand Suppl 1954;17:1–102.
23. Hitselberger WE, Witten RM. Abnormal myelograms in asymptomatic patients. J Neurosurg 1968;28:204–6.
24. Wiesel SW, Tsourmas N, Feffer HL, et al. A study of computer-assisted tomography. I. The incidence of positive CAT scans in an asymptomatic group of patients. Spine 1984;9:549–51.
25. Boden SD, McCowin PR, Davis DO, et al. Abnormal magnetic-resonance scans of the cervical spine in asymptomatic subjects. A prospective investigation. J Bone Joint Surg Am 1990;72(8):1178–84.

26. Jarvik JJ, Hollingworth W, Heagerty P, et al. The Longitudinal Assessment of Imaging and Disability of the Back (LAID Back) study. Spine (Phila Pa 1976) 2001;26(10):1158–66.
27. Hellstrom M, Jacobsson B, Sward L, et al. Radiologic abnormalities of the thoraco-lumbar spine in athletes. Acta Radiol 1990;31:127–32.
28. Weinreb JC, Wolbarsht LB, Cohen JM, et al. Prevalence of lumbosacral intervertebral disk abnormalities on MR images in pregnant and asymptomatic nonpregnant women. Radiology 1989;170:125–8.
29. Jensen MC, Brant-Zawadzki MN, Obuchowski N, et al. Magnetic resonance imaging of the lumbar spine in people without back pain. N Engl J Med 1994; 331:69–73.
30. Boos N, Rieder R, Schade V, et al. 1995 Volvo Award in clinical sciences: the diagnostic accuracy of magnetic resonance imaging, work perception, and psychosocial factors in identifying symptomatic disc herniation. Spine 1995; 20:2613–25.
31. Stadnik TW, Lee RR, Coen HL, et al. Annular tears and disk herniation: prevalence and contrast enhancement on MR images in the absence of low back pain or sciatica. Radiology 1998;206(1):49–55.
32. Weishaupt D, Zanetti M, Hodler J, et al. MR Imaging of the lumbar spine: prevalence of intervertebral disc extrusion and sequestration, nerve root compression, end plate abnormalities, and osteoarthritis of the facet joint in asymptomatic volunteers. Radiology 1998;209(3):661–6.
33. Kjaer P, Leboeuf-Yde C, Sorensen JS, et al. An epidemiologic study of MRI and low back pain in 13-year-old children. Spine 2005;30:798–806.
34. Salminen JJ, Erkintalo MO, Pentti J, et al. Recurrent low back pain and early disc degeneration in the young. Spine 1999;24:1316–21.
35. Takatalo J, Karppinen J, Niinimaki J, et al. Prevalence of degenerative imaging findings in lumbar magnetic resonance imaging among young adults. Spine 2009;34:1716–21.
36. Schmid MR, Stucki G, Duewell S, et al. Changes in cross-sectional measurements of the spinal canal and intervertebral foramina as a function of body position: in vivo studies on an open-configuration MR system. AJR Am J Roentgenol 1999;172(4):1095–102.
37. Danielson B, Willen J. Axially loaded magnetic resonance image of the lumbar spine in asymptomatic individuals. Spine 2001;26(23):2601–6.
38. Danielson B, Willen J. The diagnostic effect from axial loading of the lumbar spine during computed tomography and magnetic resonance imaging in patients with degenerative disorder. Spine 2001;26(23):2607–14.
39. Lurie J, Tosteson A, Tosteson T, et al. Reliability of magnetic resonance imaging readings for lumbar disc herniation in the Spine Patient Outcomes Research Trial (SPORT). Spine 2008;33(9):991–8.
40. Carrino J, Lurie J, Tosteson A, et al. Lumbar spine: reliability of MR imaging findings. Radiology 2009;250(1):161–70.
41. Bron J, van Royen B, Wuisman P. The clinical significance of lumbosacral transitional anomalies. Acta Orthop Belg 2007;73(6):687–95.
42. Hall FM. Back pain and the radiologist. Radiology 1980;137(3):861–3.
43. Modic M, Ross J. Lumbar degenerative disk disease. Radiology 2007;245(1):43–61.
44. Modic M, Steinberg P, Ross J, et al. Degenerative disk disease: assessment of changes in vertebral body marrow with MR imaging. Radiology 1988; 166(1 Pt 1):193–9.

45. Ohtori S, Inoue G, Ito K, et al. Tumor necrosis factor-immunoreactive cells and PGP 9. 5-immunoreactive nerve fibers in vertebral endplates of patients with discogenic low back pain and Modic type 1 or type 2 changes on MRI. Spine 2006; 31(9):1026–31.
46. Toyone T, Takahashi K, Kitahara H, et al. Vertebral bone-marrow changes in degenerative lumbar disc disease: an MRI study of 74 patients with low back pain. J Bone Joint Surg Br 1994;76:757–64.
47. Albert HB, Manniche C. Modic changes following lumbar disc herniation. Eur Spine J 2007;16(7):977–82.
48. Braithwaite I, White J, Saifuddin A, et al. Vertebral end-plate (Modic) changes on lumbar spine MRI: correlation with pain reproduction at lumbar discography. Eur Spine J 1998;7:363–8.
49. Ito M, Incorvaia K, Yu S, et al. Predictive signs of discogenic lumbar pain on magnetic resonance imaging with discography correlation. Spine 1998;23:1252–8.
50. Weishaupt D, Zanetti M, Hodler J, et al. Painful lumbar disk derangement: relevance of endplate abnormalities at MR imaging. Radiology 2001;218:420–7.
51. Lei D, Rege A, Koti M, et al. Painful disc lesion: can modern biplanar magnetic resonance imaging replace discography. J Spinal Disord Tech 2008;21:430–5.
52. O'Neill C, Kurganshy M, Kaiser J, et al. Accuracy of MRI for diagnosis of discogenic pain. Pain Physician 2008;11:311–26.
53. Kang C, Kim Y, Lee S, et al. Can magnetic resonance imaging accurately predict concordant pain provocation during provocative disc injection? Skeletal Radiol 2009;38:877–85.
54. Buttermann GR, Heithoff KB, Ogilvie JW, et al. Vertebral body MRI related to lumbar fusion results. Eur Spine J 1997;6:115–20.
55. Lang P, Chafetz N, Genant HK, et al. Lumbar spinal fusion: assessment of functional stability with magnetic resonance imaging. Spine 1990;15:581–8.
56. Chataigner H, Onimus M, Polette A. [Surgery for degenerative lumbar disc disease: should the black disc be grafted?] Rev Chir Orthop Reparatrice Appar Mot 1998;84:583–9 [in French].
57. Esposito P, Pinheiro-Franco JL, Froelich S, et al. Predictive value of MRI vertebral end-plate signal changes (Modic) on outcome of surgically treated degenerative disc disease: results of a cohort study including 60 patients. Neurochirurgie 2006;52:315–22.
58. Aprill C, Bogduk N. High-Intensity Zone: a diagnostic sign of painful lumbar disc on magnetic resonance imaging. Br J Radiol 1992;65(773):361–9.
59. Carragee EJ, Paragioudakis S, Khurana. 2000 Volvo Award Winner in Clinical Studies: lumbar high intensity zone and discography in subjects without low back problems. Spine 2000;25(23):2987–92.
60. Ricketson R, Simmons J, Hauser W. The prolapsed intervertebral disc: the high intensity zone with discography correlation. Spine 1996;21(23):2758–62.
61. Smith B, Hurwitz E, Solsberg D, et al. Interobserver reliability of detecting lumbar intervertebral disc high-intensity zone on magnetic resonance imaging and association of high-intensity zone with pain and annular disruption. Spine 1998;23(19):2074–80.
62. Pfirrmann CW, Metzdorf A, Zanetti M, et al. Magnetic resonance classification of lumbar intervertebral disc degeneration. Spine 2001;26(17):1873–8.
63. Fardon DF, Milette PC. Nomenclature and classification of the lumbar disc pathology: recommendations of the combined task forces of the North American Spine Society, American Society of Spine Radiology, and American Society of Neuroradiology. Spine 2001;26:E93–113.

64. Ross JS, Brant-Zawadzki M, Moore KR, et al. Diagnostic imaging spine. Salt Lake City (UT): Amirys; 2007.

65. Thornbury JR, Fryback DC, Turski PA, et al. Disk-cased nerve compression in patients with acute low back pain: diagnosis with MR, CT myelography, and plan CT. Radiology 1993;186:731–8.

66. van Rijn JC, Klemetso N, Reitsma JB, et al. Observer variation in the evaluation of lumbar herniated discs and root compression: spiral CT compared with MRI. Br J Radiol 2006;79:372–7.

67. Saal JA, Saal JS, Herzog RJ. The natural history of lumbar intervertebral disc extrusions treated nonoperatively. Spine 1990;15:683–6.

68. Maigne J, Rime R, Delignet B. Computed tomographic follow-up study of forty-eight cases of nonoperatively treated lumbar intervertebral disc herniation. Spine 1992;17(9):1071–4.

69. Bush K, Cowan N, Katz D, et al. The natural history of sciatica associated with disc pathology: a prospective study with clinical and independent radiologic follow-up. Spine 1992;17:1208–12.

70. Ross JS. MR imaging of the postoperative lumbar spine. Magn Reson Imaging Clin N Am 1999;7:513–24.

71. Ross JS, Robertson JT, Frederickson RC, et al. Association between peridural scar and recurrent radicular pain after lumbar discectomy: magnetic resonance evaluation. ADCON-L European Study Group. Neurosurgery 1996;38(4):855–61.

72. Geisser M, Haig A, Tong H, et al. Spinal canal size and clinical symptoms among persons diagnosed with lumbar spinal stenosis. Clin J Pain 2007; 23(9):780–5.

73. White A, Panjabi M. Clinical biomechanics of the spine. 2nd edition. Philadelphia: Lippincott-Raven; 1990.

74. Schonstrom N, Hansson T. Pressure changes following constriction of the cauda equina. An experimental study in situ. Spine 1988;13(4):385–8.

75. Schonstrom N, Lindahl S, Willen J, et al. Dynamic changes in the dimensions of the lumbar spinal canal: an experimental study in vitro. J Orthop Res 1989;7(1): 115–21.

76. Hansson T, Suzuki N, Hebelka H, et al. The narrowing of the lumbar spinal canal during loaded MRI: the effects of the disc and ligamentum flavum. Eur Spine J 2009;18(5):679–86.

77. Porter R, Ward D. Cauda equina dysfunction. The significance of two-level pathology. Spine 1992;17(1):9–15.

78. Hamanishi C, Matukura N, Fujita M, et al. Cross-sectional area of the stenotic lumbar dural tube measured from the transverse views of magnetic resonance imaging. J Spinal Disord 1994;7(5):388–93.

79. Sowa G. Facet-mediated pain. Dis Mon 2005;51:18–33.

80. Ashton IK, Ashton BA, Gibson SJ, et al. Morphological basis for back pain: the demonstration of nerve fibers and neuropeptides in the lumbar facet joint capsule but not in ligamentum flavum. J Orthop Res 1992;10(1):72–9.

81. Cavanaugh JM, Ozaktay AC, Yamashita HT, et al. Lumbar facet pain: biomechanics, neuroanatomy, and neurophysiology. J Biomech 1996;29(9):1117–29.

82. Igarashi A, Kikuchi S, Konno S, et al. Inflammatory cytokines released from the facet joint tissue in degenerative lumbar spinal disorders. Spine 2004;29(19): 2091–5.

83. Czervionke L, Fenton D. Fat-saturated MR imaging in the detection of inflammatory facet arthropathy (facet synovitis) in the lumbar spine. Pain Med 2008;9(4): 400–6.

84. Schwarzer AC, Aprill CN, Derby R, et al. Clinical features of patients with pain stemming from the lumbar zygapophysial joints. Is the lumbar facet syndrome a clinical entity. Spine 1994;19(10):1132–7.
85. Schwarzer AC, Wang SC, O'Driscoll D, et al. The ability of computed tomography to identify a painful zygapophysial joint in patients with chronic low back pain. Spine 1995;20(8):907–12.
86. Dolan AL, Ryan PJ, Arden NK, et al. The value of SPECT scans in identifying back pain likely to benefit from facet joint injection. Br J Rheumatol 1996;35: 1269–73.
87. Doyle AJ, Merrilees M. Synovial cysts of the lumbar facet joints in a symptomatic population. Spine 2004;29(8):874–8.
88. Apostolaki E, Davies AM, Evans, et al. MR imaging of lumbar facet joint synovial cyst. Eur Radiol 2000;10:615–23.
89. Metellus P, Fuentes S, Adetchessi T, et al. Retrospective study of 77 patients harbouring lumbar synovial cysts: functional and neurological outcome. Acta Neurochir 2006;148:147–54.
90. Lyons M, Atkinson J, Wharen R, et al. Surgical evaluation and management of lumbar synovial cysts: the Mayo Clinic experience. J Neurosurg 2000;93:53–7.
91. Sabers SR, Ross SR, Grogg BE. Procedure-based nonsurgical management of lumbar zygapophysial joint cyst induced radicular pain. Arch Phys Med Rehabil 2005;86:1767–71.
92. Kauppila LI, Eustace S, Kiel D, et al. Degenerative displacement of lumbar vertebrae: a 25-year follow-up study in Framingham. Spine 1998;23:1868–73.
93. Chen CK, Yeh L, Resnick R, et al. Intraspinal posterior epidural cysts associated with Baastrup's disease: report of 10 patients. AJR Am J Roentgenol 2004;183: 191–4.
94. Okada K. [Studies on the cervical facet joints using arthrography of the cervical facet joint (author's transl)]. Nippon Seikeigeka Gakkai Zasshi 1981;55(6): 563–80 [in Japanese].
95. Hamlin LM, Delaplain CB. Bone SPECT in Baastrup's disease. Clin Nucl Med 1994;19(7):640–1.
96. Tini PG, Wieser C, Zinn WM. The transitional vertebra of the lumbosacral spine: its radiological classification, incidence, prevalence, and clinical significance. Rheumatol Rehabil 1977;16(3):180–5.
97. Elster AD. Bertolotti's syndrome revisited. Transitional vertebrae of the lumbar spine. Spine 1989;14(12):1373–7.
98. Jonsson B, Stromqvist B, Egund N. Anomalous lumbosacral articulations and low back pain: evaluation and treatment. Spine 1989;14:831–4.
99. Cohen SP. Sacroiliac joint pain: a comprehensive review of anatomy, diagnosis, and treatment. Anesth Analg 2005;101:1440–53.
100. Maigne JY, Boulahdour H, Chatellier G. Value of quantitative radionuclide bone scanning in the diagnosis of sacroiliac joint syndrome in 32 patients with low back pain. Eur Spine J 1998;7:328–31.
101. Slipman CW, Sterenfeld EB, Chou LH, et al. The value of radionuclide imaging the diagnosis of sacroiliac joint syndrome. Spine 1996;21:2251–4.
102. Elgafy H, Semaan HB, Ebraheim NA, et al. Computed tomography findings in patients with sacroiliac pain. Clin Orthop 2001;382:112–8.
103. Maigne JY, Lagauche D, Doursounian L. Instability of the coccyx in coccydynia. J Bone Joint Surg Br 2000;82:1038–41.
104. Hermann K, Bollow M. Magnetic resonance imaging of the axial skeleton in rheumatoid disease. Best Pract Res Clin Rheumatol 2004;18(6):881–907.

105. Bennett D, Ohashi K, El-Khoury E. Spondyloarthropathies: ankylosing spondylitis and psoriatic arthritis. Radiol Clin North Am 2004;42:121–34.
106. Heuft-Dorenbosch L, Landewe R, Weijers R, et al. Combining information obtained from MRI and conventional radiographs in order to detect sacroiliitis in patients with recent onset inflammatory back pain. Ann Rheum Dis 2006;65: 804–8.
107. Modic MT, Feiglin DH, Piraino DW. Vertebral osteomyelitis: assessment using MR. Radiology 1985;157:157–66.
108. Maiuri F, Iaconetta G, Gallicchio B, et al. Spondylodiscitis: clinical and magnetic resonance diagnosis. Spine 1997;22:1741–6.
109. Hadjipavlou AG, Cesani-Vazquez F, Villaneuva-Meyer J. The effectiveness of gallium citrate Ga 67 radionuclide imaging in vertebral osteomyelitis revisited. Am J Orthop 1998;27:179–83.
110. Pertuiset E, Beaudreuil J, Liote F. Spinal tuberculosis in adults: a study of 103 cases in a developed country, 1980-1994. Medicine (Baltimore) 1999;78: 309–20.
111. Ward C, Latimer B, Alander D, et al. Radiographic assessment of lumbar facet distance spacing and spondylolysis. Spine 2007;32(2):85–8.
112. Belfi L, Ortiz A, Katz D. Computed tomography evaluation of spondylolysis and spondylolisthesis in asymptomatic patients. Spine 2006;31(24):E907–10.
113. Yuh WT, Zachar CK, Barloon TJ, et al. Vertebral compression fractures: distinction between benign and malignant causes with MR imaging. Radiology 1989; 172:215–9.
114. Lourie H. Spontaneous osteoporotic fracture of the sacrum. An unrecognized syndrome of the elderly. JAMA 1982;248(6):715–7.
115. Taillandier J, Langue F, Alemanni M, et al. Mortality and functional outcomes of pelvic insufficiency fractures in older patients. Joint Bone Spine 2003;70:287–9.
116. Fujii M, Abe K, Hayashi K, et al. Honda signs and variants in patients suspected of having a sacral insufficiency fracture. Clin Nucl Med 2005;30(3):165–9.
117. Grangier C, Garcia J, Howarth N, et al. Role of MRI in the diagnosis of insufficiency fractures of the sacrum and acetabular roof. Skeletal Radiol 1997;26: 517–24.

Electrodiagnostics for Low Back Pain

Alexius E.G. Sandoval, MD

KEYWORDS

- Electrodiagnostics • Electromyography
- Nerve conduction study • Lumbosacral radiculopathy
- Lumbar spinal stenosis • Low back pain

Low back pain is one of the most common chief complaints that bring a person to seek medical attention, and it is also one of the most common reasons for electrodiagnostic referral. The main purpose of electrodiagnostics in the setting of low back pain is to physiologically assess the presence of a lumbosacral radiculopathy. Lumbosacral radiculopathies most frequently occur at L5 (48%), S1 (30%), L4 (17%), L3 (5%), S2 (4%), and L2 (3%).[1,2] Electrodiagnostics and neuroimaging complement each other, with the former assessing nerve function and the latter nerve structure.[3] Although radiculopathy is a common reason for electrodiagnostic referral, the value of electrodiagnostics in assessing radicular symptoms is highly variable.[3] Nevertheless, electrodiagnostics continues to be a useful tool for the assessment of low back pain particularly when it is performed and interpreted properly.

In this article, electrodiagnostics specifically refers to electromyography (EMG) and nerve conduction studies (NCS). Somatosensory evoked potentials (SEPs) are not discussed in this article. Electrodiagnostics is not performed in isolation, but is guided by the patient's history and is used as an extension of the clinical examination.[4] The following aspects of electrodiagnostics in the context of low back pain are discussed here: objectives, patient selection, general principles, findings in common low back pain conditions, sensitivity and specificity, preoperative benefits, and limitations of electrodiagnostics.

OBJECTIVES OF ELECTRODIAGNOSTICS FOR LOW BACK PAIN

The primary objectives of electrodiagnostics for low back pain are to confirm the presence of a lumbosacral radiculopathy and to exclude other peripheral nerve conditions that may mimic radiculopathy,[5] such as plexopathy, polyneuropathy, or entrapment neuropathy.[6] The secondary objectives of electrodiagnostics are to determine the following: the nerve root levels involved, the types of underlying nerve abnormalities (whether axonal loss or demyelination, with or without conduction block), the severity, and the chronicity of radiculopathy.[5] It is not the objective of electrodiagnostics to serve as an initial screening test for low back pain.

Department of Rehabilitation Medicine, University of Washington, 1959 NE Pacific Street Box 356490, Seattle, WA 98195, USA
E-mail address: alexius@uw.edu

Phys Med Rehabil Clin N Am 21 (2010) 767–776
doi:10.1016/j.pmr.2010.06.007
1047-9651/10/$ – see front matter © 2010 Elsevier Inc. All rights reserved.

PATIENT SELECTION

The ideal patient who would most benefit from electrodiagnostics referral is either one who is a potential surgical candidate whose physical examination findings of radiculopathy do not correlate with imaging studies,[3,4] or one who has a neuroimaging abnormality with an unclear functional significance.[4]

Patients with radicular weakness and pain that already correlate with the impingement level on neuroimaging may often be managed without electrodiagnostics.[3] Patients with radicular pain and/or sensory changes but without objective motor findings often do not have detectable electrophysiologic changes on either EMG or NCS.[3]

GENERAL PRINCIPLES OF ELECTRODIAGNOSTICS

The electrodiagnostic workup for lumbosacral radiculopathy generally includes performing an EMG of the limb and paraspinal muscles and NCS, including motor and sensory studies and late responses.

EMG

The most reliable of all available electrodiagnostic methods for detecting radiculopathy is the needle EMG.[4,7] Although neuroimaging studies are usually diagnostic in the more common radiculopathies caused by structural lesions, they may be unremarkable in radiculopathies caused by infection, infiltration, demyelination, or infarction.[6]

The diagnosis of radiculopathy through EMG is based on demonstrating evidence of ongoing denervation or chronic reinnervation in at least 2 muscles innervated by the same nerve root, but innervated by different peripheral nerves.[4] EMG abnormalities must be in a myotomal distribution.[4] Clinically weak muscles should be preferentially examined during EMG.[1] Ongoing denervation is manifested by the presence of fibrillations, positive sharp waves, and reduced recruitment. Polyphasic motor unit action potentials (MUAPs) may be seen during the period of early reinnervation. Chronic reinnervation is manifested by the presence of MUAPs with long durations and large amplitudes. Not all muscles innervated by the involved root need to be abnormal on EMG. However, it is important to demonstrate that the muscles innervated by unaffected adjacent nerve roots do not have ongoing denervation or chronic reinnervation.

The optimal number of muscles that should be examined when screening for a lumbar radiculopathy is at least 5 lower extremity muscles plus a paraspinal muscle (for a total of 6 muscles).[8] If the paraspinals cannot be reliably tested, then at least 8 nonparaspinal muscles must be examined.[8] The muscles examined should be representative of the key myotomes on the extremity. Several investigators have published tables of muscles that show a high yield for detecting radiculopathy at specific root levels.[5,6,8] If a particular root is already suspect based on clinical and radiographic data, then additional muscles innervated by that root but by different peripheral nerves should be examined. While the distribution of EMG abnormalities is expected to be in a myotomal pattern, the difficulty lies in the fact that most muscles are innervated by more than one root. Thus, it is sometimes impossible to determine electrophysiologically which of 2 contiguous roots is involved.[4] For example, the L2, L3, and L4 roots overlap extensively in their muscular innervations.[4] Furthermore, EMG cannot be used to localize the exact anatomic site of a pathologic condition because a single root may be compressed by a disk or osteophyte at more than one level.[4]

For abnormalities to be seen on EMG, the underlying pathologic condition must involve motor axon loss. A purely sensory radiculopathy would have a normal EMG. Likewise, a purely demyelinating radiculopathy without axonal loss (which is rare) would also have a normal EMG. On the other hand, a demyelinating radiculopathy with conduction block would present clinically with weakness and the EMG would demonstrate decreased recruitment.[6]

The paraspinal muscles should be examined during the radiculopathy workup. The presence of ongoing paraspinal denervation, in the form of fibrillations and positive sharp waves, is an important localizing finding because it indicates that the site of nerve root abnormality is proximal to the dorsal ramus takeoff,[4] and thus situates the lesion at the root or the anterior horn cell level.[6] Unfortunately, findings of paraspinal denervation do not help determine the precise segmental level of the lesion because there is much overlap in the innervation of these back muscles. Furthermore, the presence of paraspinal denervation must be interpreted carefully because this is also seen in patients with conditions other than radiculopathy, such as motor neuron diseases and after low back surgeries and injections. Abnormal spontaneous activity in the paraspinal muscles may occur up to 4 days after a lumbar puncture or myelography.[9,10] Paraspinal EMG may be abnormal more than 3 years after lumbosacral surgery.[11] Mild degrees of paraspinal denervation may be seen in normal asymptomatic individuals, likely reflecting root injury caused by normal age-related degeneration of the spine.[4,12]

To further add to the confusion, about half of radiculopathies have normal paraspinal EMGs.[6] One explanation is the possible fascicular sparing of fibers to the dorsal rami.[6] Moreover, the absence of paraspinal denervation cannot totally exclude a radiculopathy, as the paraspinal muscles may have been spared in incomplete root lesions or the paraspinals may have already reinnervated in cases of chronic radiculopathies.[4] There are also several technical issues that may hinder the detection of paraspinal denervation, such as difficulty of the patient to either relax or activate the back muscles during EMG, or simply sampling limitations.[4]

Electrodiagnostics is a time-sensitive test; therefore, the timing of electrodiagnostics affects the results and their interpretation because of the natural history of radiculopathy. Soon after an acute nerve root injury, no abnormalities may be detected by electrodiagnostics except perhaps for reduced recruitment and/or abnormal late responses (H-reflex and F-wave). It may take 7 to 10 days for fibrillation potentials to appear in the paraspinal muscles and 3 to 6 weeks to appear in the limb muscles, with abnormal findings progressing in a proximal to distal manner.[4] It may take 6 to 26 weeks for MUAPs to display variable configurations or polyphasia,[5] indicating the start of reinnervation. Chronic reinnervation occurs months after injury and is manifested by the presence of MUAPs with long duration and large amplitude (so-called neuropathic MUAPs.) Reinnervation, like denervation, progresses in a proximal to distal manner. Reinnervation changes are first seen in the paraspinal and proximal limb muscles by around 3 months postinjury, and then are later seen in the distal muscles by around 6 months postinjury.[5] Electrodiagnostics is better suited to diagnosing subacute radiculopathies (3 weeks to 3 months from onset) rather than acute or chronic radiculopathies.[5] Thus, electrodiagnostics should ideally be performed at least 3 weeks from the onset of symptoms (not earlier) to allow time for most limb muscles to develop signs of axon loss (fibrillation potentials).[5] Otherwise, electrodiagnostics performed too early may yield inconclusive results and may require subjecting the patient to another round of tests a few weeks later.

EMG by itself can already meet most of the secondary objectives of electrodiagnostics. EMG can determine the nerve roots involved by demonstrating the myotomal distribution of abnormalities. EMG abnormalities, such as abnormal spontaneous activity (fibrillations and positive sharp waves) and neuropathic MUAPs, substantiate the existence of an underlying axonal abnormality. The severity of the radiculopathy corresponds to the gradation of abnormal spontaneous activity present and the amount of MUAP dropout.[1,13] The chronicity of the radiculopathy can be roughly estimated based on the proximal-distal distribution of abnormal EMG findings along an affected myotome, and based on the size of fibrillations (which are larger in newer lesions and smaller in older ones).[14]

NCS

NCS are usually normal in radiculopathies. Nevertheless, it is necessary to perform NCS during a radiculopathy workup to exclude other conditions that may mimic radiculopathy, such as a plexopathy, polyneuropathy, or entrapment neuropathy. For example, when assessing for L5 radiculopathy it is important to rule out a peroneal (fibular) neuropathy at the fibular neck because both conditions may present with similar signs and symptoms (foot drop and numbness on the dorsum of the foot).[6] The following NCS are commonly performed during a lumbosacral radiculopathy workup: sural and superficial peroneal (fibular) sensory studies, peroneal (fibular) and tibial motor studies (often with F-waves), and tibial H-reflexes.[1]

Sensory studies
Sensory NCS are the most important part of the NCS during a radiculopathy workup. Sensory studies are almost always normal in compressive radiculopathies because the lesion usually lies proximal to the dorsal root ganglion (DRG), thus sparing the integrity of the distal axon.[4] A normal sensory nerve action potential (SNAP) in the same distribution as sensory signs and symptoms usually indicates a radiculopathy.[6] Assessment of the SNAP helps differentiate a radiculopathy (normal SNAP) from a plexopathy or peripheral neuropathy (abnormal or absent SNAP).[5] Although this is the general rule, there are exceptions wherein an absent SNAP does not necessarily rule out a radiculopathy. For example, an L5 radiculopathy may present with an absent superficial peroneal SNAP because in up to 40% of individuals the DRG is situated in a vulnerable intraspinal canal location.[5] At the L5-S1 level, 40% to 65% of DRGs may be proximal to the intervertebral foramen and subject to compression.[15,16] Sural SNAPs may be difficult to elicit in individuals older than 60 years, which happens to be the population in which lumbar spinal stenosis is most common.[1]

Motor studies
The motor NCS are also usually normal in lumbosacral radiculopathies because only a portion of nerve fascicles within a nerve root trunk is injured in a radiculopathy,[4,5] and because there is an overlap of root innervation.[7] Rarely, the compound muscle action potential (CMAP) amplitude may be reduced when motor axon loss is severe, that is, when up to 50% of motor axons within a nerve trunk are already lost.[4,5] CMAP amplitude is considered reduced when it is less than age-related norms, or if it is equal to or less than 50% of the corresponding CMAP amplitude on the contralateral limb. Axon loss may additionally result in slowed motor nerve conduction velocity and prolonged distal latency, especially if the largest, fastest fibers are affected, but it should never be so slow and so delayed as to stray into the demyelination range.[6,7] It is always important to obtain the CMAP from a muscle that is actually innervated by the affected nerve roots, which may not always be the routinely examined distal CMAPs.

Late responses
Late responses, specifically the H-reflex and the F-wave, are part of the electrodiagnostic workup for radiculopathy. These tests are important because they assess the proximal and intraspinal segments of peripheral nerves.[5] This is their main advantage over routine NCS, which only assess the more distal portions of peripheral nerves.

H-reflex The H-reflex is named after Paul Hoffman who first evoked the response in 1918. It is a monosynaptic spinal reflex composed of an afferent 1a sensory nerve and an efferent alpha motor nerve. It is the electrodiagnostic equivalent of the clinical Achilles reflex. In the lower extremity, the H-reflex is elicited by stimulating the tibial nerve at the popliteal fossa and recording at the gastroc-soleus muscle. In this test, the S1 nerve root sensory and motor pathways are assessed.[4] Typically the H-reflex with the shortest onset latency is recorded and compared against normal controls for height.[17] The H-reflex with the shortest onset latency is usually associated with the largest amplitude as well.[17] In the case of radiculopathies, side-to-side onset latency comparisons may be more important that absolute latency prolongations.[7] Other investigators choose to measure either the H-reflex amplitude or H-amplitude ratio (abnormal H-amplitude divided by the contralateral H-amplitude).[5,7,18]

An advantage over EMG is the H-reflex's ability to diagnose early, acute S1 radiculopathy because the H-reflex becomes abnormal within days of an injury.[4] On the other hand, the H-reflex has several limitations. It is not specific for radiculopathy and may become abnormal with a lesion anywhere along the course of the tibial and sciatic nerves,[4] that is, anywhere along the sensory afferent, spinal synapse, or motor efferent pathways of the reflex.[5] Abnormal H-reflexes are seen with any abnormality that depresses the Achilles reflex, including polyneuropathy, sciatic neuropathy, lumbosacral plexopathy, and S1 radiculopathy.[6] The combination of an abnormal H-reflex and normal distal NCS cannot help differentiate between a radiculopathy and a plexopathy, but can only suggest a proximal lesion.[6] Once the H-reflex is lost it may not return even with resolution of the clinical syndrome, and thus cannot differentiate an acute from a chronic S1 radiculopathy.[4] In obese individuals the H-reflex may be technically difficult to elicit.[5] The H-reflex in normal individuals decreases with age,[7,19] and may be entirely absent in elderly individuals older than 60 years.[5]

F-wave The F-wave is named after the foot because it was first recorded from the intrinsic foot muscles. The F-wave is produced by antidromic activation of motor neurons.[7] Only the motor pathways are assessed by the F-wave.[5] An abnormal F-wave localizes a lesion in the proximal portion of the motor nerve when the routine distal motor NCS are normal.[5] The F-wave can be elicited using any motor nerve in the upper or lower extremities. Commonly assessed lower extremity F-waves are from the peroneal (fibular) and tibial innervated muscles, such as the extensor digitorum brevis and abductor hallucis brevis, respectively. These muscles are supplied by the L5-S1 roots, which are often involved in radiculopathies.[6]

The F-wave does have several limitations. It has a low overall diagnostic yield of 10% to 20% for radiculopathies,[5] and there are several reasons for this. Any focal slowing within a short segment may be diluted by normal conduction along the rest of the motor nerve pathway, resulting in a still normal F-wave. Minimal F-wave latencies assess only the fastest conducting fibers; to see an increase in the minimal F-wave latency, a lesion needs to cause focal slowing that affects all fibers equally. Most radiculopathies involve only partial axonal loss and only rarely focal demyelination. F-waves are often normal in patients with suspected radiculopathy, and even when the F-waves are abnormal, such findings are inconsequential because the EMG will also by then be abnormal and will more definitively establish the diagnosis of radiculopathy.[5,20]

ELECTRODIAGNOSTICS OF COMMON LOW BACK PATHOLOGIES CAUSING RADICULOPATHY

There are 2 common low back pathologies that cause lumbosacral radiculopathy: lumbar disk herniation and lumbar spinal stenosis. Lumbar disk herniation with radiculopathy typically presents as low back pain with prominent radicular symptoms.[3] Electrodiagnostics would classically demonstrate evidence of radiculopathy involving one or more nerve roots in an asymmetric pattern.[5] L5 radiculopathy is the most common single-level radiculopathy seen with lumbar disk herniations, followed by S1 radiculopathy.[1,2,5]

Lumbar spinal stenosis clinically presents as low back pain with neurogenic claudication.[3] Neurogenic claudication is an intermittent pain or paresthesia in the legs elicited by walking and standing, often aggravated by extension, and relieved by lying down, sitting, or walking in a forward flexed position.[1,21,22] Electrodiagnostics would usually demonstrate a chronic, bilateral, multilevel lumbosacral radiculopathy in half of these cases, with most of the remainder showing unilateral or bilateral monoradiculopathy.[4,7]

Cauda equina syndrome is also caused by lumbar central stenosis, but is more clinically severe and emergent with unilateral or bilateral lower extremity weakness, saddle anesthesia, and urinary retention.[4] Electrodiagnostic findings include polyradiculopathy with involvement of bilateral nerve roots at multiple levels.[4] Assessment of cauda equina syndrome often requires EMG of the anal sphincter to demonstrate involvement of the S2, S3, and S4 roots.[4]

SENSITIVITY AND SPECIFICITY OF ELECTRODIAGNOSTICS

Estimating the sensitivity and specificity of electrodiagnostics for radiculopathy is problematic because there is no "gold standard" for diagnosing radiculopathy against which electrodiagnostics may be compared.[7] Thus, estimates vary from study to study depending on the standard with which electrodiagnostics was compared. Studies usually estimate the sensitivity and specificity of individual components of the electrodiagnostic workup (ie, EMG, NCS, or late responses), rather than the workup as a whole.

Several studies have determined that the sensitivity of EMG in diagnosing radiculopathy is comparable to that of computed tomography (CT), magnetic resonance imaging (MRI), and myelography, with sensitivities ranging from 50% to 85% depending on the patient population studied.[4,23–25] In 2 studies of patients who underwent both EMG and CT before lumbar surgery, EMG was 100% sensitive for detecting surgically confirmed disk herniations compared with CT, which was 94% to 97% sensitive.[3,24,26] EMG can sometimes demonstrate abnormalities compatible with radiculopathy even in the absence of definitive neuroimaging findings.[3] The correlation between neuroimaging and electrodiagnostic findings is uncertain because abnormal structural changes may be seen on imaging in up to 64% of individuals who are asymptomatic.[5,27–29] Through the implementation of specific (stricter) EMG criteria, one study showed that needle EMG had a lower false-positive rate than MRI in asymptomatic older adults evaluated for lumbar spinal stenosis.[30]

In terms of the specificity of EMG for lumbar radiculopathy, Tong and colleagues[31] determined that when only positive sharp waves or fibrillations were counted as abnormal, most of the diagnostic criteria (2 limb muscles plus associated lumbar paraspinal muscle abnormal, 2 limb muscles abnormal, or 1 limb muscle plus associated lumbar paraspinal muscle abnormal) had 100% specificity.

The H-reflex is reported to have a sensitivity of 50% and a specificity of 91% for S1 radiculopathy.[7,32] Absent or asymmetrically reduced H-reflex amplitude can be found in 80% to 89% of surgically or myelographically confirmed S1 radiculopathies.[5] Haig and colleagues[33] concluded that the specificities of H-reflex absence and H-reflex asymmetry in the diagnosis of lumbar spinal stenosis were more than 90% and 100%, respectively.

The F-wave seems less useful in the assessment of radiculopathy. It has reported sensitivities of about 50% to 80% in the evaluation of lumbosacral radiculopathies.[34,35] However, these findings are not consistently replicated.[36] Haig and colleagues,[33] in their evaluation of electrodiagnostic testing for lumbar spinal stenosis, determined that F-wave absence did not occur often enough to be helpful, and concluded that F-waves seem to have no important value except where a question of polyneuropathy is entertained.

PREOPERATIVE BENEFITS OF ELECTRODIAGNOSTICS

Aside from the utility of electrodiagnostics in establishing and characterizing the diagnosis of radiculopathy, it can also help determine which patients will likely benefit from back surgery. Neuroimaging has a high false-positive rate (detecting disk herniations and spinal stenosis) in asymptomatic older adults and thus is difficult to use alone when deciding to perform back surgery.[30] By complementing the neuroimaging findings with corroborative EMG findings, the clinician is better reassured that a lesion seen on neuroimaging is indeed the pain generator.[30] A prospective, controlled, masked study compared electrodiagnosis (incorporating a paraspinal EMG mapping technique) versus MRI in the evaluation of older subjects for lumbar spinal stenosis.[37] This study showed that imaging did not differentiate symptomatic from asymptomatic persons, whereas electrodiagnosis did. The investigators concluded that radiographic findings alone were insufficient to justify treatment for spinal stenosis.

One retrospective study demonstrated that patients who were EMG positive for radiculopathy had statistically significant improvement in functional outcome (by Oswestry Disability Index) but not pain after transforaminal epidural spinal injections compared with those who were EMG negative.[38] Another study evaluated patients with lumbosacral disk herniations and radicular syndromes preoperatively with electrodiagnostics including EMG, F-waves, and dermatomal somatosensory evoked responses.[39] At 1 year postoperatively, patients who had electrophysiological abnormalities had significantly better outcomes than those who had normal studies based on a visual analog pain scale. This study concluded that neurophysiological tests may be particularly useful in cases where there was a discrepancy between clinical and imaging findings, and may be helpful when deciding whether or not to proceed with surgery.

LIMITATIONS OF ELECTRODIAGNOSTICS

The value of electrodiagnostics in the assessment of lumbosacral radiculopathy lies in its proper interpretation, taking into account the patient's history and physical examination. Consideration must also be given to the inherent individual limitations of EMG, NCS, and late responses as discussed previously. Another limitation of electrodiagnostics is that it can be technically demanding and thus operator dependent. A prospective, single-blinded, observational pilot study looked at the interrater reliability of the needle examination in lumbosacral radiculopathy at a university hospital.[40] The study concluded that there was fair interrater reliability between faculty level examiners, but poor reliability among resident-level examiners when the needle examination was used to evaluate patients with lumbar radiculopathy.

SUMMARY

Electrodiagnostics is a useful tool in the assessment of lumbosacral radiculopathy in the setting of low back pain. It serves as an extension of the clinical history and physical examination. Patients who would likely benefit the most from electrodiagnostic evaluation are those potential surgical candidates who have poor correlation between their radicular symptoms and neuroimaging. Electrodiagnostics complements neuro-imaging because the former assesses nerve physiology whereas the latter assesses nerve structure. Electrodiagnostics may aid in the decision-making process when considering surgical management for sciatica, and may aid in patient selection. Electrodiagnostics proves most useful when the findings are appreciated in the context of the patient's history and physical examination, and with the procedure's inherent limitations in mind.

REFERENCES

1. Plastaras CT. Electrodiagnostic challenges in the evaluation of lumbar spinal stenosis. Phys Med Rehabil Clin N Am 2003;14(1):57–69.
2. Grana K, Kraft G. Lumbosacral radiculopathies, distribution of electromyographic findings [abstract]. Muscle Nerve 1992;15:1204.
3. Staiger TO, Gatewood M, Wipf JE, et al. Diagnostic testing for low back pain. In: Atlas SJ, Sokol HN, editors. UpToDate. Available at: http://www.uptodate.com. Accessed October 1, 2009.
4. Atlas SJ, Nardin RA. Evaluation and treatment of low back pain: an evidence-based approach to clinical care. Muscle Nerve 2003;27(3):265–84.
5. Tsao B. The electrodiagnosis of cervical and lumbosacral radiculopathy. Neurol Clin 2007;25(2):473–94.
6. Preston DC, Shapiro BE. Radiculopathy. In: Electromyography and neuromuscular disorders. 2nd edition. Philadelphia: Elsevier; 2005. p. 459–78.
7. Fisher MA. Electrophysiology of radiculopathies. Clin Neurophysiol 2002;113(3): 317–35.
8. Dillingham TR. Electrodiagnostic approach to patients with suspected radiculopathy. Phys Med Rehabil Clin N Am 2002;13(3):567–88.
9. Webber RJ, Weingarten SI. Electromyographic abnormalities following myelography. Arch Neurol 1979;36(9):588–9.
10. Danner R. Occurrence of transient positive sharp wave like activity in the paraspinal muscles following lumbar puncture. Electromyogr Clin Neurophysiol 1982; 22(1–2):149–54.
11. See DH, Kraft GH. Electromyography in paraspinal muscles following surgery for root compression. Arch Phys Med Rehabil 1975;56(2):80–3.
12. Nardin RA, Raynor EM, Rutkove SB. Fibrillations in lumbosacral paraspinal muscles of normal subjects. Muscle Nerve 1998;21(10):1347–9.
13. Kraft G. A physiologic approach to the evaluation of lumbosacral spinal stenosis. Phys Med Rehabil Clin N Am 1998;9(2):381–9.
14. Kraft G. Fibrillation potential amplitude and muscle atrophy following peripheral nerve injury. Muscle Nerve 1990;13:814–21.
15. Hamanishi C, Tanaka S. Dorsal root ganglia in the lumbosacral region observed from the axial view of MRI. Spine 1993;18(13):1753–6.
16. Kikuchi S, Sato K, Konno S, et al. Anatomic and radiographic study of the dorsal root ganglia. Spine 1994;19(1):6–11.
17. Preston DC, Shapiro BE. Late responses. In: Electromyography and neuromuscular disorders. 2nd edition. Philadelphia: Elsevier; 2005. p. 47–58.
18. Nishida T, Kompoliti A, Janssen I, et al. H reflex in S-1 radiculopathy: latency versus amplitude controversy revisited. Muscle Nerve 1996;19(7):915–7.
19. Weintraub JR, Madalin K, Wong K, et al. Achilles tendon reflex and the H response: their correlation in 400 limbs. Muscle Nerve 1988;11(9):972.

20. Aminoff MJ. Electrophysiological evaluation of root and spinal cord disease. Semin Neurol 2002;22(2):197–9.
21. Botwin KP, Gruber RD. Lumbar spinal stenosis: anatomy and pathogenesis. Phys Med Rehabil Clin N Am 2003;14(1):1–15.
22. Penning L, Wilmink JT. Posture dependent bilateral compression of L4 or L5 roots in facet hypertrophy. Spine 1987;12(5):488–500.
23. Wilbourn A, Aminoff M. AAEM minimonograph 32: the electrodiagnostic examination in patients with radiculopathies. Muscle Nerve 1998;21:1612–31.
24. Khatri BO, Baruah J, McQuillen MP. Correlation of electromyography with computed tomography in evaluation of lower back pain. Arch Neurol 1984; 41(6):594–7.
25. Nardin RA, Patel MR, Gudas TF, et al. Electromyography and magnetic resonance imaging in the evaluation of radiculopathy. Muscle Nerve 1999;22(2): 151–5.
26. Park ES, Park CI, Kim AY, et al. Relationship between electromyography and computed tomography in the evaluation of low back pain. Yonsei Med J 1993; 34(1):84–9.
27. Boden SA, Davis DO, Dina TS, et al. Abnormal magnetic-resonance scans of the lumbar spine in asymptomatic subjects. A prospective investigation. J Bone Joint Surg Am 1990;72(3):403–8.
28. Boden SA, McCowin PR, Davis DO, et al. Abnormal magnetic-resonance scans of the cervical spine in asymptomatic subjects. A prospective investigation. J Bone Joint Surg Am 1990;72(8):1178–84.
29. Jensen MC, Brant-Zawadski MN, Obuchowski N, et al. Magnetic resonance imaging of the lumbar spine in people without back pain. N Engl J Med 1994; 331(2):69–73.
30. Chiodo A, Jaig AJ, Yamakawa KSJ, et al. Needle EMG has a lower false positive rate than MRI in asymptomatic older adults being evaluated for lumbar spinal stenosis. Clin Neurophysiol 2007;118(4):751–6.
31. Tong HC, Haig AJ, Yamakawa KSJ, et al. Specificity of needle electromyography for lumbar radiculopathy and plexopathy in 55- to 79-year-old asymptomatic subjects. Am J Phys Med Rehabil 2006;85(11):908–12.
32. Marin R, Dillingham TR, Chang A, et al. Extensor digitorum brevis reflex in normals and patients with radiculopathies. Muscle Nerve 1995;18(1):52–9.
33. Haig AJ, Tong HC, Yamakawa KSJ, et al. The sensitivity and specificity of electrodiagnostic testing for the clinical syndrome of lumbar spinal stenosis. Spine 2005; 30(23):2667–76.
34. Eisen A, Schomer D, Melmed C. An electrophysiological method for examining lumbosacral root compression. Can J Neurol Sci 1977;4(2):117–23.
35. Fisher MA. An electrophysiological appraisal of relative segmental motoneuron pool excitability in flexor and extensor muscles. J Neurol Neurosurg Psychiatr 1978;41(7):624–9.
36. Dumitru D, Zwarts MJ. Radiculopathies. In: Dumitru D, Amato AA, Zwarts M, editors. Electrodiagnostic medicine. 2nd edition. Philadelphia: Hanley & Belfus, Inc; 2002. p. 713–76.
37. Haig AJ, Geisser MF, Tong HC, et al. Electromyographic and magnetic resonance imaging to predict lumbar stenosis, low-back pain, and no back symptoms. J Bone Joint Surg Am 2007;89(2):358–66.
38. Fish DE, Shirazi EP, Pham Q. The use of electromyography to predict functional outcome following transforaminal epidural spinal injections for lumbar radiculopathy. J Pain 2008;9(1):64–70.

39. Tullberg T, Svanborg E, Isacsson J, et al. A preoperative and postoperative study of the accuracy and value of electrodiagnosis in patients with lumbosacral disc herniation. Spine 1993;18(7):837–42.
40. Kendall R, Werner RA. Interrater reliability of the needle examination in lumbosacral radiculopathy. Muscle Nerve 2006;34(2):238–41.

The Role of Exercise and Alternative Treatments for Low Back Pain

Kevin A. Carneiro, DO[a],*, Joshua D. Rittenberg, MD[b]

KEYWORDS

- Low back pain • Core stabilization
- Mechanical diagnosis and therapy • Yoga
- Acupuncture • Spinal manipulation

Low back pain is the second most common reason patients seek medical attention. Although the cost of management of this condition has increased,[1] so has the prevalence.[2] The demand for treatment methods has skyrocketed, and so have the types of treatments currently available for patients. The decision to treat a patient's low back pain with an active or passive treatment program is often a decision made by the physician in consultation with the patient.

For medical practitioners who treat patients with low back pain on a regular basis, it is clear that many patients have been treated by complementary and alternative medical (CAM) therapies. In a survey, 54% of patients with low back or neck pain used CAM therapies to treat their low back pain.[3] Low back pain is the primary reason that patients visit chiropractors, massage therapists, and acupuncturists, and it accounts for approximately 40%, 20%, and 15% of all visits, respectively, to these practitioners.[4] When insurance covers CAM treatments, the prevalence of patients using CAM providers is quite high.[5] While the previously mentioned CAM treatments can be considered, for the most part, as passive treatments, many patients seek alternative treatments that are active. Yoga, Tai Chi, and meditation are commonly sought active treatments that have their origins in Eastern traditions. This article attempts at giving plausible explanations for the use of these of these treatments for low back pain while also outlining the current state of knowledge of their effectiveness.

Physical therapy is likely the most commonly prescribed treatment for low back pain and often combined with medications, interventional techniques, and other passive

[a] Department of Physical Medicine and Rehabilitation, University of North Carolina, CB#7200, Chapel Hill, NC 27599, USA
[b] Department of Physical Medicine and Rehabilitation, Kaiser Permanente Medical Group, 3701 Broadway Avenue, 5th Floor, Oakland, CA 94611, USA
* Corresponding author.
E-mail address: kevcar99@gmail.com

Phys Med Rehabil Clin N Am 21 (2010) 777–792
doi:10.1016/j.pmr.2010.06.006
1047-9651/10/$ – see front matter © 2010 Elsevier Inc. All rights reserved.

treatments for management of low back pain, including prescription and nonprescription medications, physical therapy, and interventional techniques. Although many physicians prescribe a physical therapist-directed exercise program for their patients, the choice of what form of therapy remains unclear with the current guidelines.[6] One of the aims of this article is to describe several forms of active therapy currently used and the current state of knowledge about their role in the treatment of low back pain.

COMPLIMENTARY AND ALTERNATIVE TREATMENTS
Massage

One of the most common nonpharmacologic treatments for low back pain is massage. It is often the first treatment that patients seek out and is considered a passive treatment.[7] Among those previously using CAM, massage was rated the most helpful for their current low back pain.[7] There is a large spectrum on which specific techniques can be considered massage. The range of massage techniques can be grouped in various ways. One such grouping categorizes types of massage by the goal of treatment (**Table 1**).[8] Common massage styles and techniques include Swedish massage; cross-fiber and frictional massage; myofascial techniques, including myofascial release; and neuromuscular techniques. The list of neuromuscular techniques included trigger point therapy, muscle energy, positional release, proprioceptive neuromuscular facilitation, lymphatic, and craniosacral techniques. These techniques are employed by massage therapists but also frequently used by other manual practitioners, including osteopaths, chiropractors and physical therapists. When evaluating effectiveness of massage, it has been shown that, when compared with a relatively inexperienced masseuse, a licensed massage therapist or an experienced trained massage therapist had better outcomes.[9–11] These studies, however, have not evaluated massage techniques employed by other practitioners of manual medicine.

Theories on the pathophysiology of massage are centered primarily on the effects at the central nervous system (CNS), the peripheral nervous system, or the local muscle and tissues. At the level of the CNS, the effects of massage might be explained by using Melzack and Wall[12] gate control theory. It could be postulated that massage stimulates the large diameter afferent nerve fibers, which along with the small diameter pain transmitting nerve fibers, synapse at the dorsal horn of the spinal cord. If the afferent input from the large fibers is greater than the afferent pain input from the small fibers, then inhibition of T cells occurs and the gate closes so that pain transmission does not occur.[12] It also has been postulated that massage might stimulate the parasympathetic nervous system while decreasing the response of the sympathetic nervous system.[8] Craniosacral techniques in particular are thought to assert their influence on the autonomic system.[13]

Peripheral influence of massage has been thought to occur at the tissue level or through vasculature. Massage can be used to treat trigger points in muscles, decrease muscle tension, or loosen fibrous adhesions in fascia. Massage is also thought to decrease vascular congestion in peripheral tissues and improve lymphatic drainage.[8]

The current best synthesis of evidence of the effectiveness of massage comes from a Cochrane systematic review in 2009[8] of 13 randomized trials. Researchers concluded that massage is beneficial for patients with subacute and chronic nonspecific low back pain for improving symptoms and function. The benefits of massage were increased when combined with exercises and education.[11] When different techniques were compared, it appeared that Thai and Swedish massage were equally effective,[14] but acupressure massage was more effective than Swedish massage.[15] The notable comparison studies involved a comparison with exercise[11] and

Table 1
Taxonomy of massage treatments

Principal Goals of Treatment	Relaxation Massage	Clinical Massage	Movement Re-Education	Energy Work
Intention	Relax muscles, move body fluids, promote wellness	Accomplish specific goals such as releasing muscle spasms	Induce sense of freedom, ease, and lightness in body	Hypothesized to free energy blockages
Commonly Used Styles	Swedish massage, spa massage, sports massage	Myofascial trigger point therapy, myofascial release, strain counterstrain	Proprioceptive neuromuscular facilitation, strain counterstrain, trager	Acupressure, Reiki, polarity, therapeutic, touch, tuina
Commonly Used Techniques	Gliding, kneading, friction, holding, percussion, vibration	Direct pressure, skin rolling, resistive stretching, stretching – manual, cross-fiber friction	Contract-relax, Passive stretching, Resistive stretching, Rocking	Direction of energy, smoothing, direct pressure, holding, rocking, traction

From Furlan AD, Imamura M, Dryden T, et al. Massage for low back pain: an updated systematic review within the framework of the Cochrane Back Review Group. Spine 2009;34(16):1669–84; with permission.

acupuncture.[9] Comparing massage with exercise for pain reduction, short-term results were favored massage, but long-term results were similar. Massage was found to be superior to acupuncture for short-term function as well as long-term pain reduction and improved function.[8]

There is no current recommendation on which types of patients would benefit most from massage compared with other treatments. It is also not clear which type of massage is most efficacious. Although acupressure massage seems to be better than Swedish massage, relaxation massage has yet to be well studied. Cherkin and colleagues[16] are undertaking a trial to determine which patient characteristics would prompt a clinician to consider massage as a treatment for low back pain. They are also comparing Swedish massage with relaxation massage and usual medical care. What is clear is that massage is most efficacious when it is combined with an active exercise treatment.

Manual Spine Treatment

The origins of spinal manipulation trace back to the Chinese in 2500 BC.[17] In the United States, the emergence of manual spine techniques occurred in late 19th century, when chiropractic medicine and osteopathic medicine were born.[17,18] Founders Andrew Taylor Still and David Palmer, of osteopathy and chiropractic medicine, respectively, felt that they could influence the body's mechanisms with manipulation of joints. Osteopathy is now practiced in 47 countries,[18] and chiropractors currently perform most spine manipulation techniques in the United States.[19] Practitioners of manual therapy use techniques that range from active techniques, like muscle energy, to passive techniques, like spinal manipulation. In fact, some of the techniques described in the massage section of this article, like craniosacral manipulation and myofascial release, are used frequently by osteopaths and chiropractors. When sorting through the literature, it becomes difficult to ascertain the effectiveness of the various manual techniques because of the diversity of study populations and of the practitioners.

The techniques that are the staple of manual practitioners of low back pain are spinal manipulation and mobilization. Spinal manipulation in the literature is also called adjustment and is often synonymous with a high-velocity, low-amplitude technique (HVLA). This technique involves applying a thrusting force to distract the zygapophyseal joints slightly beyond their passive range of motion.[20] Mobilization, however, involves the application of force to the joints within the physiologic range. This is usually achieved by applying cyclical force.[1,21] These techniques have been studied in patients with acute, subacute, and chronic low back pain. Furthermore, there is literature applying these techniques to patients with various etiologies of low back pain.

Most of the evidence for the effectiveness of spinal manipulation comes from chiropractic literature. Both practitioners of spinal manipulation and referring physicians should be aware of are the red and yellow flags that accompany this form of manual therapy. Commonly cited red flags, as described by the Agency for Healthcare Research and Quality (AHCPR)[22] guidelines, include fever, unrelenting night pain or pain at rest, pain with below-knee numbness or weakness, leg weakness, loss of bowel or bladder control, progressive neurologic deficit, direct trauma, unexplained weight loss, and a history of cancer. Severe spinal stenosis and vertebral artery disease generally are considered contraindications to HVLA-type manipulation. In a review by Bronfort and colleagues,[19] the authors stated that manipulation might not be the best choice for patients who cannot increase activity/workplace duties, are physically deconditioned, and have psychosocial barriers to recovery, or yellow flags. In a recent prospective multicenter study, however, psychological factors were not found to be relevant in predicting treatment outcome.[23]

Which patients will benefit most from spinal manipulation or mobilization? To date, most of the studies on manual treatments for low back pain use mixed populations or nonspecific low back pain patients. Furthermore, few studies standardize treatment protocols. Therefore, with the current available data, one can make very few conclusions on the ideal patient who would benefit most from manual treatments. What is known is that there are certain patients who would benefit least from certain manual treatments like mobilization. Patients with acute or chronic radicular pain seem to not fare as well as those without radiating leg pain.[24] Furthermore, patients with electromyographic evidence of a lumbosacral radiculopathy do not fare as well as patients with negative electromyographic lumbosacral radiculitis when manipulation is performed under general anesthesia.[25]

There have been several reviews of manual treatments for low back pain. The most recent review of chronic low back pain was performed by Bronfort and colleagues[19] in 2008. They examined the evidence for spinal manipulation and mobilization in chronic low back pain. They defined chronic as longer than 3 months. They recommended spinal manipulation or mobilization for nonspecific low back pain. They also noted that there is fair-to-moderate evidence that spinal mobilization with stabilizing exercises is just as effective as nonsteroidal anti-inflammatory medications in the short term and long term.[19] Further, a study by Aure and colleagues[26] showed greater improvement in pain intensity, functional disability, general health, and return to work in a group receiving manual therapy versus general exercise.

A Cochrane review noted that spinal manipulation was superior to sham manipulation for short-term gain.[27] Furthermore, a chiropractic consensus article stated that for acute low back pain there is fair evidence that spinal manipulation has better short-term efficacy than mobilization and limited evidence of better short-term efficacy than exercise, ergonomic modifications, or diathermy.[21]

The best evidence of the effectiveness of osteopathic manipulative treatment (OMT) comes from a review by Licciardone and colleagues.[28] Osteopathic techniques include spinal manipulation, muscle energy technique, counterstrain, myofascial release, and osteopathy in the cranial field. As previously mentioned, techniques were very heterogeneous. The authors concluded that OMT reduces low back pain and that its level of pain reduction is greater than what could be expected from placebo. Furthermore, the effect of OMT lasted at least 3 months. When examining the individual studies, it seems that most of them were conducted in patients with subacute to chronic low back pain.

How safe are spinal manipulation techniques? An observational study noted that the common adverse effects of spinal manipulation included local discomfort (53%), headache (12%), tiredness (11%), radiating pain (10%), and dizziness (5%). The sample included patients who had received manipulative therapy of the cervical, thoracic, or lumbar spine. In addition, most symptoms occurred within 4 hours of manipulation and disappeared the same day.[29] However, there have been cases of cerebrovascular accidents and spinal cord injury associated with cervical manipulation.

The determination on which patient will respond best to manual treatment of low back pain is still not entirely clear from the current literature. One approach could be to rule out potential nonresponders first. Those with red flags would be excluded first, and those with yellow flags would warrant further deliberation. Based on the literature, it would be reasonable to be cautious when referring patients with radicular symptoms to practitioners who just perform spinal manipulation. Now, to assist in determining which patients would benefit from manual treatments of the spine, a clinical prediction rule has been formulated and is currently being studied.[30] It has been postulated that patients with acute, nonradicular, low back pain would have a more favorable response to manual treatment. In addition, patients with low fear avoidance beliefs would be better responders. This prediction rule has been validated and generalized for thrust techniques. As more outcomes research is done using this prediction rule and others like it, one might get a better sense of how manual treatments fit into low back pain treatment.

Acupuncture

Acupuncture is a widely used complementary alternative treatment for low back pain. The National Institutes for Health issued a consensus statement in 1998 endorsing acupuncture as an adjunctive or alternative treatment for low back pain. In a National Health Interview Survey conducted in 2007 by the Centers for Disease Control and Prevention, 3 million American adults responded that they had used acupuncture in the prior year for back pain.[31] A prior survey in 2002 found that 8.2 million American adults had used it during their lifetime.[32]

Acupuncture's proposed mechanism of effect is based in both Eastern and Western theory. The use of acupuncture was documented as early as the first century BC, at which time it was already an established treatment in Chinese medicine.[33] According to traditional Eastern philosophy, the human body is comprised of channels called meridians. The energy that flows through those channels is known as Qi (pronounced ch-ee). Disease states and pain occur when the flow of Qi is unbalanced. By placing needles at specific points along the meridians, balance is restored, thus addressing the disease state and achieving pain reduction or other desired therapeutic effects.

Researchers have attempted to establish a neurobiological model for its mechanism of action to provide a sounder scientific basis and gain better acceptance in the mainstream Western medical community. In fact, many skeptics consider acupuncture to be nothing more than a placebo. Although high-quality clinical studies that definitively support its use remain scarce, the body of basic science research is abundant. Manual needling and electroacupuncture have been found to produce stimulation of A-delta afferent nerve fibers, resulting in release of endorphins and other neuropeptides in the brain and other sites.[33–35] In a widely cited study by Han, acupuncture induced analgesia induced in a donor rabbit was transferred to a recipient rabbit by cerebrospinal fluid transfusion.[36] Additionally, there are several studies that demonstrate reversal of acupuncture-induced analgesia when naloxone is administered.[36–39] More recently, functional magnetic resonance imaging (fMRI) and other advanced imaging modalities have helped to demonstrate the importance of the limbic system in the analgesic effects of acupuncture.[35] Functional imaging also has helped to differentiate nonspecific placebo effects from the proposed physiologic effects of acupuncture.[40]

There have been several systematic reviews and multiple randomized controlled trials (RCTs) evaluating efficacy. According to a 2005 Cochrane review, acupuncture is effective for chronic low back pain compared with sham or no treatment, based on 35 RCTs.[41] No advantage was found compared with other conventional or alternative treatments, and acupuncture was endorsed as useful when combined with other conventional treatments. Two systematic reviews were published in 2008 with similar conclusions, aside from disagreement on whether acupuncture is proven to be superior to sham. In each systematic review, high-quality RCTs were scarce.

The German Acupuncture Trials (GERAC) randomized 1162 patients to acupuncture, sham acupuncture, or conventional therapy, defined as treatment according to German guidelines. Both acupuncture and the sham treatment were superior to conventional therapy; however, there was no difference between acupuncture and the sham treatment.[42] In a more recently published study by Cherkin, acupuncture was compared with simulated acupuncture, described as needling along nonmeridian points, and with usual care. Six hundred thirty-eight subjects were followed for up to 1 year. No difference was found between acupuncture and simulated acupuncture, although both were better than usual care. In both studies, acupuncture appeared to be efficacious, whether or not traditional points were used. However, because usual or conventional care was poorly defined and highly variable, another reasonable conclusion from this study is that needling of any kind is better than nonspecific or no care and may simply represent a placebo effect. In the same group of subjects as the Cherkin study, Sherman was unable to find consistent patient characteristics to predict a positive response to acupuncture, although patients with higher baseline dysfunction did have a better short-term response.[43] Pre-existing notions of acupuncture had no relationship with outcome in this study, although a prior study did demonstrate that positive expectations predict a good response to acupuncture compared with negative expectations.[44]

In summary, the strength of evidence supports acupuncture as an adjunctive treatment in the management of low back pain. More studies need to be done to evaluate cost-effectiveness and to definitively establish that acupuncture's benefit is more than placebo.

Tai Chi, Meditation, Yoga

In recent years, there appears to have been a surge in the number of participants of the Eastern practices of yoga, tai chi and meditation. These practices are usually led by nonhealth care practitioners in studios and health clubs. Although there are many participants who attend regular classes for lifestyle changes, there are those who are seeking out an alternative way of managing their low back pain. The practices of tai chi, meditation, and yoga can be considered active treatments where daily practice is emphasized.

Tai chi is a form of low impact exercise that has roots in China and is an integral part of traditional Chinese medicine (TCM). It has gained in popularity, particularly in older patients due to known improvement in pain and decrease in falls. However, in patients with low back pain, it is not a commonly sought-out alternative treatment.[7] The practice of tai chi consists of slow sequential controlled movements combined with deep diaphragmatic breathing.[45] It also has been described as a martial art.[7] Despite its popularity, it has not been well studied overall or specifically in patients with low back pain.[46] There is currently a randomized controlled study underway studying the effects of a tai chi program versus a wait-list control in patients with chronic low back pain.[45]

The common forms of meditation in North America are mindfulness meditation and transcendental meditation (TM). As Morone and Greco[47] describe, mindfulness meditation involves bringing nonjudgmental moment-to-moment awareness of one's thoughts, sensations, or emotions as they arise. The various practice techniques include sitting, walking, and loving-kindness. TM generally uses a sitting practice. Although patients are more knowledgeable about meditation, they are just as equally unlikely to seek out meditation as a helpful treatment for low back pain.[7] The only study of meditation in low back pain is a preliminary controlled study using an 8-week mindfulness meditation program in patients with chronic low back pain.[48] They noted improved pain acceptance and physical function after 3 months compared with the wait-list controls.

The practice of yoga in India dates back as early as 3000 BC.[49] The practice of yoga consists of physical postures (asanas), meditation, relaxation, and breathing techniques. Hatha yoga and Raja yoga are the two most popular yoga forms in the Western world. The styles that make up Hatha yoga are Viniyoga, Iyengar yoga, Bikram yoga, and Ashtanga yoga. There are approximately 15 million Hatha yoga participants in the United States.[50] Furthermore, yoga use by adults in the United States increased to more than 6% in 2007.[31,50,51] Yoga offers another active approach of treating one's back pain. It is usually directed by nonhealth care practitioners, and classes usually last 60 to 90 minutes. Although popular, there have been few randomized controlled studies that have evaluated yoga in low back pain. Just like other already mentioned treatments, there are several forms of yoga, each with their own poses and nuances that make study protocols quite difficult. However, the studies that have been published have been very favorable. All of the current prospective randomized studies have studied the effects of yoga in patients with chronic low back pain.

Iyengar is currently the most common style of yoga in the United States.[52] The practice of Iyengar yoga focuses on strict adherence to the poses. Moreover, props, such as blocks and straps, are used to maintain these yoga positions. Williams and colleagues[53] recently studied the effectiveness and efficacy of Iyengar yoga in patients with nonspecific chronic lower back pain. Study subjects underwent 24 weeks of biweekly yoga classes. Of note, back bending poses were excluded. Outcome assessments, including Oswestry Disability Questionnaire, Visual Analog Scale, and Beck Depression inventory were assessed at 12, 24, and 48 weeks. Most participants, (82%) completed the study, and adherence to the yoga classes and home practice was 88% and 87% respectively. They found that yoga made significant improvements in functional disability, pain intensity, and depression in adults with low back pain.

Another important study of yoga in patients with nonspecific chronic low back pain was performed by Sherman and colleagues[54] in 2005. The study population was middle age, middle class, working women in the Pacific Northwest. They compared the effects of Viniyoga classes to conventional therapeutic exercises and a self-care book. They described Viniyoga as a therapeutically oriented style of yoga that emphasizes safety and is easy to learn. Study subjects underwent 12 weeks of 75-minute weekly classes and were encouraged to practice at home on a daily basis. The primary outcome measures, modified Roland Disability Scale and bothersomeness of pain scale, were assessed at 6, 12, and 26 weeks. They noted that yoga was more effective than a self-care book in reducing pain and improving functional status. They also noted a nonstatistically significant decrease in pain and improved functional status as compared with the exercise group.

The mechanism by which yoga improves low back pain has yet to be fully elucidated. As stated earlier, yoga consists of physical postures (asanas), meditation, relaxation, and breathing techniques. Maintaining prolonged positions likely improves endurance of lumbar stabilizers and improves posture. Furthermore, improving flexibility in hips could also contribute to improved lumbar biomechanics. However, breathing techniques and meditation could have a significant effect on reduced pain and improved function in low back patients. It has been shown that patients with chronic low back pain exhibit altered breathing patterns during movements in which trunk stability muscles are challenged and that the changes in breathing pattern during motor control tests are not related to pain severity.[55] It also has been shown that patients with sacroiliac joint pain have impaired kinematics of the diaphragm and pelvic floor with similar motor control tests.[56] Furthermore, through motor learning strategies, diaphragm kinematics improved and were accompanied with reductions in pain and disability scores. In a study with healthy subjects, phrenic nerve stimulation of the diaphragm increased intra-abdominal pressure and enhanced spinal stiffness, without much activity of abdominal and lumbar musculature.[57]

There is currently insufficient evidence to recommend tai chi and meditation as a treatment for low back pain. There appears to be evidence to support the practice of yoga in nonspecific chronic low back pain. However, caution should be taken to avoid poses that significantly exacerbate low back pain. Similar to other treatments, there are likely predictors of response that have yet to be elucidated. Although there is likely a core stabilizing effect of yoga, altered breathing patterns probably play a role in its efficacy.

Exercise

The use of exercise in low back pain treatment is central to the management of low back pain in the physiatric approach. Currently, there is no consensus on which form of exercise is most effective when treating this complex disorder. Furthermore, a Cochrane review stated that there was little evidence that exercise is an effective treatment for acute nonspecific low back pain. The authors also stated that it may be helpful for subacute and chronic low back pain to return to normal activities and work.[58] However, the review looked primarily at studies in patients with nonspecific back pain and with nonspecific therapeutic exercise approaches. Currently, the two most common approaches to practitioner-directed spine rehabilitation involve core stabilization and the mechanical diagnosis and treatment approach (McKenzie method).

As McGill[59] has pointed out, the spine must first be stable to minimize the risk of tissue overload and damage that result from either inappropriate muscle activation or spine joint position. He also states that the risk of spine tissue damage is a function of load magnitude, directional mode of the applied load, motion repetition, spine posture, hydration level and time of day, motor control and instantaneous stability, and age and gender.[59] Changes to muscle activation and motor control, spine position, and stability are the principle ways by which a spinal stabilization program works. The goals are to re-establish motor patterns so that the spine is able to maintain stability during anticipated activities, as well as during those that are sudden. As Hodges and Jull point out, this is achieved via CNS control, which receives afferent signals from tissue mechanoreceptors and then modulates spinal stability via muscle activation.[60] They also delineate the strategies for spinal control as feed-forward or feedback strategies. Feed-forward strategies involve responding to an anticipated perturbation by activating certain muscles. Feedback strategies involve activation of muscles in response to a sudden perturbation in the system.

Stabilizing muscles in the lumbar spine have been grouped into local and global muscles. Bergmark[61] describes global muscles as larger, superficial muscles that attach from the pelvis to the thorax. These include rectus abdominis, internal and external obliques, and the erector spinae. They move the spine with a large moment arm. Local muscles cross one or a few segments, attach directly to the vertebrae, and are responsible for control of intervertebral motion. Muscles include lumbar multifidus, transverse abdominis, intertransversarii, interspinales, and posterior fibers of psoas.[60]

It has been shown that the transverses abdominis and the lumbar multifidi contract before distal limb movement and that, in patients with low back pain, this anticipatory contraction is delayed.[62–67] It also has been shown that patients with low back pain exhibit lumbar multifidi atrophy.[68–72] Lumbar segmental stabilizing programs have been shown to lead to faster and more complete recovery of the multifidi. It also has been suggested that excessive activity in the superficial (global) muscles might be in response to poor intersegmental control.[73] One of the goals of a stabilization program is to activate the deep local muscles and decrease the activity of the global muscles. The pattern of re-educating the transversus abdominus and the lumbar multifidi has been described by Richardson and colleagues.[74]

The decision to use a stabilization program in a patient with low back pain can be made using the current evidence of chronicity of the low back pain and by using clinical prediction rules. In acute low back pain, segmental stabilizing exercises have been shown to be as effective in reducing pain and disability as general practitioner care after 4 weeks of treatment.[75] However, there is moderate evidence that segmental stabilizing exercises are more effective in reducing long-term recurrence of low back pain, at 1- and 3-year follow-up, than treatment by general practioner.[76] There are currently no randomized controlled trials for lumbar stabilization exercises in subacute low back pain. There is moderate evidence that a lumbar stabilization program can be effective in reducing pain and disability in patients with chronic low back pain from spondylolysis or spondylolisthesis for both short and long term.[76] A clinical prediction rule was devised by Hicks and colleagues.[77] Prognostic factors associated with clinical success with a stabilization exercise program included positive prone instability test, age less than 40 years, aberrant movements, straight leg raise greater than 91°, and presence of lumbar hypermobility. It further decreased lumbar multifidus activation, but no transversus abdominis activation was associated with factors predictive of clinical success with a stabilization exercise program.

The mechanical diagnosis and therapy method (MDT) is another well studied treatment for low back pain. It uses a diagnostic algorithm to categorize patients into one of three subgroups for a more specific treatment approach. The assessment process looks at mechanical and symptomatic responses to movement and positioning. The three subgroups (clinical patterns) include the postural syndrome, dysfunction syndrome, and derangement syndrome.[78] In brief, the postural syndrome is one in which the patient has a full and pain-free range of motion. However, he or she has symptoms with sustained end-range loading. The dysfunction syndrome is when there is a loss in the range of motion caused by shortened structures (ie, scarring, fibrosis, nerve root adherence). There is also a limited and symptomatic end range of motion. The derangement syndrome is when there is a mechanically impeded end range that is perceived by the patient to be an obstruction, which may or may not be painful. In this case, a direction of rigidity often is contrasted by a direction of instability.[78] The subtle difference in the previously mentioned syndromes prompts different treatment paradigms. Practitioners of the MDT method receive specialized training through the McKenzie Institute.

A key component of the MDT approach involves establishing a directional preference. A directional preference in the lumbar spine occurs when repeated movements in a single direction reduces or abolishes axial lumbar pain or causes peripheral or leg pain to retreat proximally (centralization).[78] Both centralization and directional preference assessments have been studied in patients with low back pain. Long and colleagues[79] noted that a subgroup that exhibited a directional preference had better outcomes (decreased pain, less medication use, decreased disability) when prescribed exercises that match each individual's directional preference than with the opposite or a nondirectional treatment. The ability to centralize symptoms also has been used to predict success in treatment and create a clinical prediction tool.[80] It has been shown that a subgroup of patients who centralized symptoms experienced greater improvements in disability than subjects who received a stabilization program. Centralization also has been shown to be of a predictor of outcome and to predict chronic pain and disability at 1 year.[81]

Although the effectiveness of exercise for low back pain treatment has been shown to be equivocal,[58] Delitto[82] points out that it is because of the failure of researchers to adequately account for the importance of subgrouping. Core stabilization and MDT treatments have been shown to be effective in certain populations with low back pain. However, further research is needed to improve on choosing the appropriate patients for these active treatments.

DISCUSSION AND SUMMARY

A systematic literature review showed that positive patient expectations were associated with better health outcomes.[83] It also has been shown that in patients with low back pain, general expectations for improvement but not specific expectations of chosen therapies were significant for changes in disability.[84] That same study showed that the association between general expectations and outcome was substantially higher when physicians directed care versus patient choice. The authors postulated that a component of positive expectations may be confidence that a health care provider will choose the appropriate intervention to heal the patient. Due to the increasing prevalence of low back pain, there are more treatments than ever for this condition. Using evidence-based outcomes to determine the benefits of these diverse treatments is the role of a spine specialist. Furthermore, knowledge about CAM treatments is important given patient expectations and satisfaction with these treatments.[85] The determination of whether a patient should pursue an active or passive treatment program also should be made. Medical practitioner-directed active treatments that have been shown to be effective for the treatment of low back pain include physical therapy-directed exercise programs (core stabilization and MDT). Based on the current literature, it appears that yoga is the most effective nonphysician-directed active treatment approach to nonspecific low back pain. Acupuncture is a medical practitioner-directed passive treatment that has been shown to be a good adjunct treatment. More randomized controlled studies are needed to support both CAM treatments and exercise in the treatment of low back pain.

REFERENCES

1. Martin BI, Turner JA, Mirza SK, et al. Trends in health care expenditures, utilization, and health status among US adults with spine problems, 1997–2006. Spine 2009;34(19):2077–84.
2. Freburger JK, Holmes GM, Agans RP, et al. The rising prevalence of chronic low back pain. Arch Intern Med 2009;169(3):251–8.
3. Wolsko PM, Eisenberg DM, Davis RB, et al. Patterns and perceptions of care for treatment of back and neck pain: results of a national survey. Spine 2003;28(3): 292–7 [discussion: 298].
4. Cherkin DC, Deyo RA, Sherman KJ, et al. Characteristics of visits to licensed acupuncturists, chiropractors, massage therapists, and naturopathic physicians. J Am Board Fam Pract 2002;15(6):463–72.
5. Lind BK, Lafferty WE, Tyree PT, et al. The role of alternative medical providers for the outpatient treatment of insured patients with back pain. Spine 2005;30(12): 1454–9.
6. Chou R, Huffman LH. Nonpharmacologic therapies for acute and chronic low back pain: a review of the evidence for an American Pain Society/American College of Physicians clinical practice guideline. Ann Intern Med 2007;147(7): 492–504.

7. Sherman KJ, Cherkin DC, Connelly MT, et al. Complementary and alternative medical therapies for chronic low back pain: what treatments are patients willing to try? BMC Complement Altern Med 2004;4:9.

8. Furlan AD, Imamura M, Dryden T, et al. Massage for low back pain: an updated systematic review within the framework of the Cochrane Back Review Group. Spine 2009;34(16):1669–84.

9. Cherkin DC, Eisenberg D, Sherman KJ, et al. Randomized trial comparing traditional Chinese medical acupuncture, therapeutic massage, and self-care education for chronic low back pain. Arch Intern Med 2001;161(8):1081–8.

10. Hernandez-Reif M, Field T, Krasnegor J, et al. Lower back pain is reduced and range of motion increased after massage therapy. Int J Neurosci 2001;106(3–4): 131–45.

11. Preyde M. Effectiveness of massage therapy for subacute low-back pain: a randomized controlled trial. CMAJ 2000;162(13):1815–20.

12. Melzack R, Wall PD. The challenge of pain. New York: Penguin Books; 1988.

13. Green C, Martin CW, Bassett K, et al. A systematic review of craniosacral therapy: biological plausibility, assessment reliability and clinical effectiveness. Complement Ther Med 1999;7(4):201–7.

14. Chatchawan U, Thinkhamrop B, Kharmwan S, et al. Effectiveness of traditional Thai massage versus Swedish massage among patients with back pain associated with myofascial trigger points. J Bodyw Mov Ther 2005;9(4):298–309.

15. Franke A, Gebauer S, Franke K, et al. [Acupuncture massage vs Swedish massage and individual exercise vs group exercise in low back pain sufferers–a randomized controlled clinical trial in a 2 × 2 factorial design]. Forsch Komplementarmed Klass Naturheilkd 2000;7(6):286–93 [in German].

16. Cherkin DC, Sherman KJ, Kahn J, et al. Effectiveness of focused structural massage and relaxation massage for chronic low back pain: protocol for a randomized controlled trial. Trials 2009;10:96.

17. Wiese G, Callender A. History of spinal manipulation. In: Haldeman S, Dagenais S, Budgell B, et al, editors. Principles and practice of chiropractic. 3rd edition. New York: McGraw-Hill; 2005. p. 5–22.

18. Gevitz N. The DOs. Baltimore (MD): JHU Press; 2004.

19. Bronfort G, Haas M, Evans R, et al. Evidence-informed management of chronic low back pain with spinal manipulation and mobilization. Spine J 2008;8(1): 213–25.

20. Haldeman S, Phillips R. Spinal manipulative therapy in the management of low back pain. In: Hadler N, Frymoyer J, Ducker T, et al, editors. The adult spine: principles and practice. New York: Raven Press; 1991. p. 1581–605.

21. Lawrence DJ, Meeker W, Branson R, et al. Chiropractic management of low back pain and low back-related leg complaints: a literature synthesis. J Manipulative Physiol Ther 2008;31(9):659–74.

22. Bigos S, Bowyer O, Braen G, et al. Acute low back problems in adults: clinical practice guideline 14. AHCPR Pub. No. 95-0642. Rockville (MD): US Department of Health and Human Service, Agency for Health Service, Agency for Health Care Policy and Research; 1994. AHCPR Publication # 95–0642.

23. Leboeuf-Yde C, Rosenbaum A, Axén I, et al. The Nordic Subpopulation Research Programme: prediction of treatment outcome in patients with low back pain treated by chiropractors—does the psychological profile matter? Chiropr Osteopat 2009;17:14.

24. Postacchini F, Facchini M, Palieri P. Efficacy of various forms of conservative treatment in low back pain. Neurol Orthop 1988;6:28–35.

25. Siehl D, Olson DR, Ross HE, et al. Manipulation of the lumbar spine with the patient under general anesthesia: evaluation by electromyography and clinical–neurologic examination of its use for lumbar nerve root compression syndrome. J Am Osteopath Assoc 1971;70(5):433–40.
26. Aure OF, Nilsen JH, Vasseljen O. Manual therapy and exercise therapy in patients with chronic low back pain: a randomized, controlled trial with 1-year follow-up. Spine 2003;28(6):525–31 [discussion: 531–2].
27. Assendelft WJ, Morton SC, Yu EI, et al. Spinal manipulative therapy for low back pain. Cochrane Database Syst Rev 2004;1:CD000447.
28. Licciardone JC, Stoll ST, Fulda KG, et al. Osteopathic manipulative treatment for chronic low back pain: a randomized controlled trial. Spine 2003;28(13): 1355–62.
29. Senstad O, Leboeuf-Yde C, Borchgrevink C. Frequency and characteristics of side effects of spinal manipulative therapy. Spine 1997;22(4):435–40 [discussion: 440–1].
30. Childs JD, Fritz JM, Flynn TW, et al. A clinical prediction rule to identify patients with low back pain most likely to benefit from spinal manipulation: a validation study. Ann Intern Med 2004;141(12):920–8.
31. Barnes PM, Bloom B, Nahin RL. Complementary and alternative medicine use among adults and children: United States, 2007. Natl Health Stat Report 2008; 12:1–23.
32. Barnes PM, Powell-Griner E, McFann K, et al. Complementary and alternative medicine use among adults: United States, 2002. Adv Data 2004;343:1–19.
33. Kaptchuk TJ. Acupuncture: theory, efficacy, and practice. Ann Intern Med 2002; 136(5):374–83.
34. Lewis K, Abdi S. Acupuncture for lower back pain: a review. Clin J Pain 2010; 26(1):60–9.
35. Wang S, Kain ZN, White P. Acupuncture analgesia: I. The scientific basis. Anesth Analg 2008;106(2):602–10.
36. Han JS, Terenius L. Neurochemical basis of acupuncture analgesia. Annu Rev Pharmacol Toxicol 1982;22:193–220.
37. Ernst M, Lee MH. Influence of naloxone on electro-acupuncture analgesia using an experimental dental pain test. Review of possible mechanisms of action. Acupunct Electrother Res 1987;12(1):5–22.
38. Tsunoda Y, Sakahira K, Nakano S, et al. Antagonism of acupuncture analgesia by naloxone in unconscious man. Bull Tokyo Med Dent Univ 1980;27(2):89–94.
39. Mayer DJ, Price DD, Rafii A. Antagonism of acupuncture analgesia in man by the narcotic antagonist naloxone. Brain Res 1977;121(2):368–72.
40. Dhond RP, Kettner N, Napadow V. Neuroimaging acupuncture effects in the human brain. J Altern Complement Med 2007;13(6):603–16.
41. Furlan AD, van Tulder M, Cherkin D, et al. Acupuncture and dry needling for low back pain: an updated systematic review within the framework of the cochrane collaboration. Spine 2005;30(8):944–63.
42. Haake M, Müller H, Schade-Brittinger C, et al. German Acupuncture Trials (GERAC) for chronic low back pain: randomized, multicenter, blinded, parallel-group trial with 3 groups. Arch Intern Med 2007;167(17):1892–8.
43. Sherman KJ, Cherkin DC, Ichikawa L, et al. Characteristics of patients with chronic back pain who benefit from acupuncture. BMC Musculoskelet Disord 2009;10:114.
44. Linde K, Witt CM, Streng A, et al. The impact of patient expectations on outcomes in four randomized controlled trials of acupuncture in patients with chronic pain. Pain 2007;128(3):264–71.

45. Hall AM, Maher CG, Latimer J, et al. A randomized controlled trial of tai chi for long-term low back pain (TAI CHI): study rationale, design, and methods. BMC Musculoskelet Disord 2009;10:55.
46. Manheimer E, Wieland S, Kimbrough E, et al. Evidence from the Cochrane Collaboration for Traditional Chinese Medicine Therapies. J Altern Complement Med 2009;15(9):1001–14.
47. Morone NE, Greco CM. Mind-body interventions for chronic pain in older adults: a structured review. Pain Med 2007;8(4):359–75.
48. Morone NE, Rollman BL, Moore CG, et al. A mind–body program for older adults with chronic low back pain: results of a pilot study. Pain Med 2009;10(8): 1395–407.
49. Sorosky S, Stilp S, Akuthota V. Yoga and pilates in the management of low back pain. Curr Rev Musculoskelet Med 2008;1(1):39–47.
50. Saper RB, Eisenberg DM, Davis RB, et al. Prevalence and patterns of adult yoga use in the United States: results of a national survey. Altern Ther Health Med 2004;10(2):44–9.
51. Birdee GS, Legedza AT, Saper RB, et al. Characteristics of yoga users: results of a national survey. J Gen Intern Med 2008;23(10):1653–8.
52. Jacobs BP, Mehling W, Avins AL, et al. Feasibility of conducting a clinical trial on Hatha yoga for chronic low back pain: methodological lessons. Altern Ther Health Med 2004;10(2):80–3.
53. Williams KA, Petronis J, Smith D, et al. Effect of Iyengar yoga therapy for chronic low back pain. Pain 2005;115(1–2):107–17.
54. Sherman KJ, Cherkin DC, Erro J, et al. Comparing yoga, exercise, and a self-care book for chronic low back pain: a randomized, controlled trial. Ann Intern Med 2005;143(12):849–56.
55. Roussel N, Nijs J, Truijen S, et al. Altered breathing patterns during lumbopelvic motor control tests in chronic low back pain: a case-control study. Eur Spine J 2009;18(7):1066–73.
56. O'Sullivan PB, Beales DJ. Changes in pelvic floor and diaphragm kinematics and respiratory patterns in subjects with sacroiliac joint pain following a motor learning intervention: a case series. Man Ther 2007;12(3):209–18.
57. Hodges PW, Eriksson AE, Shirley D, et al. Intra-abdominal pressure increases stiffness of the lumbar spine. J Biomech 2005;38(9):1873–80.
58. van Tulder MW, Koes B, Malmivaara A. Outcome of non-invasive treatment modalities on back pain: an evidence-based review. Eur Spine J 2006;15(Suppl 1):S64–81.
59. McGill S. Lumbar spine stability: mechanism of injury and restabilization. In: Liebenson C, editor. Rehabilitation of the spine: a practitioner's manual. 2nd edition. Baltimore (MD): Lippincott Williams & Wilkins; 2006. p. 93–111.
60. Hodges P, Jull GA. Spinal segmental stabilization training. In: Liebenson C, editor. Rehabilitation of the spine: a practitioner's manual. 2nd edition. Baltimore (MD): Lippincott Williams & Wilkins; 2006. p. 585–611.
61. Bergmark A. Stability of the lumbar spine. A study in mechanical engineering. Acta Orthop Scand Suppl 1989;230:1–54.
62. Hodges PW, Richardson CA. Inefficient muscular stabilization of the lumbar spine associated with low back pain. A motor control evaluation of transversus abdominis. Spine 1996;21(22):2640–50.
63. Hodges PW, Richardson CA. Contraction of the abdominal muscles associated with movement of the lower limb. Phys Ther 1997;77(2):132–42 [discussion: 142–4].

64. Hungerford B, Gilleard W, Hodges P. Evidence of altered lumbopelvic muscle recruitment in the presence of sacroiliac joint pain. Spine 2003;28(14): 1593–600.
65. MacDonald D, Moseley GL, Hodges PW. Why do some patients keep hurting their back? Evidence of ongoing back muscle dysfunction during remission from recurrent back pain. Pain 2009;142(3):183–8.
66. Hodges PW. Changes in motor planning of feedforward postural responses of the trunk muscles in low back pain. Exp Brain Res 2001;141(2):261–6.
67. Hodges PW, Moseley GL, Gabrielsson A, et al. Experimental muscle pain changes feedforward postural responses of the trunk muscles. Exp Brain Res 2003;151(2):262–71.
68. Yoshihara K, Shirai Y, Nakayama Y, et al. Histochemical changes in the multifidus muscle in patients with lumbar intervertebral disc herniation. Spine 2001;26(6): 622–6.
69. Zhao WP, Kawaguchi Y, Matsui H, et al. Histochemistry and morphology of the multifidus muscle in lumbar disc herniation: comparative study between diseased and normal sides. Spine 2000;25(17):2191–9.
70. Yoshihara K, Nakayama Y, Fujii N, et al. Atrophy of the multifidus muscle in patients with lumbar disk herniation: histochemical and electromyographic study. Orthopedics 2003;26(5):493–5.
71. Kang CH, Shin MJ, Kim SM, et al. MRI of paraspinal muscles in lumbar degenerative kyphosis patients and control patients with chronic low back pain. Clin Radiol 2007;62(5):479–86.
72. Mengiardi B, Schmid MR, Boos N, et al. Fat content of lumbar paraspinal muscles in patients with chronic low back pain and in asymptomatic volunteers: quantification with MR spectroscopy. Radiology 2006;240(3):786–92.
73. Cholewicki J, McGill SM. Mechanical stability of the in vivo lumbar spine: implications for injury and chronic low back pain. Clin Biomech (Bristol, Avon) 1996; 11(1):1–15.
74. Richardson CA, Jull GA. Muscle control–pain control. What exercises would you prescribe? Man Ther 1995;1(1):2–10.
75. Hides JA, Richardson CA, Jull GA. Multifidus muscle recovery is not automatic after resolution of acute, first-episode low back pain. Spine 1996;21(23): 2763–9.
76. Rackwitz B, de Bie R, Limm H, et al. Segmental stabilizing exercises and low back pain. What is the evidence? A systematic review of randomized controlled trials. Clin Rehabil 2006;20(7):553–67.
77. Hicks GE, Fritz JM, Delitto A, et al. Preliminary development of a clinical prediction rule for determining which patients with low back pain will respond to a stabilization exercise program. Arch Phys Med Rehabil 2005;86(9):1753–62.
78. McKenzie R. McKenzie spinal rehabilitation methods. In: Liebenson C, editor. Rehabilitation of the spine: a practitioner's manual. 2nd edition. Baltimore (MD): Lippincott Williams & Wilkins; 2006. p. 330–51.
79. Long A, Donelson R, Fung T. Does it matter which exercise? A randomized control trial of exercise for low back pain. Spine 2004;29(23):2593–602.
80. Browder DA, Childs JD, Cleland JA, et al. Effectiveness of an extension-oriented treatment approach in a subgroup of subjects with low back pain: a randomized clinical trial. Phys Ther 2007;87(12):1608–18 [discussion: 1577–9].
81. Werneke M, Hart DL. Centralization phenomenon as a prognostic factor for chronic low back pain and disability. Spine 2001;26(7):758–64 [discussion: 765].

82. Delitto A. Research in low back pain: time to stop seeking the elusive "magic bullet". Phys Ther 2005;85(3):206–8.
83. Mondloch MV, Cole DC, Frank JW. Does how you do depend on how you think you'll do? A systematic review of the evidence for a relation between patients' recovery expectations and health outcomes. CMAJ 2001;165(2):174–9.
84. Myers SS, Phillips RS, Davis RB, et al. Patient expectations as predictors of outcome in patients with acute low back pain. J Gen Intern Med 2008;23(2): 148–53.
85. Eisenberg DM, Post DE, Davis RB, et al. Addition of choice of complementary therapies to usual care for acute low back pain: a randomized controlled trial. Spine 2007;32(2):151–8.

Pharmacologic Treatment for Low Back Pain: One Component of Pain Care

Timothy J. Lee, MD

KEYWORDS

- Low back pain • Acetaminophen
- Nonsteroidal anti-inflammatory drugs • Muscle relaxants
- Antidepressants • Antiepileptics • Opioids

Low back pain (LBP) is a highly prevalent health problem. Most adults experience LBP, pain in the lumbar region with or without leg pain (sciatica), at some time in their lives. Classification of LBP is generally based on duration of pain (acute or chronic) and location of pain (nonspecific or secondary). LBP is defined as acute when it lasts less than 1 month, subacute when it lasts 1 to 3 months, and chronic when it lasts longer than 3 months. About 90% of patients presenting to primary care with LBP have nonspecific LBP, which is LBP that cannot be attributed to a specific cause, such as infection, tumor, or fracture.[1,2] Up to 90% of patients with acute nonspecific LBP have improvement of symptoms within 3 months; however, recurrence rates are high, and a number of patients may develop some degree of chronic LBP. This article addresses the pharmacologic treatment of nonspecific LBP and not the treatment of secondary LBP. This article also discusses the most commonly prescribed oral medications for LBP but not the less commonly prescribed pharmacologic treatments, such as transdermal and intrathecal therapy.

The evidence on pharmacologic treatment of LBP comes from clinical trials that have multiple limitations, including short-term trials only, selected trial populations that may not reflect clinical practices, trials using single treatments, and trials measuring pain reduction without evidence of improved functioning. Also, acute LBP is frequently self-limiting, and thus, nearly any treatment administered in the acute phase may seem to be effective. The most commonly prescribed oral medications for LBP include acetaminophen and nonsteroidal anti-inflammatory drugs (NSAIDs), muscle relaxants, antidepressants, antiepileptics, and opioids. Current evidence

VA Puget Sound, 1660 South Columbian Way, Seattle, WA 98108, USA
E-mail address: timothylee@live.com

Phys Med Rehabil Clin N Am 21 (2010) 793–800
doi:10.1016/j.pmr.2010.06.013
1047-9651/10/$ – see front matter © 2010 Published by Elsevier Inc.

pmr.theclinics.com

shows that these medications all have equal efficacy in reducing pain, provide only partial pain reduction at best,[3] and are each associated with different adverse side effects. Evidence supports the efficacy of short-term analgesic therapy for LBP; however, the safety and efficacy of long-term analgesic therapy is not clear. Therefore, current evidence-based guidelines recommend limiting the duration of use for most medications in the treatment of LBP.[4]

PHARMACOLOGIC TREATMENT OF LBP
Acetaminophen and NSAIDS

Because studies show all analgesics to have equal efficacy in pain reduction, it is recommended that the agents with least risk of harm be used first. Therefore, acetaminophen or NSAIDs are recommended as first-line agents for LBP. A systematic review found no clear difference between acetaminophen and NSAIDs for pain relief in patients with LBP. Acetaminophen, unlike NSAIDs, is not known to be associated with myocardial infarction or gastrointestinal bleeding and may be preferable for patients at risk of these conditions. All NSAIDs appear to be equivalent in efficacy for acute LBP, so the choice of agent may be based on patient preference and cost.

Recommendation
Evidence supports a short course of acetaminophen or NSAIDs for acute or chronic LBP. Long-term use should be avoided.[4]

Muscle Relaxants

Muscle relaxants are divided into 2 categories:

1. Antispastic agents, baclofen, tizanidine, dantrolene, and diazepam, are not recommended for nonspecific LBP. These agents are indicated for spasticity related to central nervous system injury, such as multiple sclerosis.
2. Antispasmodic agents, cyclobenzaprine, methocarbamol, metaxalone, and carisoprodol, may be used short-term (2 weeks) for acute LBP. Long-term use is not recommended.

Evidence from clinical trials regarding muscle relaxants is limited because of short-term trials, poor methodological design, and small numbers of patients. There is no clear evidence that one muscle relaxant is superior to another, so the choice of agent should be based on risk of side-effects, drug interactions, and cost. Adverse effects, particularly dizziness and drowsiness, are consistently reported with all muscle relaxants. Cyclobenzaprine (Flexeril) has been the most heavily studied muscle relaxant with proven short-term effectiveness. Cyclobenzaprine 5 mg is as effective as 10 mg, with fewer adverse effects.[4] The sedative properties of cyclobenzaprine may benefit patients with sleep disturbance. Methocarbamol (Robaxin) is less sedating but has also been less studied. Metaxalone (Skelaxin) has not been studied since the 1970s. One fair-quality study showed no difference between metaxalone and placebo. Carisoprodol (Soma) is metabolized to meprobamate (sedative controlled substance) with addiction potential. Benzodiazepines also have addiction potential and are not recommended for the treatment of muscle spasm. The only trial evaluating a benzodiazepine available in the United States found no difference between diazepam and placebo for muscle spasm.

Recommendation
Evidence supports a short course (2 weeks) of antispasmodic agents, such as cyclobenzaprine or methocarbamol, for acute LBP. Long-term use is not recommended.

All muscle relaxants should be used with caution in older patients. Carisoprodol and diazepam should not be used for LBP, because of their addiction potential and lack of efficacy over other muscle relaxants.

Antidepressants

Tricyclic medications (amitriptyline, nortriptyline, desipramine) have been shown in randomized trials to provide a small pain reduction in patients with chronic LBP without clinical depression.[4] These trials did not show functional improvements and side effects occurred in more than 20% of patients. The analgesic effect from tricyclics is believed to be because of inhibition of norepinephrine reuptake rather than serotoninergic activity. Selective serotonin-reuptake inhibitors (SSRIs) have not been shown to be more effective than placebo in patients with chronic LBP. Antidepressants with serotonin-norepinephrine reuptake inhibitor (SNRI) effects, such as bupropion (Wellbutrin), venlafaxine (Effexor), and duloxetine (Cymbalta), have been shown to provide analgesia for certain conditions; however, there are few studies on their use for LBP.

Recommendation

Evidence supports the use of tricyclic medications for chronic low LBP in patients who have not responded to first-line agents. These medications should be started at a low dosage; for example, amitriptyline 10 to 25 mg at bedtime, increased by 10 to 25 mg per week, up to 75 to 150 mg at bedtime or as tolerated. Limited evidence exists on the efficacy of SNRIs for LBP. Evidence does not support the use of SSRIs for LBP.

Depression is common in patients with LBP; as many as 50% of individuals with chronic LBP may have comorbid depression. Clinicians need to address and treat depression appropriately. Studies have shown that treating pain and depression together results in better outcomes than treating either one alone.[5,6] The patient should be informed of the impact that pain can have on mood and vice versa, and thus, the importance of treating both together. This holds true for other comorbid mental health disorders, such as posttraumatic stress disorder and anxiety.

Antiepileptic Medications

The efficacy of antiepileptic medications for subacute or chronic LBP is based on a few small studies. The precise mechanism of their analgesic effect remains unclear. These agents are thought to limit neuronal excitation, and their sites of action include receptors and sodium and calcium ion channels. Gabapentin (Neurontin) for chronic sciatic pain was evaluated in 2 small short-term trials. There was some evidence of effect for gabapentin titrated to 3600 mg/d; however, the trial lacked a double-blind design. Adverse events reported with gabapentin include drowsiness, loss of energy, and dizziness. Gabapentin for spinal stenosis was evaluated in one small trial. The addition of gabapentin titrated to 2400 mg/d to a regimen of supervised exercise therapy, lumbar supports, and NSAIDs in patients with spinal stenosis and neurogenic claudication resulted in some pain improvement.[4]

Recommendation

Gabapentin may be tried for chronic LBP in selected patients (eg, those with spinal stenosis and neurogenic claudication or evidence of nerve root pain) who have not responded to first-line agents. Starting at a low dosage, it should be increased as tolerated; for example, 100 to 300 mg at bedtime, increased by 100 mg every 3 days, up to 1800 to 3600 mg/d taken in divided doses 3 times daily. Other antiepileptic drugs, such as carbamazepine (Tegretol), pregabalin (Lyrica), and lamotrigine (Lamictal), are not recommended for LBP given the limited evidence.

Opioids

Two systematic reviews and meta-analyses of opioid use for chronic LBP identified few high quality or long-term trials. There are no published trials on the safety and efficacy of long-term opioid therapy for LBP. One systematic review of opioid use for LBP showed a lack of evidence of long-term therapy because the trials were short-term with mean study duration of 8 weeks only.[7] In addition, this review showed that substance use disorders were common in patients taking opioids for chronic LBP. One meta-analysis found that opioid medications compared with placebo or non-opioid analgesics did not significantly reduce pain in patients with chronic LBP. Tramadol, an SNRI combined with a weak opioid, has been shown to be minimally more effective than placebo for improving pain and function. Clinical trials on opioid therapy for chronic LBP often do not show functional improvement and rarely quantify the risk of adverse events, such as abuse or addiction. A recent study observed an increased risk of opioid overdoses in patients receiving higher prescribed doses of opioids for pain.[8] This study showed more overdoses among patients diagnosed as suffering from depression or substance abuse or concurrently receiving benzodiazepines. Patients with mental and substance use disorders are at higher risk for developing opioid misuse[9] and yet some studies have found that opioid prescribing is more strongly associated with the presence of mental and substance use disorders than with pain severity or clinical findings.[10]

In the 1980s, opioids were largely limited to cancer and acute pain. In 1986, Dr Russell Portenoy, a cancer pain expert, published a review of 38 patients on chronic opioids and concluded that chronic opioid therapy can be safe for patients with noncancer pain. During the 1990s, Portenoy and others encouraged the use of opioids for chronic pain, equating effective pain treatment with opioid therapy and using the terms undertreatment, pseudoaddiction, and "opiophobia." Clinicians were informed that opioid therapy had no ceiling and that it was appropriate to escalate "to effect," regardless of the amounts prescribed. In 1995 Purdue Pharma introduced OxyContin, claiming it had low abuse potential. In the last decade opioid prescribing for chronic pain has increased dramatically and during this time there has been a dramatic rise in opioid-related abuse, overdoses, and deaths.[11] A public outcry in 2001 over OxyContin-related deaths, lead to investigations and in 2007 top executives of Purdue Pharma pleaded guilty to claiming OxyContin had low abuse potential when they had no evidence to support this. Portenoy has admitted to misgivings about how he and others used the research.

Opioids are now the most commonly prescribed medication in the United States,[8] there has been no evidence that opioids for LBP improve functional disability or self-assessed health status,[12] and prescription opioid-related abuse, overdoses, and deaths have become a public health crisis.

Recommendation

Evidence supports the use of short-term opioid therapy for severe acute LBP. There are no quality studies looking at the safety and efficacy of long-term opioid therapy for LBP. Therefore, long-term opioid therapy must be used with caution and close oversight and to help rehabilitation toward clear and established treatment goals. The use of an opioid treatment agreement informing the patient of safe and appropriate use of opioid therapy can be helpful. Routine urine drug testing is recommended for safety reasons. Regular reassessment is recommended to monitor treatment adherence and progress toward treatment goals. Continuing opioid therapy needs to be contingent on active treatment participation and clear improvements in function and quality of life. Opioid therapy needs to be discontinued when there is evidence of treatment failure or repeated unsafe behavior, such as active substance use disorder.

When opioids are taken on a daily basis for pain, it is recommended that they be taken on a time-contingent rather than pain-contingent or as-needed basis and that long-acting opioids be used to provide more sustained analgesia. Daily use of short-acting opioids or "breakthrough" dosing of opioids is generally not recommended for chronic pain, because of the short duration of benefit and the development of roller-coaster serum levels. Recent evidence shows that larger prescribed opioid doses for chronic pain can result in a greater risk of overdosing on opioids, and therefore, prescribing within a low to moderate daily dosage range may be important. Recently published guidelines on the use of opioid therapy for chronic pain suggest limiting daily opioid doses to a maximum of 120 mg to 180 mg of morphine or its equivalent and to refer patients for additional help before escalating opioid doses further.[13]

DISCUSSION

Most adults experience LBP at some point in their lives, the recurrence rates are high, and a number may end up with some degree of chronic LBP. Only a small proportion of individuals develop disabling chronic LBP, and it is this group who account for most health-care and social costs associated with LBP.[14] It is estimated that 5% of people with LBP account for 75% of the costs associated with LBP. Risk factors for developing disabling chronic LBP have been identified in prospective studies. In these studies, psychological factors proved to be predictive of pain treatment outcomes and displayed more predictive power than biomedical or biomechanical variables.[15] In a systematic review of prospective studies, psychological factors, such as catastrophic thoughts and beliefs, fear-avoidance behaviors, depression, and work dissatisfaction were shown to be strongly associated with the development of disabling chronic LBP.[15] These psychological factors must be considered when prescribing medications for LBP.

As discussed in the article on psychosocial issues, psychological factors have been associated with poor outcomes in LBP treatment. All individuals with chronic pain are coping with their condition; however, some may be using coping strategies that become counterproductive or maladaptive for them. Pain-related catastrophizing and fear-avoidance behaviors, considered to be forms of maladaptive coping, have been strongly associated with poor treatment outcomes and the development of disabling chronic LBP.[16,17] Early identification of risk factors known to contribute to poor treatment response and progression of disabling chronic LBP followed by treatment directed at these factors has the potential to reduce disabling chronic LBP, thereby reducing the personal suffering and disability as well as the negative social and economic impact of LBP on society. For example, if catastrophizing beliefs and fear-avoidance behaviors are identified, the treatment plan can include, In addition to pharmacologic treatment, education and methods aimed at helping the individual restructure catastrophic beliefs and at beginning gradual and paced goal-directed activity despite pain.

Individuals who have risk factors for a poor treatment outcome are generally considered to have "complex" LBP. Those with complex LBP often present as being overwhelmed by their pain symptoms and with marked functional impairment. Individuals with complex chronic LBP are best served by a comprehensive treatment approach that is informed by a biopsychosocial model. This model views chronic pain as a complex experience that affects and is influenced by an individual's physical, emotional, cognitive, and social health.[18] Psychosocial variables, including pain-related beliefs and cognitions, are seen as having an important impact on pain-related outcomes. Comprehensive pain care uses the principles of chronic disease management and often involves multidisciplinary and multimodal treatments emphasizing adaptive self-management. Primary treatment goals are to improve long-term health, activity, and quality of life. Key components of comprehensive pain care include patient education, pharmacologic therapy, physical therapy and exercise, cognitive-behavioral therapy and social services.

In contrast to pharmacologic treatment, comprehensive pain care is strongly supported by evidence to be effective and cost-effective for long-term results in chronic pain, at improving return to work, and reducing additional surgery and health-care use.[19] A major problem has been that third-party payers do not reimburse many of the cost-effective components of comprehensive pain care. This problem has resulted in the closure of comprehensive multidisciplinary pain programs around the country and the expansion of pain clinics that deliver only escalating pharmacologic treatments, advanced diagnostics and expensive spinal procedures that have limited evidence of long-term efficacy for chronic LBP and contribute significantly to the high health-care costs associated with LBP.

Comprehensive pain care may be viewed as time-consuming and costly by providers, including primary care providers, who are frequently impeded by large patient panels, short clinic visits, and limited capacity for follow-up and monitoring.

Pharmacologic treatment has become the quicker, easier way to try coping with these patients. Comprehensive pain care, however, does not need to involve elaborate and expensive specialty services. Much can be accomplished in the form of brief education and adaptive self-management support during clinic encounters or phone contacts. Currently, a new health-care initiative is being implemented, which may be helpful for primary care providers—the Patient-Centered Medical Home—which uses principles of comprehensive care, such as collaboration and teamwork in the primary care setting, to assist patients in their self-management of chronic pain.

Studies have shown that collaborative care in the primary care setting results in significant improvements in chronic pain treatment outcomes.[5,6]

When initiating long-term pharmacologic treatment, efforts should be directed at engaging the patient in comprehensive pain care. These efforts involve listening to their story and validating and normalizing their experience, while recommending and supporting healthy and adaptive responses to their chronic pain. When LBP has persisted longer than 3 months, the aim of pain management needs to shift from cure of pain to recovery of health and function. The patient needs to be informed that although cure of their chronic pain is not possible, much can be done to help them improve their pain control, mobility, and quality of life. Patients are informed that medications can provide only partial pain reduction at best, that each involves different benefit-to-harm profiles, and that all are best used in a rehabilitation context to improve longterm health and activity. Patients are informed of the many influences on pain, suffering, and disability and of the importance of approaching chronic pain from a biopsychosocial perspective.

Patients learn that acceptance of chronic pain is not giving up rather it is choosing to engage in valued activity despite persisting pain. Acceptance of chronic pain is not a passive but an active step in the process of change, and it has been strongly associated with improved treatment outcomes. Patients are taught that in the context of chronic pain, it is normal for pain intensity to fluctuate and to increase with activity and that "hurt is not the same as harm." Patients learn that they change their coping and self-management strategies away from passive and avoidance behaviors toward more active and adaptive behaviors, such as engaging slowly and steadily in valued activities while still experiencing pain.

In summary, current evidence supports the efficacy of short-term pharmacologic treatment for LBP. Evidence on the efficacy and safety of long-term pharmacologic treatment for LBP is limited, and therefore, when medications are used for long-term treatment of LBP, it is recommended that they be used with caution, monitoring, and in a rehabilitative context. Patients with evidence of complex chronic LBP are best served by a comprehensive pain-care approach emphasizing adaptive self-management to improve long-term health, activity, and quality of life.

REFERENCES

1. Van Tulder M, Assendelft W, Koes B, et al. Spinal radiographic findings and nonspecific low back pain. A systematic review of observational studies. Spine 1997;22:427–34.
2. Pengel LH, Herbert RD, Maher CG, et al. Acute low back pain: systematic review of its prognosis. BMJ 2003;327:323.
3. Machado L, Kamper S, Herbert R, et al. Analgesic effects of treatments for nonspecific low back pain: a meta-analysis of placebo-controlled randomized trials. Rheumatology 2009;48:520–7.
4. Chou R, Hoyt-Huffman L. Medications for acute and chronic low back pain: a review of the evidence for an American Pain Society/American College of Physicians clinical practice guidelines. Ann Intern Med 2007;147:505–14.
5. Kroenke K, Bair M, Damush T, et al. Optimized antidepressant therapy and pain self-management in primary care patients with depression and musculoskeletal pain: a randomized controlled trial. JAMA 2009;301(20):2099–110.
6. Dobscha S, Corson K, Perrin N, et al. Collaborative care for chronic pain in primary care: a cluster randomized trial. JAMA 2009;301(12):1242–52.
7. Maretell BA, et al. Systemic review: opioid treatment for chronic back pain: prevalence, efficacy, and association with addiction. Ann Intern Med 2007;146(2):116–27.
8. Dunn K, Saunders K, Rutter C, et al. Opioid prescriptions for chronic pain and overdose: a cohort study. Ann Intern Med 2010;152:85–92.
9. Turk D. Predicting opioid misuse by chronic pain patients: a systematic review and literature synthesis. Clin J Pain 2008;24(6):497–592.
10. Sullivan M, Edlund M, Zhang L, et al. Association between mental health disorders, problem drug use, and regular prescription opioid use. Arch Intern Med 2006;166:2087–93.
11. Kuehn BM. Opioid prescriptions soar: increase in legitimate use as well as abuse. JAMA 2007;297:249–51.
12. Martin B, Deyo R, Mirza S, et al. Expenditures and health status among adults with back and neck problems. JAMA 2008;299(6):656–64.
13. Chou R, Fanciullo G, Fine P, et al. Clinical guidelines for the use of chronic opioid therapy in chronic noncancer pain. J Pain 2009;10(2):113–30.
14. Hashemi L, Webster B, Clancy E, et al. Length of disability and cost of workers' compensation low back pain claims. J Occup Environ Med 1997;39:937–45.
15. Linton S. A review of psychological risk factors in back and neck pain. Spine 2000;25:1148–56.
16. Foster NE, Bishop A, Thomas E, et al. Illness perceptions of low back pain patients in primary care: what are they, do they change and are they associated with outcome? Pain 2008;136(1–2):177–87.
17. Pincus T, Vogel S, Burton A, et al. Fear avoidance and prognosis in back pain: a systematic review and synthesis of current evidence. Arthritis Rheum 2006; 54:3999–4010.

18. Gallagher R. Biopsychological pain medicine and mind-brain-body-science. Phys Med Rehabil Clin N Am 2004;15(4):855–82, vii.

19. Gatchel R, Okifuji A. Evidence-based scientific data documenting the treatment and cost-effectiveness of comprehensive pain programs for chronic nonmalignant pain. J Pain 2006;7(11):779–93.

Chronic Low Back Pain and Psychosocial Issues

James E. Moore, PhD[a,b,*]

KEYWORDS

• Psychosocial • Cognitive behavioral • Low back pain
• Interdisciplinary

Chronic low back pain is one of the most common and costly health-care problems today[1–3] in terms of medical care expenses and in lost productivity, disability payments, and personal suffering.[4–7] The prevalence and economic impact of low back pain are tremendous and seems to be increasing.[6–8] For example, in a survey of North Carolina households, chronic low back pain with impairment increased from 3.9% in 1992 to 10.2% in 2006.[9] Speculation about possible contributors to this increase have included rising rates of obesity, depression, physical and psychosocial work demands, and increased awareness and reporting of low back pain.[8] Health-care expenditure for imaging studies, spinal injections, spinal surgeries, and prescription opioids has continued to increase despite the absence of convincing evidence of efficacy.[10] Direct annual health-care expenditure for low back pain in the United States reached $90.7 billion in 1998.[7] Disability benefits and lost productivity add billions more. Although low back pain episodes often improve quickly, a substantial minority continue to experience chronic or recurrent back pain and significant disability.[11–13]

Despite the high prevalence of back pain and the enormous personal and societal costs, the health-care system response has not been satisfactory. The traditional biomedical approach to back pain has been particularly inadequate. There is poor correlation between pain and disability on the one hand and diagnostic studies reflecting the nature and severity of injury on the other.[14,15] Many biomedical treatments in common practice today are not supported by improved outcomes,[10,16] and despite advances in medical technology, back pain disability has continued to increase.[17] The failure of the biomedical model to yield improved outcomes for chronic low back pain led to the adoption of a biopsychosocial model recognizing the reciprocal influences of cognitive, emotional, behavioral, and social/environmental factors as

[a] Rehabilitation Institute of Washington, 4300 Aurora Avenue North, Suite 100, Seattle, WA 98103, USA
[b] Department of Psychiatry and Behavioral Sciences, University of Washington School of Medicine, Seattle, WA, USA
* Rehabilitation Institute of Washington, 4300 Aurora Avenue North, Suite 100, Seattle, WA 98103.
E-mail address: jmoore@rehabwashington.com

Phys Med Rehabil Clin N Am 21 (2010) 801–815
doi:10.1016/j.pmr.2010.06.005
1047-9651/10/$ – see front matter © 2010 Elsevier Inc. All rights reserved.

well as biomedical ones.[18] The biopsychosocial model as applied to pain conditions was initially influenced most significantly by Wilbert Fordyce, who developed the first chronic pain treatment based on psychological principles[19] and who presented a behavioral model for the treatment of chronic pain.[20] His application of the principles of operant conditioning to the treatment of chronic pain paved the way for current cognitive behavioral and interdisciplinary pain rehabilitation approaches. In the last 40 years, there has been continued growth in the research and application of biopsychosocial concepts in chronic pain.[21,22] This article reviews common psychosocial issues related to chronic low back pain, including factors that influence the onset of low back pain and the transition from acute to chronic pain. The research on chronic low back pain strongly suggests that psychosocial factors are at least as important as biomedical ones in predicting and influencing the course of pain.[14,15,23]

The biopsychosocial approach to low back pain focuses on the complex interplay of cognitive, emotional, behavioral, and social/environmental factors and how they interact with the biomedical factors of injury, nociception, and pain perception. Psychosocial factors influence the initial onset of low back pain, the transition of low back pain to a chronic condition, the maintenance of chronic pain, and the responsiveness to treatment.

PSYCHOSOCIAL FACTORS INFLUENCING PAIN ONSET

A purely biomedical model would not assume that psychosocial factors have any influence on the onset of new pain; only that nociception results in a pain experience proportional to the severity of injury. There are numerous prospective studies that have identified various psychosocial factors that can influence the onset of pain. Unfortunately, there is inconsistency among these studies because of the employment of widely differing measures, settings, and subject populations. In addition, many psychosocial constructs share common variance, thus creating significant measurement redundancy. Depending on the number, selection, and order of variables entered into multivariate analyses, the results can yield contradictory conclusions regarding the psychosocial factors that impact low back pain.

Fear Avoidance

The concept of fear-avoidance beliefs grew from a model of exaggerated pain perception,[24] suggesting that individuals fall along a continuum ranging from a tendency to confront a painful experience by remaining active to a tendency to avoid movement and activity because of pain-related fear. Avoidance of activity is thought to contribute to disuse, deconditioning, and pain-related disability.[25–27]

Research demonstrates that fear-avoidance beliefs predict the future onset of new low back pain. That is, pain-free individuals who believe that physical or work activities should be avoided when in pain or that such activity is dangerous have a greater likelihood of developing low back pain in the future.[28–30] Similar findings demonstrate a relationship between pain catastrophizing, pain-related fear, and fear-avoidance beliefs with the onset of new low back pain.[31,32] Noting the presence of fear-avoidance beliefs in pain-free individuals, Leeuw and colleagues[33] suggest that these beliefs may be a vulnerability factor for the inception of new low back pain, perhaps by influencing how ambiguous physical sensations are interpreted.

Workplace Factors

Dissatisfaction with work is predictive of new onset of low back pain. Studies longitudinally following subjects who were pain-free or had only minor prior episodes of low back pain found that dissatisfaction with work status, perceived inadequacy of income, and performance of unskilled or manual tasks were associated with future medical consultations for low back pain.[34,35] Perceived lack of social support from a supervisor or coworkers was associated with the future reporting of low back pain in several studies.[32,36–41] Workers who report having limited control over their work,[41] an excessive workload,[31] or low job satisfaction[37,39,42] have increased risk of future back pain.

Psychological Distress

Elevated levels of psychological distress in pain-free individuals have been associated with future episodes of low back pain.[31,43] In a longitudinal study that followed occupationally active adults over a 12-year period, researchers found that level of emotional distress at baseline predicted long-term low back disability.[44]

Abuse History

It is extremely difficult to conduct a prospective study to determine the effect of abuse on the subsequent onset of low back pain, although at least one study has done just that. Linton[45] assessed the history of prior physical or sexual abuse in a group of women who reported some or no spinal pain at the time of initial assessment. One year later, for those without pain at baseline, prior physical but not sexual abuse was associated with new occurrences of spinal pain. Physical and sexual abuse were associated with increased episodes of functional problems at one-year follow-up for this group. For the group reporting pain at baseline, neither physical nor sexual abuse predicted pain or disability at follow-up. Because a history of abuse may be associated with family dysfunction or psychopathology, it is difficult to make a clear connection between abuse versus other psychosocial factors and subsequent pain problems.

PSYCHOSOCIAL FACTORS INFLUENCING CHRONIC PAIN AND DISABILITY

Numerous cognitive, emotional, behavioral, and environmental factors can affect the transition from acute to chronic pain. Cognitive factors, such as pain catastrophizing, recovery expectations, and fear-avoidance pain beliefs, have demonstrated an association with the development of chronic pain.[46–53] Emotional factors, such as depression, anxiety, distress, anger, and pain-related fear, have also been implicated in this process.[46,54,55] Behavioral factors, including pain behavior, avoidance behavior, and passive coping style, interact with social, cultural, financial, and other environmental factors to influence this transition.[17,20]

Within a Fear-Avoidance Model

One way to review the interaction of cognitive, emotional, behavioral, and social/environmental factors is within one of the more dominant models of chronic pain development, the fear-avoidance model. In this model, the experience of pain is met with cognitive appraisal of the meaning and significance of pain. If pain is appraised as a benign experience, as from muscle soreness or minor strain, the individual is less likely to experience fear and more likely to maintain or quickly resume normal activities, which in turn can lead to rapid recovery. Conversely, if pain is appraised as a sign of severe injury or dangerous medical condition, that is, if the individual engages in catastrophic pain cognitions, the individual is likely to become fearful. Pain-related fear leads to avoidance of movement or activities that the individual believes will cause greater pain, further injury, or repeat injury. Avoidance of movement and activity can lead to a downward spiral of progressive deconditioning and increased pain and the development of disability, helplessness, and depression.

Pain catastrophizing, an exaggerated and dysfunctional negative appraisal of pain as a threat, is the cognitive precursor to pain-related fear. Cognitive appraisal includes other cognitions, such as expectations of recovery, belief in the need for passive treatments, and cognitive coping style. High fear-avoidance beliefs and negative recovery expectations contribute to the transition to chronic pain and disability.[46,47,50–53,56] Appraisal of pain as a threat also is likely to trigger increased attention, anticipation, or hypervigilance to pain, which can result in increased brain activity in pain-sensitive brain regions and increased intensity of pain.[57–59] Catastrophic pain cognitions and higher levels of fear-avoidance beliefs are associated with exaggerated predictions of pain severity, less tolerance for physical activities, and higher levels of self-reported disability.[56,60,61]

The pain-related fear resulting from catastrophic pain cognitions and fear-avoidance beliefs can produce many avoidance behaviors. These might include lack of movement or activity and abnormal postures or movement patterns designed to avoid pain, such as limping, guarding, and bracing. These avoidance behaviors can be operantly reinforced by their effect on reducing or controlling pain. Avoidance of movement can minimize pain and reduce pain-related fear, each a positive consequence reinforcing avoidance behavior. Over time, avoidance behaviors can become highly resistant to extinction. Indeed, if avoidance is the predominant response, there is limited opportunity to learn that movement or activity is possible without negative consequences. Avoidance behaviors can be reinforced via other consequences, including attention and support from family, avoidance of responsibilities or an unpleasant work environment, or financial compensation.

Continued pain-avoidance behaviors ultimately result in loss of strength, endurance, and flexibility and, in very chronic situations, can result in severe health consequences, such as obesity, cardiovascular disease, and Type II diabetes. It also probably leads to increasing pain severity and loss of ability to engage in the functional and rewarding activities of life. Often, when chronic pain sufferers realize that they are not recovering as initially expected and, in fact, are declining further into pain and disability, their depression and other forms of emotional distress become severe.[62,63]

Each person may develop fear-avoidance beliefs in different ways. Starting in childhood, one suffers minor and sometimes more serious injuries and typically experiences pain many times during one's life. Each pain experience is a learning opportunity that may serve to shape one's belief systems. How parents and others respond to a child in pain may teach that child that pain is a normal part of life and nothing to be feared, or conversely, that pain is a signal that something could be seriously wrong, thus requiring concern and attention. Someone who participates in competitive sports may learn that minor pains should be ignored and should not affect athletic performance. Those performing heavy labor jobs may similarly learn that pain is a normal and routine part of life and can usually be ignored. Each person also has vicarious learning experiences from observing role models respond to painful experiences. These can be members of the family or community, professional athletes, or characters from television and films. Fear-avoidance beliefs develop in many ways and exist even before the onset of pain.

Fear-avoidance beliefs might also be influenced by health-care providers who have developed their own systems of fear-avoidance beliefs. Providers with high levels of fear-avoidance beliefs are more likely to advise patients to avoid painful movements, more likely to recommend sick leave as a valuable treatment for pain, and less likely to encourage patients to maintain as many normal physical activities as are tolerable.[64,65] These recommendations are contrary to most current back-pain guidelines that recommend advising patients to remain active. Providers who caution patients to avoid movement and activity or who keep them out of work until pain improves are probably reinforcing greater pain-related fear and worry in their patients.

Reinforcement of Pain Behavior

Another variable contributing to the transition to chronic pain involves the degree to which pain behavior is reinforced. According to operant theory, behavior that produces positive consequences for the individual will probably increase in frequency, whereas behavior that is punished or ignored is likely to decrease in frequency or extinguish. Dysfunctional pain cognitions, such as belief in the need for passive treatments, the thought that movement is dangerous, or the expectation of long-term disability, can also be influenced by environmental contingencies. Spouses, family members, friends, and others can inadvertently reinforce dysfunctional pain behaviors or cognitions by attention, sympathy, assistance with tasks, or other solicitous responses. Whether a consequence is positive or not depends on the perspective of each individual. For some individuals, for example those that highly value their independence, offers of assistance might be perceived as negative consequences. To the extent that there are positive consequences for an individual following pain behaviors, those behaviors are likely to continue happening.

Financial reinforcement may be a factor when pain has resulted from an industrial injury and there may be disability payments or a pending future financial settlement. Most people who are disabled by back pain experience associated financial loss and, therefore, have an incentive for recovery. However, if disability income while off work closely approximates what would be earned if on the job, pain behavior might be reinforced by the combination of work avoidance and financial compensation, especially with a dissatisfied employee. Patients with limited formal education who were earning a high income performing skilled heavy labor may receive more disability income than they can ever hope to receive if they return to work at a lighter-duty job. This can certainly maintain pain behaviors.

Sometimes it is hard to understand the ways in which pain behavior is being reinforced. It can be reinforced by positive consequences or by avoidance or escape from negative situations. It might involve a spouse who was previously distant but is now more attentive and affectionate. It might be a mother who enjoys being a homemaker, and who can spend time with her children because of her low back pain disability, but who otherwise could not afford to be unemployed. It might be a worker bored with the job and dissatisfied with the income who is hoping to be retrained for an easier and better-paying occupation. It might be a middle-aged worker in a highly stressful job requiring long work hours who also has taken on the care of an elderly parent and whose pain behavior is reinforced via escape from an overly stressful lifestyle. It could also be an unhappy husband who now has an acceptable reason to turn back unwanted sexual advances from his spouse. A psychological evaluation for chronic low back pain seeks to identify via behavioral analysis how pain behavior is being operantly maintained.

As mentioned earlier, pain behaviors, such as limping, guarding, bracing, reclining, and not exercising, or other behaviors designed to avoid pain can be directly reinforced by the reduction of pain and the pain-related fear associated with certain movements or activities. These avoidance behaviors may be appropriate following an acute injury, thus allowing healing to occur. Continuing to avoid normal movement patterns after complete healing is one of the primary causes for continued pain and disability. It is common for secondary pain problems to result from sustained abnormal movements or inactivity. The longer pain behaviors continue, the more likely that they will become influenced by external contingencies, such as attention, sympathy, or assistance from others.

Medical providers can become the source of reinforcement for pain behaviors and thus contribute to the development of chronic pain. Attention and concern from caring medical professionals can be a powerful source of reinforcement for many individuals. If the provider encourages excessive avoidance of physical activity, extended time off work, ongoing use of opioid medication, and suspension of normal household responsibilities, the provider may be reinforcing pain behavior and disability. Patients' beliefs and pain cognitions are also susceptible to operant reinforcement. Ordering unnecessary tests or referring the patient for another opinion may reinforce the belief that something serious might have been missed. Being uncertain while reassuring a patient ("I don't think it is necessary to get a surgical opinion; it is very unlikely that you have anything wrong that would require surgery") can reinforce beliefs that it is still possible that something serious has been missed. Telling patients to "take it easy" or "listen to your body" might reinforce their belief that it is dangerous to be physically active or that pain is a sign of injury.

Depression

Depression is common in chronic low back pain.[63,66,67] The prevalence tends to be 2 to 3 times greater than in the general population.[68] In patients with substantial disability associated with pain, such as those seen in pain clinics, the prevalence is far greater, affecting most patients.[66] Depression increases with greater pain severity, when there is more than one pain problem, when pain is unexplained by medical findings, and when pain becomes chronic. When depression coexists with a chronic medical condition, there is greater functional impairment, more symptoms without identified pathology, greater health-care use, and higher costs.[69]

For coexisting pain and depression, most evidence suggests that depression develops after the onset of pain, often after it becomes apparent that pain is not resolving.[62] Acute pain typically does not produce depression, because it is likely that the acutely injured person expects recovery to occur and pain to resolve. When pain becomes chronic and is accompanied by disability, financial loss, and negative social consequences, the person in pain responds with a range of cognitions, some of which can trigger depression. Those with more positive cognitive coping skills may not develop depression. Banks and Kerns[63] presented a diathesis stress model of pain and depression wherein each individual may have preexisting psychological characteristics, including negative schemas, attributions leading to learned helplessness, and skills deficits that can predispose to the development of depression. When an individual with more negative psychological characteristics experiences chronic pain, impairment and disability associated with pain, and perceived invalidating responses from others, they are at greater risk of depression. Conversely, persons with more positive cognitive schemas, better coping skills, and a validating and supportive social environment may weather chronic pain without severe emotional distress.

Although for most co-occurring pain and depression, depression is a response to pain and associated life changes, it can also exist before pain.[62] Although the findings are not consistent across studies, there are data that suggest that depression may predispose someone to the onset of low back pain.[70] An individual who is already clinically depressed at the time of injury or who has a history of recurrent depression may have more negative cognitive schemas, a more passive coping style, and fewer psychological and social resources to cope effectively with an injury.

The diagnosis of depression is often missed, especially in an individual presenting with complaints of pain.[71,72] Physicians have limited time to address medical and psychological issues, and the psychological ones, if addressed, usually are addressed briefly.[72] Patients with strong somatization tendencies are often unaware of their own depression, and others do not report depressive symptoms because of the perceived social stigma of a mental health problem or their fear that pain complaints would be discounted as arising from psychological problems.

Even when depression is correctly diagnosed, treatment is usually inadequate.[73] The first-line approach to treatment of major depression in recent years has been anti-depressant medication, choosing antidepressant medication or psychotherapy, specifically cognitive behavioral or interpersonal therapy, or medication and psychotherapy. The choice of treatment options has been left to patient and clinician preference or cost considerations. However, the efficacy of antidepressants has been brought into question by extensive literature reviews. These reviews included published and unpublished studies and suggested some selective reporting of research results, with those demonstrating efficacy of antidepressants much more likely to be published than those showing negative or questionable results.[74,75] These studies raise serious questions about the value of antidepressants for most depressed individuals. Recent reviews have found little antidepressant benefit for mild and moderate depression but suggested more serious depression was somewhat responsive to antidepressant medications.[74,76] These results suggest that treating depressed individuals with antidepressants alone may be a poor alternative to other treatments with known efficacy, such as cognitive behavioral therapy. Despite the limited scientific support for the use of antidepressants in most patients, providers and patients believe strongly in their efficacy, perhaps because of a combination of significant placebo response, extensive marketing, and biased reporting in the literature.

The real danger in only prescribing antidepressants is the risk that patients may not accept responsibility for resolving their depression. For patients with chronic low back pain, there may be many negative life changes contributing to depression, including occupational disability, financial stress, sleep disruption, negative health consequences, relationship distress, sexual dysfunction, family role changes, and limitations in social, recreational, and household activities. It is no wonder that depression is so common. To expect medication alone to improve mood in the face of all these changes is not realistic. Conversely, cognitive behavioral therapy can help develop cognitive coping strategies and behavioral action plans to resolve many of these problems.

PSYCHOSOCIAL TREATMENT OF CHRONIC LOW BACK PAIN

The evidence for efficacy of cognitive behavioral therapy for chronic low back pain is still somewhat clouded by the wide range of treatments included under that rubric, some of which are probably much more effective than others. However, this psychologically based intervention has the most empiric support for the treatment of patients with low back pain.[23,77] Cognitive behavioral therapy recognizes that a reciprocal interaction exists among an individual's thoughts, feelings, behaviors, and biomedical factors that in turn interact with the social environment. As discussed earlier, catastrophic thoughts may result in pain-related fear and avoidance behavior and ultimately, in a downward spiral of increased pain, disability, and emotional distress. Cognitive behavioral therapy is typically focused on identifying, challenging, and changing dysfunctional pain cognitions to reduce emotional distress and the person's tendency to avoid normal and appropriate activity or to engage in dysfunctional behavior.

Cognitive Restructuring

Cognitive behavioral therapy begins with educating patients to recognize that their fear or other emotional responses to pain or to every event in their lives is a direct consequence of their cognitive appraisal of the situation. The therapist then assists the patient in identifying their assumptions, interpretations, or other thoughts that produce negative emotions or behaviors. These thoughts might involve the appraisal of pain as arising from a serious or dangerous injury or disease, an expectation that it will get progressively worse or become disabling, or the belief that health-care providers are failing to diagnose or treat the condition effectively or that family members are uncaring or disbelieving. These and numerous other dysfunctional cognitions can obviously lead to emotional reactions, such as fear, anger, despair, and depression. Thoughts might also include beliefs that physical activity is dangerous, that regaining prior physical capacities is impossible, or that rehabilitation treatment will be ineffective or harmful. Once patients are able to recognize the thought processes that account for their emotional reactions, they are assisted in determining if those specific thoughts are completely rational and supported by the available evidence, or whether they are based on distorted and dysfunctional beliefs and assumptions. They are then taught strategies to revise irrational cognitions, with the expected outcome being more appropriate emotional consequences.

Interpreting pain or other events in a more logical or rational fashion can also result in adaptive behavioral changes. For example, if movement is thought to be safe and beneficial rather than dangerous and likely to cause pain or injury, the behavioral response of movement or exercise becomes more probable. If patients perceive providers as trying their best rather than as disinterested and uncaring, they are more likely to work collaboratively with providers and follow the advice given. If patients think that they are helpless or powerless to influence the recovery process, there is likely to be less active coping effort than if they believe that their actions will improve pain or function. Cognitive behavioral therapy for chronic pain is typically designed to help patients adopt beliefs, such as "It is safe and beneficial for me to remain physically active even if I have some pain," "My pain does not mean I am causing further injury," "There are things I can do to control my pain and to improve my ability to be active; I am not helpless," and "Just because I have back pain, it does not mean I cannot have an enjoyable life."

Exposure Therapy

In addition to changing cognitions to bring about more positive emotions and behaviors, it is possible to change behavior to produce corresponding adaptive cognitive and emotional changes. The most effective way to overcome an irrational fear is to confront or expose oneself to the feared stimulus. For example, dog-phobic children could be helped to overcome fear by gradually exposing them to dogs, starting with a small gentle dog and gradually introducing somewhat larger and friskier dogs. With each experience, the children are likely to learn that most dogs are not dangerous and will start to have less catastrophic thoughts regarding dogs. As beliefs about dogs are altered from thinking them dangerous to seeing them as friendly, fear diminishes. This process could also be viewed within a classical conditioning model in which a feared stimulus (dogs) is repeatedly paired with a benign response (lack of aggression); the fear response should gradually extinguish.

In someone with chronic low back pain who is afraid to walk briskly, lift a child, or ride more than a few minutes in a vehicle, the treatment of choice would be exposure. A provider operating from a cognitive behavioral perspective could help a patient develop a plan to progressively confront these feared situations. The process would include a plan to start with slow short walks, lifting very light objects, or riding or just sitting very briefly in a vehicle. The individual can gradually increase walking distance and speed, lifting of heavier objects, and longer trips in a vehicle as confidence in their safety increases. With enough experience performing an activity without injury or major pain flare-up, fear and avoidance tendencies would be expected to extinguish.

Exposure strategies may be particularly helpful for individuals with high fear-avoidance beliefs. High fear avoidance is associated with high levels of self-reported disability, a tendency to overpredict the pain resulting from a particular behavioral activity, and a lower level of physical performance.[56,60,61,78] In fact, pain-related fear was a better predictor of performance than was pain. The tendency to overpredict the pain resulting from an activity is corrected when the task is actually performed. The highly fear-avoidant individual is subsequently able to accurately predict pain from that particular activity but continues to overpredict the level of pain that a new task would produce. Generalization of corrected pain prediction does not appear to readily occur, implying that it might be necessary to systematically arrange exposure in vivo to a wide variety of tasks for which the patient reports fear-avoidance beliefs.

Vlaeyen and colleagues[79,80] have compared the benefits of a graded exercise program with the benefits of exposure therapy. They found that pain-related fear was only diminished during exposure therapy, that is, actually performing the activity patients found threatening. Performing a graded general conditioning program was not as effective in reducing specific pain-related fears. The implication is that exposure to perceived threatening activities should be part of any treatment for chronic low back pain.

Cognitive Behavioral Education

Cognitive behavioral educational programs to address fear-avoidance beliefs and help patients plan for gradually increased activity and exposure to activities that elicit fear have yielded improvements in subacute and chronic low back pain samples.[81-85] These brief and inexpensive interventions designed to help patients learn self-management strategies yielded improvements in pain, function, and pain-related fear. As with other cognitive behavioral treatments, this type of intervention can yield long-lasting benefits.[84,85] Despite guidelines that recommend encouraging as many normal activities as the patient can tolerate, physicians typically have too little time during a standard office visit to adequately educate, reassure, and collaborate with patients in planning ways to increase activities.[72] Shortly after an office visit for low back pain during which patients were presumably reassured about the safety and benefits of physical activity, most continue to report beliefs that something dangerous is wrong with their backs, that unnecessary movement should be avoided, and that movement could cause a serious problem.[86] This suggests that there is still much room for improvement in reassuring patients and encouraging resumption of normal activities.

INTERDISCIPLINARY TREATMENT OF CHRONIC LOW BACK PAIN

Pain and disability that continue beyond normal healing time and have not responded to appropriate conservative or surgical treatments may require an interdisciplinary pain rehabilitation program, especially when the medical and psychological complexity of the pain problem increases.

Haldorsen and colleagues[87] explored the issue of matching work-disabled patients to the right intensity of treatment. Patients were categorized into 3 groups based on prognosis for returning to work (good, medium, poor). The composite prognosis rating was determined through a combination of physical examination and performance and psychological measures. Patients were then randomly assigned to ordinary treatment; light multidisciplinary treatment (education to reduce fear and encourage activity, provision of an individualized exercise program, and, in some cases, referral to a physical therapist or psychologist); or an extensive multidisciplinary treatment program (a 4-week program involving meeting 6 hours per day, 5 days per week and including cognitive behavioral therapy, education, a comprehensive exercise program, and, sometimes, workplace interventions). Patients with a good prognosis for return to work did equally well with each treatment. Patients with a medium prognosis did equally well in either of the multidisciplinary treatments but not the ordinary treatment. Patients with poor prognoses only benefited from the extensive multidisciplinary program. These findings support the notion that more complicated patients, physically and psychologically, require more intensive and interdisciplinary treatments, with the most complex group requiring treatment consistent with an interdisciplinary pain rehabilitation program. In a review by Guzman in 2001, intensive multidisciplinary biopsychosocial rehabilitation improved pain and function in patients off work for more than 3 months with chronic low back pain; less intensive treatments were not effective.

There is now strong evidence for the efficacy of interdisciplinary rehabilitation programs for chronic low back pain.[16,23,88–92] Reviews have indicated that for nonradicular low back pain, interdisciplinary pain rehabilitation probably has better or at least equal outcomes to more invasive interventions, such as injections or surgery that also carry greater risk of iatrogenic consequences and greater cost.[16,91,92] Recent evidenced-based guidelines from the American Pain Society and the American College of Physicians have strongly recommended intensive interdisciplinary rehabilitation for subacute and chronic low back pain.[16,23,89]

Interdisciplinary pain rehabilitation programs usually treat patients 5 full days each week for about 4 weeks, often with follow-up visits. Programs typically use an inter disciplinary team of physicians, pain psychologists, physical therapists, occupational therapists, vocational rehabilitation counselors, and nurses. Treatment most often is based on cognitive behavioral principles and is designed to reduce fear-avoidance beliefs and other dysfunctional pain cognitions. Treatment reduces avoidance behavior by involving patients in an individualized graded exercise program to improve strength, flexibility, endurance, and body mechanics and by using as much patient-specific exposure therapy as is feasible in a clinical setting. There are significant cognitive behavioral educational components, including cognitive restructuring and behavioral coping strategies, for managing pain and the emotional sequelae of pain, such as depression, anger, and anxiety. Programs are generally designed to provide the education and skills that patients require to independently manage pain in the future.

SUMMARY

Chronic low back pain cannot be optimally understood or managed without recognition of the psychosocial factors that influence the onset and maintenance of pain and the individual's response to treatment. From a cognitive behavioral perspective, to adequately treat low back pain, the cognitive, emotional, behavioral, and social factors must be considered in addition to the biomedical ones. Cognitive behavioral therapy can help alter dysfunctional pain cognitions; avoidance and other maladaptive behaviors; the emotional sequelae of pain, including fear, depression, and anger; and the environmental contingences maintaining pain and disability. When these psychosocial issues are significant, it is unlikely that they will respond favorably to any single modality treatment; rather, they are likely to require an intensive interdisciplinary pain rehabilitation approach.

REFERENCES

1. Cypress BK. Characteristics of physician visits for back symptoms: a national perspective. Am J Public Health 1983;73(4):389–95.
2. Carey TS, Evans A, Hadler N, et al. Care-seeking among individuals with chronic low back pain. Spine 1995;20:312–7.
3. Hart LG, Deyo RA, Cherkin DC. Physician office visits for low back pain: frequency, clinical evaluation, and treatment patterns from a U.S. national survey. Spine 1995;20:11–9.
4. Frymoyer JW, Cats-Baril WL. An overview of the incidences and costs of low back pain. Orthop Clin North Am 1991;2:263–71.
5. Rizzo JA, Abbott TA, Berger ML. The labor productivity effects of chronic backache in the United States. Med Care 1998;36:1471–88.
6. Dagenais S, Caro J, Haldeman S. A systematic review of low back pain cost of illness studies in the United States and internationally. Spine J 2008;8(1): 8–20.
7. Luo X, Pietrobon R, Sun SX, et al. Estimates and patterns of direct health care expenditures among individuals with back pain in the United States. Spine 2004;29(1):79–86.
8. Manchikanti L, Singh V, Datta S, et al. Comprehensive review of epidemiology, scope, and impact of spinal pain. Pain Physician 2009;12:E35–70.
9. Freburger JK, Holmes GM, Agans RP, et al. The rising prevalence of chronic low back pain. Arch Intern Med 2009;169(3):251–8.
10. Deyo RA, Mirza SK, Turner JA, et al. Overtreating chronic back pain: time to back off? J Am Board Fam Med 2009;22(1):62–8.
11. Von Korff M, Saunders K. The course of back pain in primary care. Spine 1996; 21:2833–9.
12. Von Korff M, Deyo RA, Cherkin D, et al. Back pain in primary care: outcomes at one year. Spine 1993;18:855–62.
13. Carey TS, Garrett JM, Jackman A, et al. Recurrence and care seeking after acute back pain: results of a long-term follow-up study. Med Care 1999;37:157–64.
14. Carragee EJ, Alamin TF, Miller JL, et al. Discographic, MRI and psychosocial determinants of low back pain disability and remission: a prospective study in subjects with benign persistent back pain. Spine J 2005;5(1):24–35.
15. Boos N, Semmer N, Elfering A, et al. Natural history of individuals with asymptomatic disc abnormalities in magnetic resonance imaging: predictors of low back pain-related medical consultation and work incapacity. Spine 2000;25(12): 1484–92.
16. Chou R, Loeser JD, Owens DK, et al. Interventional therapies, surgery, and interdisciplinary rehabilitation for low back pain. Spine 2009;34(10):1066–77.
17. Fordyce WE, editor. Back pain in the workplace: management of disability in nonspecific conditions. Seattle (WA): IASP Press; 1995. p. 1–6.
18. Engel GL. The need for a new medical model: a challenge for biomedicine. Science 1977;196(4286):129.
19. Fordyce WE, Fowler R, DeLateur B. An application of behavior modification technique to a problem of chronic pain. Behav Res Ther 1968;6:105–7.

20. Fordyce WE. Behavioral methods for chronic pain and illness. St Louis (MO): C V Mosby; 1976.

21. Turk DC. Biopsychosocial perspective on chronic pain. In: Gatchel RJ, Turk DC, editors. Psychological approaches to pain management. New York: Guilford Press; 1996. p. 3–32.

22. Turk DC, Okifuji A. Psychological factors in chronic pain: evolution and revolution. J Consult Clin Psychol 2002;70(3):678–90.

23. Chou R, Huffman LH. Nonpharmacologic therapies for acute and chronic low back pain: a review of the evidence for an American Pain Society/American College of Physicians clinical practice guideline. Ann Intern Med 2007;147: 492–504.

24. Lethem J, Slade PD, Troup JDG, et al. Outline of a fear-avoidance model of exaggerated pain perception: I. Behav Res Ther 1983;21:401–8.

25. Vlaeyen JW, Kole-Snijders AM, Boeren RG, et al. Fear of movement/(re)injury in chronic low back pain and its relation to behavioral performance. Pain 1995;62: 363–72.

26. Vlaeyen JW, Linton SJ. Fear-avoidance and its consequences in chronic musculoskeletal pain: a state of the art. Pain 2000;85:317–32.

27. Waddell G, Newton M, Henderson I, et al. A fear-avoidance beliefs questionnaire (FABQ) and the role of fear-avoidance beliefs in chronic low back pain and disability. Pain 1993;52:157–68.

28. Linton SJ, Buer N, Vlaeyen JW, et al. Are fear avoidance beliefs related to the inception of an episode of back pain? A prospective study. Psychol Health 1999;14:1051–9.

29. Jensen JN, Albertsen K, Borg V, et al. The predictive effect of fear-avoidance beliefs on low back pain among newly qualified health care workers with and without previous low back pain: a prospective cohort study. BMC Musculoskelet Disord 2009;10:117.

30. Van Nieuwenhuyse A, Somville PR, Cronbez G, et al. The role of physical workload and pain related fear in the development of low back pain in young workers: evidence from the BelCoBack study; results after one year of follow up. Occup Environ Med 2006;63:45–52.

31. Linton SJ. Do psychological factors increase the risk for back pain in the general population in both a cross-sectional and prospective analysis? Eur J Pain 2005; 9(4):355–61.

32. Van Nieuwenhuyse A, Fatkhutdinava L, Verbeke G, et al. Risk factors for first-ever low back pain among workers in their first employment. Occup Med 2004;54(8): 513–9.

33. Leeuw M, Goossens ME, Linton SJ. The fear-avoidance model of musculoskeletal pain: current state of scientific evidence. J Behav Med 2007;30(1):77–94.

34. Papageorgiou AC, Macfarlane GJ, Thomas E, et al. Psychosocial factors in the workplace – do they predict new episodes of low back pain?: evidence from the South Manchester Back Pain study. Spine 1997;22(10):1137–42.

35. Papageorgiou AC, Croft PR, Thomas E, et al. Psychosocial risks for low back pain: are these related to work? Ann Rheum Dis 1998;57:500–2.

36. Eriksen W, Bruusgaard D, Knardahl S. Work factors as predictors of intense or disabling low back pain; a prospective study of nurses' aides. Occup Environ Med 2004;61:398–404.

37. Hoogendoorn WE, van Poppel MN, Bongers PM, et al. Systematic review of psychosocial factors at work and private life as risk factors for back pain. Spine 2000;25(16):2114–25.

38. Hoogendoorn WE, Bongers PM, de Vet HC, et al. Psychosocial work characteristics and psychological strain in relation to low-back pain. Scand J Work Environ Health 2001;27(4):258–67.

39. Hoogendoorn WE, Bongers PM, de Vet HC, et al. High physical work load and low job satisfaction increase the risk of sickness absence due to low back pain: results of a prospective cohort study. Occup Environ Med 2002;59(5): 323–8.

40. Linton SJ. Occupational psychological factors increase the risk for back pain: a systematic review. J Occup Rehabil 2001;11(1):53–66.

41. Clays E, De Bacquer D, Leynen F, et al. The impact of psychosocial factors on low back pain: longitudinal results from the Belstress study. Spine 2007;32(2):262–8.

42. Bigos SJ, Battié MC, Spengler DM, et al. A prospective study of work perceptions and psychosocial factors affecting the report of back injury. Spine 1991;16:1–6.

43. Croft PR, Papagiorgiou AC, Ferry S, et al. Psychologic distress and low back pain. Evidence from a prospective study in the general population. Spine 1995; 20(24):2731–7.

44. Brage S, Dandanger I, Nygard JF. Emotional distress as a predictor for low back disability. Spine 2007;32(2):269–74.

45. Linton SJ. A prospective study of the effects of sexual or physical abuse on back pain. Pain 2002;96(3):347–51.

46. Boersma K, Linton SJ. Psychological processes underlying the development of a chronic pain problem: a prospective study of the relationship between profiles of psychological variables in the fear-avoidance model and disability. Clin J Pain 2006;22(2):160–6.

47. Schultz IZ, Crook JM, Berkowitz J, et al. Biopsychosocial multivariate predictive model of occupational low back disability. Spine 2002;27(23):2720–5.

48. Schultz IZ, Crook J, Meloche GR, et al. Psychosocial factors predictive of occupational low back disability: towards development of a return-to-work model. Pain 2004;107:77–85.

49. Foster NE, Thomas E, Bishop A, et al. Distinctiveness of psychological obstacles to recovery in low back pain patients in primary care. Pain 2010;148(3):398–406.

50. Iles RA, Davidson M, Taylor NF. Psychosocial predictors of failure to return to work in non-chronic non-specific low back pain: a systematic review. Occup Environ Med 2008;65:507–17.

51. Iles RA, Davidson M, Taylor NF, et al. Systematic review of the ability of recovery expectations to predict outcomes in non-chronic non-specific low back pain. J Occup Rehabil 2009;19(1):25–40.

52. Grotle M, Vollestad NK, Brox JI. Clinical course and impact of fear-avoidance beliefs in low back pain. Spine 2006;31(9):1038–46.

53. Turner JA, Franklin G, Fulton-Kehoe D, et al. Worker recovery expectations and fear-avoidance predict work disability in a population-based workers' compensation back pain sample. Spine 2006;31(6):682–9.

54. Linton SJ. A review of psychological risk factors in back and neck pain. Spine 2000;25(9):1148–56.

55. Pincus T, Vogel S, Burton AK, et al. Fear avoidance and prognosis in back pain. Arthritis Rheum 2006;54(12):3999–4010.

56. Crombez G, Vlaeyen JW, Heuts PH, et al. Pain-related fear is more disabling than pain itself: evidence on the role of pain-related fear in chronic back pain disability. Pain 1999;80:329–39.

57. Ploghaus A, Tracey I, Gati JS, et al. Dissociating pain from its anticipation in the human brain. Science 1999;284:1979–81.

58. Porro CA, Baraldi P, Pagnoni G, et al. Does anticipation of pain affect cortical nociceptive systems? J Neurosci 2002;22(8):3206–14.
59. Wager TD, Rilling JK, Smith EE, et al. Placebo induced changes in fMRI in the anticipation and experience of pain. Science 2004;303:1162–7.
60. Crombez G, Vervaet L, Baeyens F, et al. Do pain expectancies cause pain in chronic low back patients? A clinical investigation. Behav Res Ther 1996;34: 919–25.
61. Crombez G, Eccleston C, Vlaeyen JW, et al. Exposure to physical movements in low back pain patients: restricted effects of generalization. Health Psychol 2002; 21:573–8.
62. Fishbain D, Cutler R, Rosomoff H, et al. Chronic pain-associated depression: antecedent or consequence of chronic pain? A review. Clin J Pain 1997;13: 116–37.
63. Banks SM, Kerns RD. Explaining high rates of depression in chronic pain: a diathesis-stress framework. Psychol Bull 1996;119:95–110.
64. Linton SJ, Vlaeyen J, Ostelo R. The back pain beliefs of health care providers: are we fear-avoidant? J Occup Rehabil 2002;12:223–32.
65. Coudeyre E, Rannou F, Tubach F, et al. General practitioners' fear-avoidance beliefs influence their management of patients with low back pain. Pain 2006; 124:330–7.
66. Bair MJ, Robinson RL, Katon W, et al. Depression and pain comorbidity: a literature review. Arch Intern Med 2003;163:2433–45.
67. Romano JM, Turner JA. Chronic pain and depression; does the evidence support a relationship? Psychol Bull 1985;97:18–34.
68. Demyttenaere K, Bruffaerts R, Lee S, et al. Mental disorders among persons with chronic back or neck pain: results from the World Mental Health Surveys. Pain 2007;129(3):332–42.
69. Katon W, Sullivan M, Walker E. Medical symptoms without identified pathology: relationship to psychiatric disorders, childhood and adult trauma, and personality traits. Ann Intern Med 2001;134:917–25.
70. Carroll LJ, Cassidy JD, Cote P. Depression as a risk factor for onset of an episode of troublesome neck and low back pain. Pain 2004;107:134–9.
71. Katon W, Sullivan MD. Depression and chronic medical illness. J Clin Psychiatry 1990;51(Suppl 6):3–11.
72. Turner JA, LeResche L, Von Korff M, et al. Back pain in primary care: patient characteristics, content of initial visit, and short-term outcomes. Spine 1998;23:463–9.
73. Kessler RC, Berglund P, Demler O, et al. The epidemiology of major depressive disorder: results from the national comorbidity survey replication (NCS-R). JAMA 2003;289:3095–105.
74. Kirsch I, Deacon BJ, Huedo-Medina TB, et al. Initial severity and antidepressant benefits: a meta-analysis of data submitted to the food and drug administration. PLoS Med 2008;5(2):0260–8.
75. Turner EH, Matthews AM, Linardatos E, et al. Selective publication of antidepressant trials and its influence on apparent efficacy. N Engl J Med 2008;358:252–60.
76. Fournier JC, DeRubeis RJ, Hollon SD, et al. Antidepressant drug effects and depression severity. JAMA 2010;303(1):47–53.
77. Hoffman BM, Papas RK, Chatkoff DK, et al. Meta-analysis of psychological interventions for chronic low back pain. Health Psychol 2007;26(1):1–9.
78. McCracken LM, Gross RT, Sorg PJ, et al. Prediction of pain in patients with chronic low back pain: effects of inaccurate prediction and pain-related anxiety. Behav Res Ther 1993;31:647–52.

79. Vlaeyen JW, de Jong J, Geilen M, et al. Graded exposure in vivo in the treatment of pain-related fear: a replicated single-case experimental design in four patients with chronic low back pain. Behav Res Ther 2001;39:151–66.
80. Vlaeyen JW, de Jong J, Geilen M, et al. The treatment of fear of movement/(re)-injury in chronic low back pain: further evidence on the effectiveness of exposure in vivo. Clin J Pain 2002;18:251–61.
81. Moore JE, Von Korff M, Cherkin D, et al. A randomized trial of a cognitive-behavioral program for enhancing back pain self care in a primary care setting. Pain 2000;88:145–53.
82. Von Korff M, Moore JE, Lorig K, et al. A randomized trial of a layperson-led self-management group intervention for back pain patients in primary care. Spine 1999;23.2608–15.
83. Linton SJ, Andersson T. Can chronic disability be prevented? A randomized trial of a cognitive-behavioral intervention and two forms of information for patients with spinal pain. Spine 2000;25(21):2825–31.
84. Linton SJ, Nordin E. A 5-year follow-up evaluation of the health and economic consequences of an early cognitive behavioral intervention for back pain: a randomized, controlled trial. Spine 2006;31(8):853–8.
85. Lamb SE, Hansen Z, Lall R, et al. Group cognitive behavioral treatment for low-back pain in primary care: a randomized controlled trial and cost-effectiveness analysis. Lancet 2010;375:916–23.
86. Von Korff M, Moore JE. Stepped-care for back pain: activating approaches for primary care. Ann Intern Med 2001;134:911–7.
87. Haldorsen EM, Grasdal AL, Skouen JS. Is there a right treatment for a particular patient group? Comparison of ordinary treatment, light multidisciplinary treatment, and extensive multidisciplinary treatment for long-term sick listed employees with musculoskeletal pain. Pain 2002;95:49–63.
88. Guzman J, Esmail R, Karjalainnen K, et al. Multidisciplinary rehabilitation for chronic low back pain: systematic review. BMJ 2001;322:1511–6.
89. Chou R, Qaseem A, Snow V, et al. Diagnosis and treatment of low back pain: a joint clinical practice guideline from the American College of Physicians and the American Pain Society. Ann Intern Med 2007;147:478–91.
90. Flor H, Fydrich T, Turk DC. Efficacy of multidisciplinary pain treatment centers: a meta-analytic review. Pain 1992;49:221–30.
91. Turk DC. Clinical effectiveness and cost effectiveness of treatment for patients with chronic pain. Clin J Pain 2002;18:355–65.
92. Turk DC, Burwinkle TM. Clinical outcomes, cost-effectiveness, and the role of psychology in treatments for chronic pain sufferers. Prof Psychol Res Pr 2005; 36(6):602–10.

Interventions for Low Back Pain: Conclusions

The interventional procedures available to help diagnose and treat low back pain are numerous and expanding. With a growing population that is living longer, the incidence of low back pain will likely increase. New technology will continue to emerge in attempts to improve both evaluation and treatment of low back pain. Interventions and devices, however, do not undergo the same rigorous Food and Drug Administration approval process required for new pharmaceuticals to prove safety and efficacy. Devices and interventions for the spine evolve from physioanatomic theories of pain generation and are approved for use based on similar procedures and/or devices already in existence. They are most often used in clinical practice before establishing efficacy or long-term safety. This is true not only for the common interventions used currently but also for emerging treatments and treatments that have previously fallen out of favor only to return with a new twist (eg, chemonucleolysis, intradiscal steroid injection, coblation nucleoplasty, intradiscal electrothermal therapy, percutaneous intradiscal radiofrequency therapy, and biacuplasty).[1] These may be legitimate treatments for low back pain, but further trials demonstrating their efficacy are needed to validate their use. Physiatrists treating low back pain should be cognizant that each procedure has a unique set of diagnostic and therapeutic capabilities, risks, limitations, and evidence of efficacy before integrating them into a comprehensive rehabilitation management plan. Indiscriminate use of interventions exposes patients to unnecessary risks and contributes to the socioeconomic burden of health care costs. Practitioners should endeavor to corroborate evidence-based treatments and support well-designed research. The results of these efforts will not only improve the quality of care for our patients but also provide a basis to negotiate reimbursement with third-party payers.

Alison Stout, DO
Department of Rehabilitation
University of Washington
Seattle, WA, USA

Department of Rehabilitation
VA Puget Sound HCS, 117-RCS
1660 South Columbian Way
Seattle, WA 98108, USA

E-mail address:
sportsandspinedoc@yahoo.com

REFERENCE

1. Chou R, Atlas SJ, Stanos SP, et al. Nonsurgical interventional therapies for low back pain: a review of the evidence for an American Pain Society clinical practice guideline. Spine (Phila Pa 1976) 2009;34(10):1070–93.

Phys Med Rehabil Clin N Am 21 (2010) 817
doi:10.1016/j.pmr.2010.08.003
1047-9651/10/$ – see front matter © 2010 Elsevier Inc. All rights reserved.

pmr.theclinics.com

Interventional Treatment for Low Back Pain: General Risks

Arthur Hartog, MD, PhD

KEYWORDS

• Spinal injection • Complications • Risks • Epidural
• Low back pain • Low back pain treatment

The commonly performed spinal procedures, such as epidural injections, spinal nerve blocks, zygapophysial joint (z-joint) interventions, and discography, are reported to be safe. However, diagnostic and therapeutic spinal interventions can lead to serious complications, although their incidence seems to be low. Knowledge of potential complications is still required to minimize risks.

This article describes the risks associated with the most commonly performed procedures, precautions that can be taken to minimize these risks, and treatment options available once complications have occurred.

INFECTION

The incidence of infectious complications after spinal injections is reported as 1%–2%. Most infections are minor, but severe complications, such as epidural abscess, meningitis, osteomyelitis, septic z-joint arthritis, and discitis, have been reported.[1–8] The predominant mechanism for infections is considered to be the introduction of *Staphylococcus aureus* from the skin to the spinal structures, although cases have been reported in which gram-negative aerobes and anaerobes were identified, presumably after accidental intestinal penetration.

Apart from meticulous sterile technique for preventing infectious complications after spinal injections, the standard use of prophylactic antibiotics has been recommended, but only for discography.[9]

Early diagnosis and treatment are essential to minimize the chance of a poor outcome. General signs of infection may include severe back pain, fever, chills, and malaise. Other signs may vary depending on the underlying pathology, such as meningeal irritation for meningitis or progressive neurologic deficit for an epidural abscess. Diagnostic tests should be chosen based on the suspected pathology and often

---

DC|Pain Center Rotterdam, Vasteland 10, 3011 BL Rotterdam, The Netherlands
E-mail address: ahartog@diagnostischcentrum.com

Phys Med Rehabil Clin N Am 21 (2010) 819–823
doi:10.1016/j.pmr.2010.06.008
1047-9651/10/$ – see front matter © 2010 Elsevier Inc. All rights reserved.

include magnetic resonance imaging (MRI) and blood tests, such as complete blood count, erythrocyte sedimentation rate, and C-reactive protein. Specific tests, such as cerebrospinal fluid (CSF) analysis, may be indicated.

Appropriate treatment, such as administration of antibiotics or surgery, should be initiated as soon as possible.

ALLERGY

Allergic and anaphylactic reactions to commonly used medications for spinal injections are very rare. However, such reactions have been described after the administration of contrast media, local anesthetics, and corticosteroids, most often in the 2 hours after the epidural injection.[10] Symptoms may vary from mild ones, such as light-headedness and nausea, to convulsions and compete cardiovascular and respiratory collapse.

A careful history of previous allergic reactions should be taken before all spinal injections. Hemodynamic and respiratory monitoring and full resuscitation equipment, including antihistamine medication, should be readily available.

CORTICOSTEROIDS

Corticosteroids injected into spinal structures have systemic side effects. These include flushes, facial erythema, rash, pruritus, headache, dizziness, insomnia, elevated temperature, irregular menses, mood swings, gastrointestinal discomfort, epidural lipomatosis, and fluid retention.

A significant effect of a spinal injection with corticosteroids is adrenal suppression, which usually lasts 4 to 7 days after a single epidural injection but the effects can last for up to 5 weeks.[11]

Hyperglycemia after spinal corticosteroid injections is rarely of clinical importance. However, in diabetic patients, the elevation of blood glucose is usually more pronounced. There are reports that the severity of glucose increase is related to the level of hemoglobin A1c at the time of injection.[12] Diabetic patients should be informed of the possible blood glucose increase, which may require adjustment of their insulin dose.

Current evidence seems to favor the use of nonparticulate preparations for spinal injections over particulate ones, especially for epidural injections. The use of particulate steroid preparations in lumbar and cervical spinal injections has been shown to be associated with severe morbidity, such as spinal cord infarction presumably by arterial embolisation.[13–15] In an animal study, direct injection with particulate steroid into the vertebral artery resulted in severe neurologic deficits, whereas no deficits were found when nonparticulate steroids were used.[16] Furthermore, a comparative study showed no statistical or clinical difference in pain relief effectiveness between cervical transforaminal particulate triamcinolone and nonparticulate dexamethasone.[17]

BLEEDING

The spine, particularly the epidural space, is a densely vascularized structure. Therefore, all spinal injections carry an inherent risk of bleeding complications. The incidence of clinically significant spinal hematomas is very low, but they have been shown to be associated with severe morbidity.[18–21]

An increased bleeding tendency is associated with a higher risk of epidural hematoma, but epidural hematoma can develop in any patient after spinal procedures.[19,22] An increased bleeding tendency is often encountered in patients with coagulation disorders, such as hemophilia or von Willebrand disease, in those taking anticoagulants, or in those with liver or renal disease. It is essential that patients with an increased bleeding tendency are identified by taking a complete history on coagulation disorders, use of anticoagulants, easy bruising, and prolonged bleeding after dental procedures.

Appropriate blood tests are required once a coagulation disorder is suspected. Based on the outcome of these tests, referral to a hematologist for further analysis and treatment may be necessary.

Guidelines for patients on anticoagulants who are proposed for spinal procedures have been described elsewhere.[23,24] Generally, anticoagulants are put on hold, and with warfarin, an international normalized ratio of 1.4 is the general standard. However, when injections have a low associated risk of bleeding, there is some controversy regarding the discontinuation of nonsteroidal anti-inflammatory medications (NSAIDs) or even therapeutic anticoagulation.

Early diagnosis and treatment of spinal hematoma is important, because the outcome is highly dependent on the time interval between the onset of symptoms and the initiation of treatment.[22] Symptoms include unexpected duration or spread of sensory or motor deficit, unexplained spinal or radicular pain, and bladder or bowel dysfunction. Symptoms may present immediately postprocedure or be delayed for several days.[25,26]

MRI is the preferred imaging modality if a spinal hematoma is suspected. Once the diagnosis of spinal hematoma is made, immediate referral to a neurosurgical facility is mandatory, because treatment generally involves surgical decompression.

CARDIOVASCULAR RESPONSE

The injection of local anesthetics into spinal structures has the potential to cause a significant cardiovascular response. Mechanisms involved are sympathetic block, which can result in hypotension, and vagal stimulation, which may result in bradycardia.[27]

Accidental intravascular injection of a large dose of local anesthetic can result in cardiovascular toxicity, with severe hypotension occurring as a result of decreased cardiac output and peripheral vascular resistance. Signs of central nervous system toxicity, such as tinnitus, numbness of the tongue, and seizures, are usually seen before cardiovascular collapse when lidocaine is used, but not necessarily when bupivacaine is used.

Inadvertent intrathecal administration of an epidural dose of local anesthetics can result in a high spinal block, or, ultimately, a total spinal block. The associated cardiovascular and respiratory collapse generally require hemodynamic support with intravenous fluids and catecholamines. Tracheal intubation and mechanical ventilation may be required until spontaneous ventilation returns.

POSTDURAL PUNCTURE HEADACHE

Postdural puncture headache (PDPH) is characterized by a positional headache after dural puncture that worsens when the patient assumes an upright position. The headache is commonly perceived in the frontal and occipital areas and is relieved when lying down. Other symptoms, such as nausea and vomiting, may also be present. The onset of symptoms typically occurs within 48 hours to 3 days after the dural puncture.[28,29] These symptoms are annoying and can be debilitating but are usually benign. However, after dural puncture, severe complications, such as subdural hematoma, cerebral herniation, and death, have been described.[30]

The exact mechanisms involved in PDPH are unclear, but it is thought that leakage of CSF causes a drop in CSF pressure resulting in traction on the intracranial structures and venodilatation.[31]

The incidence of unintentional dural puncture during lumbar epidural injections is reported to be 0.5%,[32] thought to be inversely related to the interventionist's experience. Once the dura is punctured, the incidence of PDPH is related to the size of the needle, with an increased incidence when a thicker needle is used.

PDPH will resolve without treatment within 7 days in 72% of patients and within 6 weeks in 85%.[31] Treatment consists of supportive measures, such as rehydration or use of caffeine and acetaminophen or NSAIDs. Patients have usually found a prone position to be the most comfortable. In some cases, an epidural blood patch may be considered, in which up to 30 mL of the patient's blood is injected into the epidural space.[31]

UROLOGICAL COMPLICATIONS

Epidural injection of local anesthetics or opioids may result in urinary retention.[33] However, this complication is very rare with the commonly used doses.

REFERENCES

1. Dougherty JH Jr, Fraser RA. Complications following intraspinal injections of steroids. Reports of two cases. J Neurosurg 1978;48:1023–5.
2. Shealy CN. Dangers of spinal injections without proper diagnosis. JAMA 1966; 197:1104–6.
3. Chan ST, Leung S. Spinal epidural abscess following steroid injection for sciatica. Case report. Spine 1989;14:106–8.
4. Gutknecht DR. Chemical meningitis following epidural injection of corticosteroids. Am J Med 1987;82:570.
5. Tham EJ, Stoodley MA, Macintyre PE, et al. Back pain following postoperative epidural analgesia: an indicator of possible spinal infection. Anaesth Intensive Care 1997;25:297–301.
6. Goucke CR, Graziotti P. Extradural abscess following local anesthetic and steroid injection for chronic low back pain. Br J Anaesth 1990;65:427–9.
7. Cooper AB, Sharpe MD. Bacterial meningitis and cauda equina syndrome after epidural steroid injections. Can J Anaesth 1996;43:471–4.
8. Weingarten TN, Hooten WM, Huntoon MA. Septic facet joint arthritis after a corticosteroid facet injection. Pain Med 2006;7:52–6.
9. Bogduk N, Aprill C, Derby R. Discography. In: White AH, editor. Spine care: diagnosis and treatment. St Louis (MO): C V Mosby; 1995. p. 219–36.
10. Simon DL, Kunz RD, German JD, et al. Allergic or pseudoallergic reaction following epidural steroid deposition and skin testing. Reg Anesth 1989;14: 253–5.
11. Manchikanti L. Role of neuraxial steroids in interventional pain management. Pain Physician 2002;5:182–99.
12. Younes M, Neffati F, Touzi M, et al. Systemic effects of epidural and intra-articular glucocorticoid injections in diabetic and non-diabetic patients. Joint Bone Spine 2007;74:472–6.
13. Kennedy DJ, Dreyfuss P, Aprill CN, et al. Paraplegia following image-guided transforaminal lumbar spine epidural steroid injection: two case reports. Pain Med 2009;10:1389–94.

14. Scanlon GC, Moeller-Bertram T, Romanowsky SM, et al. Cervical transforaminal epidural steroid injections: more dangerous than we think? Spine 2007;32: 1249–56.
15. Muro K, O'Shaughnessy B, Ganju A. Infarction of the cervical spinal cord following multilevel transforaminal epidural steroid injection: case report and review of the literature. J Spinal Cord Med 2007;30:385–8.
16. Guarino A. Perils of depomedrol injections into the vertebral artery - an animal study. Pain Med 2008;9:99.
17. Dreyfuss P, Baker R, Bogduk N. Comparative effectiveness of cervical transforaminal injections with particulate and nonparticulate corticosteroid preparations for cervical radicular pain. Pain Med 2006;7:237–42.
18. Abram SE, O'Connor TC. Complications associated with epidural steroid injections. Reg Anesth 1996;21:149–62.
19. Wulf H. Epidural anaesthesia and spinal hematoma. Can J Anaesth 1996;43: 1260–71.
20. Williams KN, Jackowski A, Evans PJ. Epidural haematoma requiring surgical decompression following repeated cervical epidural steroid injections for chronic pain. Pain 1990;42:197–9.
21. Bose B. Quadriparesis following cervical epidural steroid injections: case report and review of the literature. Spine J 2005;5:558–63.
22. Vandermeulen EP, van Aken H, Vermijlen J. Anticoagulants and spinal-epidural anesthesia. Anesth Analg 1994;79:1165–77.
23. Horlocker TT, Wedel DJ, Benzon H, et al. Regional anesthesia in the anticoagulated patient: defining the risks (the second ASRA Consensus Conference on neuraxial anesthesia and anticoagulation). RAPM 2003;28:172–97.
24. Layton FL, Kallmes DF, Horlocker TT. Recommendations for anticoagulated patients undergoing image-guided spinal procedures. Am J Neuroradiol 2006; 27:467–71.
25. Rodriguez Y, Baena R, Gaena P, et al. Spinal epidural hematoma during anticoagulant therapy. A case report and review of the literature. J Neurosurg Sci 1995; 39:87–94.
26. Horlocker TT, Wedel DJ, Schlicting JL. Postoperative epidural analgesia and oral anticoagulant therapy. Anesth Analg 1994;79:89–93.
27. Brown DL. Spinal, epidural and caudal anesthesia. In: Miller RD, editor. Anesthesia. 5th edition. Philadelphia: Churchill Livingstone; 2000. p. 1491–519.
28. Leibold RA, Yealy DM, Coppola M, et al. Post-dural-puncture headache: characteristics, management, and prevention. Ann Emerg Med 1993;22:1863–70.
29. Reynolds F. Dural puncture and headache. BMJ 1993;306:874–6.
30. Eerola M, Kaukinen L, Kaukinen S. Fatal brain lesion following spinal anaesthesia. Report of a case. Acta Anaesthesiol Scand 1981;25:115–6.
31. Turnbull DK, Shepherd DB. Post-dural puncture headache: pathogenesis, prevention and treatment. Br J Anaesth 2003;91:718–29.
32. Bromage PR. Complications and contraindications. In: Bromage PR, editor. Epidural analgesia. Philadelphia: WB Saunders; 1978. p. 654–711.
33. Armitage EN. Lumbar and thoracic epidural. In: Wildsmith JA, Armitage EN, editors. Principles and practice of regional anaesthesia. New York: Churchill Livingstone; 1987. p. 109.

Epidural Steroid Injections for Low Back Pain

Alison Stout, DO[a,b,*]

KEYWORDS

- Epidural steroid • Spine intervention • Lumbar
- Transforaminal • Interlaminar • Caudal • Low back pain
- Low back pain treatment

The injection of glucocorticoid medication into the epidural space to treat low back pain has been around since the early 1950s.[1] By the 1960s, initial reports in the United States described treatment for sciatica using the caudal and interlaminar (IL) approaches.[2,3] In the middle 1970s, injections via the transforaminal (TF) approach alongside the nerve root were described in combination with fluoroscopic radiographic guidance.

The premise of injecting glucocorticoid and anesthetic medication into the epidural space is that it will decrease pain and inflammation at the site of injection. Axial low back pain has many possible sources, but one of the main suspected etiologies is the intervertebral disc. Pain from the disc has been attributed to disc disruption and inflammation. Annulus fibrosis derangement and nucleus pulposus herniation induce an inflammatory response in the dura, nerve roots, dorsal root ganglion, and the spinal cord, with notable elevation of phospholipase A2 activity.[4] In extracts from human disc herniations, phospholipase A2 activity was found to be 20 to 10,000 times greater than any other human source.[4] Specimens from human herniated discs have also demonstrated increased levels of matrix nitric oxide, metalloproteinase activity, prostaglandin E2, and interleukin-6.[5,6] These and other immunohistochemical substances contribute to increased inflammation and pain transmission. The hypothesis is that the glucocorticoid medication interrupts the inflammatory cascade and inhibits neural transmission by nociceptive C fibers. The pathoanatomical basis of disc-mediated pain is more completely detailed in the anatomy article by Vora and colleagues elsewhere in this issue.

---

[a] Spine and Musculoskeletal Medicine, Rehabilitation Care Services, Veterans Administration, Puget Sound, WA, USA
[b] Department of Rehabilitation, University of Washington, Seattle, WA 98195, USA
* Rehabilitation Care Services, VA Puget Sound HCS, 117-RCS, 1660 South Columbian Way, Seattle, WA 98108.
E-mail address: stouta@uw.edu

Phys Med Rehabil Clin N Am 21 (2010) 825–834
doi:10.1016/j.pmr.2010.08.001
1047-9651/10/$ – see front matter © 2010 Published by Elsevier Inc.

GENERAL INDICATIONS

Epidural steroid injection (ESI) has been used to treat various spinal disorders. It is primarily and most effectively used to treat radicular symptoms. Currently, there is a paucity of evidence to support the use of ESIs for the treatment of axial low back pain associated with conditions such as postlaminectomy syndrome, degenerative disc disease, annular tears, lumbar spinal stenosis (LSS), spondylosis, and spondylolisthesis. The aim of this article is review some of the available literature on the use of ESIs for axial low back pain. The use of ESIs for radicular pain will be reviewed in detail in the upcoming *Physical Medicine and Rehabilitation Clinics of North America* State of the Art Review on Radiculopathy.

Although there is a theoretical basis for lumbar epidural injections for the treatment of low back pain, their value remains controversial. The last decade has been characterized by a more detailed look at the efficacy of epidural steroids, with a large number of systematic reviews, but relatively few randomized controlled trials (RCTs). Adding to the controversy is the dramatic increase in lumbosacral injections documented in the Medicare population from 1994 to 2001.[7] Additionally, less than half of the epidural injections in this database study were performed for sciatica or radiculopathy, where the greatest evidence of benefit is available.[7] Approximating the total cost of an ESI performed in an ambulatory surgery center with fluoroscopy in 2008 at $2850 plus $275 for supplies,[8] it is obvious why the rise in injection rates has been implicated as a main cause for rise in health care expenditures for low back pain.

COMPLICATIONS OF ESIs

The general risks of lumbar spine interventions are discussed in an article by Dr Hartog elsewhere in this issue. Risks specific to lumbar ESIs can be catastrophic, but infrequent.[9] Transient complications encountered with lumbar ESIs can be caused by adverse effects of glucocorticoids, including but not limited to insomnia, impaired glucose control, facial flushing, and hypertension. Procedural complications include vasovagal reactions, nausea, and increased back or leg pain.[9] Published case reports of more serious complications include infection, hematoma, intravascular injection of medication resulting in spinal cord injury, direct nerve trauma, subdural injection, air embolism, disc entry, urinary retention, and hypersensitivity reactions.[9] In 2008, a review of lumbar IL and TF ESI concluded that most if not all complications could be avoided by sterile precautions, careful technique, and a thorough understanding of the anatomy and fluoroscopic contrast patterns.[10]

Knowledge of epidural anatomy and its translation to fluoroscopic anatomy is key to preventing complications and is fully described in the article on anatomy by Vora and colleagues elsewhere in this issue. The epidural space contains the spinal nerve roots and their dural sleeves, the internal vertebral venous plexus, loose areolar tissue, segmental blood supply, adipose tissue, and lymphatics. The location of the dura is an obvious consideration, and the vascular structures are equally if not more important. The epidural veins form an arcuate pattern, positioned laterally at the level of each vertebral body. This is an important consideration for ESIs, as venous puncture is more likely to occur laterally than with midline approaches.[11] Intra-arterial injection has been implicated in paraplegia following lumbosacral TF injection of particulate steroid.[12] The artery of Adamkewicz is the largest radiculomedullary artery and major supplier of the anterior spinal artery in the lumbar region. The artery enters the spinal canal through a single intervertebral foramen between T9 and L2 in 85% of individuals and is located on the left side 63% of the time.[12–14] However, radiculomedullary arteries can enter the spinal canal at any lumbosacral level, and paraplegia after TF injection has been reported as caudally as the S1 level.[15] The specifics of anatomic considerations are discussed further in the section on procedural techniques.

ESI APPROACHES, EVIDENCE, AND EFFICACY

Techniques available to access the lumbosacral epidural space include the caudal, IL, and TF approach. In the lumbosacral spine, the TF route has become more common as epidural corticosteroids administered by other, and often nonimage-guided, routes have been reported as not as effective as claimed in uncontrolled studies.[16–18] Prospective studies by Derby and colleagues[19] in the 1990s described improved outcomes using the TF route for radicular pain.[20] Despite the body of evidence that supports the use of fluoroscopy and the possible advantage of the TF approach, there is significant variation in the method for ESI. This makes the study of the overall effectiveness of ESIs difficult, as techniques are not equivalent. The following is an overview of the literature and is not intended to serve as a reference for conducting the procedures.

Fluoroscopy

The use of fluoroscopic guidance for TF epidural needle placement is considered standard of care. Fluoroscopy is used in conjunction with radiopaque contrast to establish correct placement without intravascular injection. With IL and caudal approaches, needle placement sometimes is made without fluoroscopic guidance. It should be noted, however, that inaccurate needle placement occurs in 35% to 53% of caudal and 17% to 30% of IL injections performed without fluoroscopic guidance.[21–24]

Injectate

There are no standardized practices for the type and volume of medication administered via an epidural injection, and there is significant variation across disciplines and institutions. A steroid/local anesthetic mixture is the most commonly used for ESI in both academic institutions and private practices. A few practices add other medications such as opioids or clonidine, and sometimes anesthetic alone is injected.[25] The volume of the injectate varies based on the approach used. Generally, volumes do not exceed 2 to 3 mL for TF and 3 to 4 mL for IL ESIs, although up to 6 to 10 mL for IL ESIs, and 20 mL for a caudal approach have been reported.[26] Some argue that larger volumes may dilute the injectate and lessen effects at a specific target.

Caudal

Technique
Caudal ESIs were popularly used especially before the routine use of fluoroscopy because of the ease of access via palpable anatomic landmarks and a lower risk of dural puncture. Because the access point for this procedure is more distal to the presumed pathology in most cases, slightly larger volumes of injectate often are instilled. The typical target is pathology at the L5-S1 level, as medication rarely disperses cranial to this level.[27] Some physicians, however, have developed techniques using an epidural catheter to reach more cranially via a caudal entry point.

Patients are placed in the prone position, and the caudal space is identified using palpation of the sacral hiatus and fluoroscopy. The spinal needle is introduced through the sacral hiatus, and accurate needle placement is ensured using radiopaque contrast and fluoroscopy. To lessen the chance of dural puncture, the needle should not be advanced more cranial than S3 given that the dural sac typically ends at the S2 level. Real-time or "live" fluoroscopy is used to rule out placement in an epidural vein, although some techniques also use a test dose of lidocaine with epinephrine. Once placement is verified, the medication is slowly injected. Post-injection wash-out views on fluoroscopy are used to confirm spread of the injectate to the target level.

Evidence

There have been six RCTs on caudal ESIs for the treatment of sciatica, three of which have included a diagnosis of low back pain.[8] Unfortunately, none of these studies were performed with fluoroscopy.[28–30] One study showed significantly decreased pain after three ESIs, although results were confounded by treatments outside the study protocol.[28]

For the diagnosis of lumbar spinal stenosis (LSS), which often includes symptoms of neurogenic claudication or radicular pain with or without low back pain, caudal injections were recently studied. In 2008, 40 patients were randomized to fluoroscopically guided caudal injection with either 9 mL lidocaine and 2 mL normal saline, or 9 mL lidocaine, 6 mg betamethasone, and 2 mL normal saline.[31] Multiple injections were allowed throughout the 12-month follow-up period. Success was defined as at least a 50% decrease in numeric pain rating scale and a 40% decrease in the Oswestry Disability Index. There were equivalent results, with approximately 60% success in both the anesthetic alone and the anesthetic plus betamethasone groups at 12 months.[31] A significant weakness of this study includes unlimited injections throughout the follow-up period, with an unknown amount of time between last injection and follow-up points and a nonstandard intention-to-treat analysis. Additionally, the level of stenosis being targeted was not reported.

There is not sufficient evidence for the use of caudal ESIs in the treatment of axial low back pain with our without radicular pain. There is also insufficient evidence to support the use of caudal ESIs for the treatment of LSS.

IL

Technique

The IL technique achieves access to the epidural space preferably one spinal segment below the suspected pathology using a paramedian or midline approach. The route of the needle from superficial to deep includes the skin, subcutaneous tissue, paraspinal muscles (paramedian approach) or interspinous ligament (midline approach), ligamentum flavum, then entry into the epidural space. Some practitioners avoid the IL approach if there has been surgery at the site of intended injection, especially laminectomy, given derangement of the anatomy and a higher risk of dural puncture. The most common means to identify entry into the epidural space is the loss of resistance technique, which can be lost with epidural scarring. Fluoroscopy with radiopaque contrast is used to confirm epidural placement and exclude vascular flow.

Evidence

There are two controlled studies and one observational study for the treatment with IL ESI for axial low back pain.[8] Serrao and colleagues[32] compared ESI with intrathecal midazolam and found no significant difference at 2-month follow-up. An earlier RCT included 39 patients with axial low back pain and radicular symptoms treated with ESI or interspinous saline. There was significant improvement in the steroid group at 1- and 3-month follow-up; however, specific results for low back pain are not known, and fluoroscopy was not used.[33] There is also an observational study that reported pain improvement of 25% to 35% of subjects for greater than 1 year after either one TF or IL ESI.[34] Without a control group, however, and a large drop out rate, these results are difficult to interpret. There is insufficient evidence for the use of nonfluoroscopically guided IL ESIs for the treatment of axial low back pain.

For the treatment of LSS, there is a single, small, randomized controlled study on a single fluoroscopically guided IL ESI. In 2009, Koc and colleagues[35] compared IL ESI with a physical therapy control for the treatment of LSS. Patients had both lower extremity and axial low back pain. The ESI was targeted to the most stenotic level via epidural catheter. The therapy group had 2 weeks of inpatient physical therapy, and all groups (including a third control arm) received diclofenac and a home exercise program. All groups had significant improvements in visual analog scale and Roland Morris Disability Inquiry at up to 6-month follow-up. The ESI group was superior only at 2 weeks.[35] There are some who argue that a single epidural injection may not be sufficient, and that better outcomes may be possible with including up to three injections if pain returns. Currently, however, there is inconclusive evidence for IL ESIs for the treatment of LSS.

There are several studies on IL ESIs for the treatment of failed back surgery syndrome (FBSS), also known as postlaminectomy syndrome. These patients usually are symptomatic of axial low back pain and radicular symptoms, and treatment effect is not specified for one or the other in most of the literature. In 1989, Rocco and colleagues[36] studied 22 patients still symptomatic after laminectomy and randomized them to receive epidural lidocaine with triamcinolone or morphine, or both. After three IL injections at the location of the patients' pain, there was no difference between groups, suggesting no benefit of epidural steroid. Nonetheless, it is unknown if fluoroscopic guidance was used, and there was no clear control group. Another study on recurrent low back pain after laminectomy randomized 206 patients to nonfluoroscopically guided IL injection with anesthetic plus methylprednisolone or indomethicin, or both.[37] All groups had decreased average pain at 2 weeks, and there was no further follow-up. The short-term follow-up is a major limitation of this study and precludes any interpretation of results. Additionally, the injection was done above the level of operation and presumed source of pain. Many would argue that medication flow in the epidural space is predominately cranial, and epidural injection should always be from below the target level to maximize medication delivery to the presumed source of pain.[38] There is no evidence for the use of nonfluoroscopically guided IL ESI for the treatment of low back pain in FBSS. There are no available studies for the treatment of FBSS with fluoroscopically guided IL ESI.

Overall, there are many studies on the use of IL ESIs performed without fluoroscopic guidance that do not show any conclusive benefit for the treatment of axial low back pain in general, or in the setting of LSS or FBSS. One small study suggests that a single, large-volume, fluoroscopically guided IL ESI is not superior to physical therapy in the treatment of LSS.

Transforaminal

Technique
The TF approach is considered to be more specific, delivering the injectate directly to the site of pathology at the ventral epidural space next to the disc, the dorsal root ganglion, and the nerve root. The technique involves using fluoroscopy to identify a subpedicular target within the intervertebral foramen. The needle is advanced to achieve a perineural location in the so-called "safe triangle" that lies just below the pedicle and above the dural sleeve of the target nerve root. Precautions are taken to avoid advancing the needle tip medial to the six o'clock position of the pedicle in the AP (anteroposterior) view to avoid dural puncture.

Technique to target the S1 nerve root in its foramen is somewhat analogous to the subpedicular approach at lumbar levels. The target point for an S1 TF ESI is on the caudal border of the S1 pedicle, just dorsal to the internal opening of the S1 anterior sacral foramen. The needle is inserted into the posterior sacral foramen just short of the floor of the sacral canal and lateral to the six o'clock position of the pedicle.[39]

Real-time or ("live") fluoroscopy or digital subtraction angiography is used to rule out vascular flow. The anesthetic is injected first, and a pause of 60 to 90 seconds is conducted to monitor for central nervous system adverse effects, which are generally thought of as reversible (seizures, transient paresis, and respiratory depression), and an additional indicator of intravascular injection. The corticosteroid or other medication is then injected and post-injection "wash-out" images are taken to confirm flow of the medication to the target.

Selective nerve root block

In practice and in the literature, the terms selective nerve root block (SNRB) and TF ESI are often used interchangeably. The term SNRB describes a highly selective TF injection in which the interventionalist anesthetizes a single specific nerve root/dorsal root ganglion to confirm or refute it as the source of pain.[40] The selective nature of the nerve root block applies if the injectate/anesthetic travels only to the target nerve root and not medially into the epidural space. It has recently been demonstrated, however, that with as little as 0.5 cc of contrast directed via SNRB at L4 and L5, epidural flow to an adjacent level can be seen.[41] With standard doses of 1 to 2 mL of anesthetic used, these injections are likely often nonselective or at least only partially selective.

Evidence

For radicular pain, there are two recent RCTs supporting the efficacy of TF ESI. Decreased surgical rates and decreased pain scores at 12-month follow-up have been noted.[42,43] There are no RCTs on the use of TF ESIs for the management of axial low back pain in isolation. There are no studies on TF ESI for the treatment of primarily axial low back pain in FBSS.

There have been several studies on the treatment of LSS with TF ESI. They show favorable response, but include patients with axial low back pain and significant radicular pain, making interpretation specifically for the treatment of low back pain difficult.[42,44,45] For axial low back pain in isolation, Lee and colleagues[46] compared treatment with TF versus IL ESIs in 102 subjects with LSS and 103 with herniated nucleus pulposus. Success was defined as a decrease in the numeric pain rating scale of at least 2 points and patient satisfaction. All groups showed significant improvement. The LSS patients treated with TF ESI showed statistically significant greater success than those treated with IL ESI.[46] There was not a significant difference in the rate of success between the TF and IL routes in those with herniated nucleus pulposus. The fact that all groups significantly improved suggests that ESIs may be effective for the treatment of axial low back pain caused by herniated disc or LSS. The lack of a control group, however, significantly limits this conclusion. What can be concluded is that TF ESI is likely superior to IL ESI in the treatment of axial low back pain caused by LSS.

IL Versus TF

Injectate flow

The primary contention for using the TF approach in preference to the IL approach is that it delivers the medication directly to the ventral epidural space, in closer proximity to the presumed target of the disc or dorsal root ganglion. Studies evaluating contrast patterns generally support this concept in the lumbar spine.

Botwin and colleagues[38] evaluated the contrast patterns in lumbar IL injections in 2004 and found that approximately one-third revealed ventral contrast flow, and 16% were bilateral. In contrast, Manchikanti and colleagues[47] evaluated lumbar TF ESI flow patterns and demonstrated ventral epidural filling in 88% of the procedures and nerve root sleeve filling in 97% of procedures. These two studies suggest better epidural flow to the anterior structures with TF approach. Conversely, a prospective evaluation of contrast flow patterns with fluoroscopically guided lumbar ESI compared the lateral parasagittal IL (PIL) approach with the TF approach. The PIL approach was superior to the TF approach for placing contrast into the ventral epidural space, with reduction in fluoroscopy times and improved spread.[48] In general, a more lateral approach, TF or PIL, will be more likely to produce ventral flow than a midline or paramedian IL injection. This may differ from the cervical spine, as a recent analysis of contrast patterns for cervical IL epidural injections using the midline approach found rate of ventral epidural spread from this posterior approach was 56.7% with 1 cc and 90% with 2 cc of injectate.[49]

Evidence

The effectiveness of TF versus IL ESIs has been compared, and the results are mixed. Schaufele evaluated the effectiveness of TF versus IL ESI for the treatment of symptomatic lumbar disc herniations and found TF injections resulted in better short-term pain improvement and fewer long-term surgical interventions than the IL ESI.[50] Ackerman and Ahmad[51] compared TF, IL, and caudal approaches for treating lumbar disc herniations and found that pain relief was significantly more effective with TF injections. As noted in the discussion of TF ESI evidence, treatment with TF versus IL ESIs was compared in patients with axial low back pain, 102 with LSS, and 103 with herniated nucleus pulposus.[46] All groups showed significant improvement, but the LSS patients treated with TF ESI showed statistically significant greater improvement than those treated with IL ESI.[46] There was not, however, a significant difference in success between techniques in those with herniated nucleus pulposus. The evidence suggests that TF ESI may be more effective than IL ESI for treating axial low back pain, especially in LSS. It should be noted, however, that neither the TF nor the IL technique has been shown to have clear benefit over control for the treatment of axial LBP.

ESI SUMMARY

Although the literature collectively demonstrates that lumbosacral ESIs may be effective in treating radicular pain caused by herniated nucleus pulposus or lumbar central stenosis, there is insufficient evidence for the routine use of lumbar ESI for treating subacute or chronic axial low back pain. There may be a role for ESIs in specific diagnoses, such as LSS, although conclusive evidence is currently lacking. Some physicians have suggested that though ESIs may not be therapeutic for axial low back pain, they may be considered as a diagnostic tool to determine whether structures within the epidural space are contributing to a patient's pain in an effort to help guide other treatments. Whether for diagnostic or therapeutic purposes, ESIs should not be a primary treatment for axial low back pain and further evidence to confirm efficacy is needed before they are considered for the routine use within a comprehensive rehabilitation treatment plan.

REFERENCES

1. Lievre JA, Bloch-Michel H, Attali P. [Epidural hydrocortisone in the treatment of sciatica]. Rev Rhum Mal Osteoartic 1955;22(9–10):696–7 [in French].
2. Benzon HT. Epidural steroid injections for low back pain and lumbosacral radiculopathy. Pain 1986;24(3):277–95.
3. Gardner WJ, Goebert HW Jr, Sehgal AD. Intraspinal corticosteroids in the treatment of sciatica. Trans Am Neurol Assoc 1961;86:214–5.
4. Saal JS, Franson RC, Dobrow R, et al. High levels of inflammatory phospholipase A2 activity in lumbar disc herniations. Spine (Phila Pa 1976) 1990;15(7):674–8.

5. Furusawa N, Baba H, Miyoshi N, et al. Herniation of cervical intervertebral disc: immunohistochemical examination and measurement of nitric oxide production. Spine (Phila Pa 1976) 2001;26(10):1110–6.

6. Kang JD, Georgescu HI, McIntyre-Larkin L, et al. Herniated cervical intervertebral discs spontaneously produce matrix metalloproteinases, nitric oxide, interleukin-6, and prostaglandin E2. Spine (Phila Pa 1976) 1995;20(22):2373–8.

7. Friedly J, Chan L, Deyo R. Increases in lumbosacral injections in the Medicare population: 1994 to 2001. Spine (Phila Pa 1976) 2007;32(16):1754–60.

8. DePalma MJ, Slipman CW. Evidence-informed management of chronic low back pain with epidural steroid injections. Spine J 2008;8(1):45–55.

9. Botwin KP, Gruber RD, Bouchlas CG, et al. Complications of fluoroscopically guided caudal epidural injections. Am J Phys Med Rehabil 2001;80(6):416–24.

10. Goodman BS, Posecion LW, Mallempati S, et al. Complications and pitfalls of lumbar interlaminar and transforaminal epidural injections. Curr Rev Musculoskelet Med 2008;1:212–22.

11. Raj P, editor. Pain medicine a comprehensive review. St Louis (MO): Mosby; 1996. p. 188–9.

12. Houten JK, Errico TJ. Paraplegia after lumbosacral nerve root block: report of three cases. Spine J 2002;2(1):70–5.

13. Conners J, Wojack J. Interventional neuroradiology: strategies and practical techniques. Philadelphia: WB Saunders Company; 1999.

14. Boll DT, Bulow H, Blackham KA, et al. MDCT angiography of the spinal vasculature and the artery of Adamkiewicz. AJR Am J Roentgenol 2006;187(4):1054–60.

15. Kennedy DJ, Dreyfuss P, Aprill CN, et al. Paraplegia following image-guided transforaminal lumbar spine epidural steroid injection: two case reports. Pain Med 2009;10(8):1389–94.

16. Bogduk N, Christophidis N, Cherry D, et al. Epidural use of steroids in the management of back pain and sciatica of spinal origin. Report of the working party on epidural use of steroids in the management of back pain. Canberra (Australia): National Health and Medical Research Council; 1993.

17. Kepes ER, Duncalf D. Treatment of backache with spinal injections of local anesthetics, spinal and systemic steroids. A review. Pain 1985;22(1):33–47.

18. Koes BW, Scholten RJ, Mens JM, et al. Efficacy of epidural steroid injections for low back pain and sciatica: a systematic review of randomized clinical trials. Pain 1995;63(3):279–88.

19. Derby R, Kine G, Saal JA, et al. Response to steroid and duration of radicular pain as predictors of surgical outcome. Spine (Phila Pa 1976) 1992;17(Suppl 6):S176–83.

20. Lutz GE, Vad VB, Wisneski RJ. Fluoroscopic transforaminal lumbar epidural steroids: an outcome study. Arch Phys Med Rehabil 1998;79(11):1362–6.

21. Renfrew DL, Moore TE, Kathol MH, et al. Correct placement of epidural steroid injections: fluoroscopic guidance and contrast administration. AJNR Am J Neuroradiol 1991;12(5):1003–7.

22. Stitz MY, Sommer HM. Accuracy of blind versus fluoroscopically guided caudal epidural injection. Spine (Phila Pa 1976) 1999;24(13):1371–6.

23. White AH, Derby R, Wynne G. Epidural injections for the diagnosis and treatment of low-back pain. Spine (Phila Pa 1976) 1980;5(1):78–86.

24. Mehta M, Salmon N. Extradural block. Confirmation of the injection site by X-ray monitoring. Anaesthesia 1985;40(10):1009–12.

25. Cluff R, Mehio AK, Cohen SP, et al. The technical aspects of epidural steroid injections: a national survey. Anesth Analg 2002;95(2):403–8.

26. Chen B, Stitik T. Epidural steroid injections. Emedicine. Available at: http://emedicine.medscape.com/. Accessed February 20, 2010.
27. Bryan B, Lutz C, Lutz G. Fluoroscopic assessment of epidural contrast spread after caudal injection. Proceedings of the International Spine Intervention Society Annual Scientific Meeting. Las Vegas, July, 1999.
28. Mathews JA, Mills SB, Jenkins VM, et al. Back pain and sciatica: controlled trials of manipulation, traction, sclerosant and epidural injections. Br J Rheumatol 1987;26(6):416–23.
29. Brievik H, Hsla P, Molnar I, et al. Treatment of chronic low back pain and sciatica. Comparison of caudal epidural injections of bupivacaine and methylprednisolone with bupivacaine followed by saline. Adv Pain Res Ther 1976;1:927–32.
30. Yates DW. A comparison of the types of epidural injection commonly used in the treatment of low back pain and sciatica. Rheumatol Rehabil 1978;17(3): 181–6.
31. Manchikanti L, Cash KA, McManus CD, et al. Preliminary results of a randomized, equivalence trial of fluoroscopic caudal epidural injections in managing chronic low back pain: part 4—spinal stenosis. Pain Physician 2008;11(6):833–48.
32. Serrao JM, Marks RL, Morley SJ, et al. Intrathecal midazolam for the treatment of chronic mechanical low back pain: a controlled comparison with epidural steroid in a pilot study. Pain 1992;48(1):5–12.
33. Helliwell M, Roberson J, Ellia R. Outpatient treatment of low back pain and sciatica by a single extradural corticosteroid injection. Br J Clin Pract 1985;39:228–31.
34. Buttermann GR. The effect of spinal steroid injections for degenerative disc disease. Spine J 2004;4(5):495–505.
35. Koc Z, Ozcakir S, Sivrioglu K, et al. Effectiveness of physical therapy and epidural steroid injections in lumbar spinal stenosis. Spine (Phila Pa 1976) 2009;34(10):985–9.
36. Rocco AG, Frank E, Kaul AF, et al. Epidural steroids, epidural morphine and epidural steroids combined with morphine in the treatment of postlaminectomy syndrome. Pain 1989;36(3):297–303.
37. Aldrete JA. Epidural injections of indomethacin for postlaminectomy syndrome: a preliminary report. Anesth Analg 2003;96(2):463–8.
38. Botwin KP, Natalicchio J, Hanna A. Fluoroscopic guided lumbar interlaminar epidural injections: a prospective evaluation of epidurography contrast patterns and anatomical review of the epidural space. Pain Physician 2004;7(1):77–80.
39. Bogduk N. International Spine Intervention Society practice guidelines for spinal diagnostic and treatment procedures. 1st edition. San Francisco (CA): Library of Congress Cataloging in Publication Data; 2004.
40. Furman MB, Lee TS, Mehta A, et al. Contrast flow selectivity during transforaminal lumbosacral epidural steroid injections. Pain Physician 2008;11(6):855–61.
41. Vassiliev D. Spread of contrast during L4 and L5 nerve root infiltration under fluoroscopic guidance. Pain Physician 2007;10(3):461–6.
42. Riew KD, Yin Y, Gilula L, et al. The effect of nerve-root injections on the need for operative treatment of lumbar radicular pain. A prospective, randomized, controlled, double-blind study. J Bone Joint Surg Am 2000;82(11):1589–93.
43. Vad VB, Bhat AL, Lutz GE, et al. Transforaminal epidural steroid injections in lumbosacral radiculopathy: a prospective randomized study. Spine (Phila Pa 1976) 2002;27(1):11–6.
44. Ng L, Chaudhary N, Sell P. The efficacy of corticosteroids in periradicular infiltration for chronic radicular pain: a randomized, double-blind, controlled trial. Spine (Phila Pa 1976) 2005;30(8):857–62.

45. Botwin KP, Gruber RD, Bouchlas CG, et al. Fluoroscopically guided lumbar trans-formational epidural steroid injections in degenerative lumbar stenosis: an outcome study. Am J Phys Med Rehabil 2002;81(12):898–905.

46. Lee JH, An JH, Lee SH. Comparison of the effectiveness of interlaminar and bilateral transforaminal epidural steroid injections in treatment of patients with lumbosacral disc herniation and spinal stenosis. Clin J Pain 2009;25(3):206–10.

47. Manchikanti L, Cash KA, Pampati V, et al. Evaluation of lumbar transforaminal epidural injections with needle placement and contrast flow patterns: a prospective, descriptive report. Pain Physician 2004;7(2):217–23.

48. Candido KD, Raghavendra MS, Chinthagada M, et al. A prospective evaluation of iodinated contrast flow patterns with fluoroscopically guided lumbar epidural steroid injections: the lateral parasagittal interlaminar epidural approach versus the transforaminal epidural approach. Anesth Analg 2008;106(2):638–44.

49. Kim KS, Shin SS, Kim TS, et al. Fluoroscopically guided cervical interlaminar epidural injections using the midline approach: an analysis of epidurography contrast patterns. Anesth Analg 2009;108(5):1658–61.

50. Schaufele MK, Hatch L, Jones W. Interlaminar versus transforaminal epidural injections for the treatment of symptomatic lumbar intervertebral disc herniations. Pain Physician 2006;9(4):361–6.

51. Ackerman WE 3rd, Ahmad M. The efficacy of lumbar epidural steroid injections in patients with lumbar disc herniations. Anesth Analg 2007;104(5):1217–22.

Sacroiliac Joint and Lumbar Zygapophysial Joint Corticosteroid Injections

David J. Kennedy, MD[a],*, Max Shokat, DO[a],
Christopher J. Visco, MD[b]

KEYWORDS

- Sacroiliac joint • Lumbar zygapophysial joints
- Corticosteroid injection • Intra-articular corticosteroid injection

The sacroiliac joint (SIJ) and the lumbar zygapophysial joints (z-joints) are both innervated diarthrodial synovial articulations. They have been repeatedly shown to be potential pain generators.[1–3] These joints both have demonstrated pain-referral patterns based on pain diagrams from joint distension with saline, joint electrical stimulation, and pain relief obtained from image-guided anesthetic blocks.[2,4,5] These specific pain-referral patterns are beyond the scope of this article and are covered elsewhere.

The ability to diagnose either the z-joint or the SIJ joint as the primary pain generator on historical features, physical examination, and/or diagnostic imaging is not absolute.[6,7] Studies have mainly focused on anesthetic block as the standard and best diagnostic test, specifically with dual comparative anesthetic blocks giving the highest diagnostic yield.[6] A dual comparative anesthetic block requires the patient to undergo the same block on separate occasions, with a different local anesthetic at each occasion. A positive result is one in which the patient obtains short-lasting relief with the use of a short-acting anesthetic and longer relief with the use of a long-acting anesthetic.[8] Using this method, the prevalence of z-joint pain approaches 30% in older patients.[9] Sacroiliac joint pain prevalence is not as clear in the literature, and has reported rates ranging from 13% to 63%.[10]

[a] Department of Orthopaedics and Rehabilitation, University of Florida College of Medicine, PO Box 112727, Gainesville, FL 32611, USA
[b] Department of Rehabilitation and Regenerative Medicine, Columbia University College of Physicians and Surgeons, 180 Fort Washington Avenue, HP 199, New York, NY 10032, USA
* Corresponding author.
E-mail address: kennedj@ortho.ufl.edu

Phys Med Rehabil Clin N Am 21 (2010) 835–842
doi:10.1016/j.pmr.2010.06.009
1047-9651/10/$ – see front matter © 2010 Elsevier Inc. All rights reserved.

Injectable corticosteroids are often used in other inflammatory and noninflammatory musculoskeletal conditions, such as tendinitis, tenosynovitis, arthritis, and other musculoskeletal complaints. Intra-articular corticosteroid injections may decrease pain by other potential mechanisms, including the decrease of prostaglandin and leukotriene synthesis, polymorphic nucleocyte migration, modulation of peripheral nociceptor neurons and direct membrane stabilization mechanism, modulation of spinal cord dorsal horn cells, and might even possibly have a slight anesthetic effect.[11–13] It is for these reasons that corticosteroid injections are widely used for SIJ- and z-joint–mediated pain. In fact, the injection of corticosteroid in the lumbar z-joints is one of the most common pain procedures performed in the United States.[14]

Despite the widespread use, there is scant literature on the efficacy of intra-articular corticosteroid injections to treat either SIJ or z-joint pain. Multiple factors may contribute to this, including poor patient selection criteria, as well as potential large systemic effects from the injection of a corticosteroid. Furthermore, there are no studies using dual anesthetic blocks as selection criteria before the injection of corticosteroids. Often the patient selection is based on history, clinical examination, and correlation with imaging findings. This article reviews the literature for the basis of therapeutic intra-articular injection of corticosteroid in the SIJ and the lumbar z-joints.

PROCEDURE GUIDANCE

The accuracy of these injections has been shown to be quite low when using only anatomic landmark guidance without the assistance of any type of image guidance.[7] A variety of image guidance options have been used to ensure accurate needle placement, including fluoroscopy, ultrasound, and computed tomography (CT scans). Fluoroscopic guidance for spine procedures has a few specific benefits, one being the ability to visualize contrast flow in "real time" to help avoid an intravascular injection or otherwise unwanted location for the needle tip as it is being directed to the target location. Second, the confirmation of the needle in the intra-articular space can be accomplished under fluoroscopy by use of a small amount of contrast. Ultrasound guidance and CT guidance have also been used. These procedures confirm an intra-articular injection by guiding the bevel deep to the capsule in the case of diarthrodial joints; however, the major pitfall of using these forms of guidance is the inability to visualize vascular flow of an injection. Without image guidance, the procedure cannot specifically be labeled an SIJ or z-joint injection.

As evidenced by this issue of *Physical Medicine and Rehabilitation Clinics of North America,* there are a large number of potential pain generators in the lumbar spine. Needle localization becomes important as we seek to be clear and communicate the exact procedure we are performing. For instance, is it the intra-articular SIJ that was injected, the posterior ligamentous structures, or both? It becomes imperative to correctly identify the primary pain generator to target an intervention. This is all despite the poor correlation between accuracy and efficacy in corticosteroid injections. The literature is profuse with studies on nonspecific low-back pain. The addition of nonspecific (nonguided) treatments to the mix does not improve our clinical acumen. Algorithms have been proposed for the diagnosis and treatment of back pain, but fail to recognize the subtle and varied individual differences in patients, and generally poor treatment effect of many of these procedures.[15] Subgrouping patients by clinical characteristics, physical examination maneuvers, imaging studies, and possibly diagnostic blocks can help to correctly identify a treatment subgroup.

This is particularly the case when a specific joint may be targeted, as in a therapeutic injection as an adjunct to a comprehensive treatment plan.

THE SACROILIAC JOINT

The SIJ is a diarthrodial joint that receives innervation from the lumbosacral nerve roots and has demonstrated nociceptive and proprioceptive afferent units.[16] It is an established potential source of buttock pain with or without lower extremity pain.[17,18] Pain-referral patterns have been established based on provocation and analgesic response with a local anesthetic in both asymptomatic volunteers and patients with pain.[5,19,20]

There is currently no accepted gold standard for the diagnosis of SIJ-mediated pain on either clinical examination or interventional procedure.[16] Similar to most joint disorders, imaging studies collectively have had limited utility and poor correlation with symptoms. The lone exception is the bone scan, which has demonstrated a high specificity but low sensitivity for sacroiliitis.[21]

Studies evaluating physical examination provocative maneuvers have had mixed results when compared with image-guided intra-articular injection of local anesthetic. Using greater than 90% pain relief with this procedure, Dreyfuss and colleagues[22] demonstrated the single most sensitive physical examination maneuver was point of maximal pain over the sacral sulcus with a sensitivity of 60%. Later studies have shown increased sensitivity and specificity with a combination of physical examination maneuvers, but still less than those diagnosed with an intra-articular injection of a local anesthetic.[23,24]

Because the historical features, physical examination, and imaging often leave the diagnosis in doubt, some have taken to using image-guided, intra-articular injection of anesthetics to further aide in the diagnosis. There have been multiple studies on the use of a single diagnostic injection, and the false positive range being 20% to 54% for uncontrolled single blocks.[9] This has further led to the use of dual diagnostic injections with either a placebo or comparative local anesthetics with differing duration of action to confirm SIJ pain. Collectively, these studies demonstrate the level of evidence of diagnostic SIJ injections to be moderate, but higher than provocative physical examination maneuvers. Using controlled, comparative diagnostic injections, the prevalence of SIJ pain has been demonstrated at 10% to 27%.[7] Because there is no collectively agreed on gold standard diagnostic test for SIJ-mediated pain, a combination of multiple physical examination maneuvers and controlled local anesthetic instillation may currently be the best tools available to identify the SIJ as the primary pain generator.

When reviewing the literature on intra-articular corticosteroids, the lack of a gold standard for the diagnosis of SIJ-mediated pain and the requirement of image guidance must both be taken into consideration. To date, there have been only 4 randomized controlled trials and 14 observational reports on the efficacy of intra-articular steroid injections into the SIJ. The recurring issue with most of these studies is the appropriate selection of patients. Selection criteria are frequently made on historical features and physical examination only, and occasionally with a single diagnostic block. Despite this lack of rigor in patient selection, lasting improvements in pain, disability, and work status have been demonstrated in therapeutic SIJ corticosteroid injections in those who had pain relief following a single diagnostic anesthetic injection into the SIJ.[25]

Studies have also primarily evaluated patients with spondyloarthropathy, and most had follow-up that did not extend beyond 6 months. These studies demonstrate a positive effect of corticosteroid injections in those with SIJ-mediated pain in spondyloarthropathy; however, the literature is less clear in those without spondyloarthropathy. In addition, if strict criteria are set for the requirement of comparative blocks in combination with provocative physical examination maneuvers, none of the studies to date are sufficient. This lack of robust literature has led some to state there is no evidence supporting or refuting the use of therapeutic intra-articular injections of corticosteorids for SIJ-mediated pain.[16]

Another controversial issue concerning the SIJ is the potential discrepancy between the location of the pain and the location of the injection. The joint space is thought to have ventral and dorsal innervation; additionally, the pain may be coming from the synovial joint itself versus periarticular soft tissues, specifically the ligaments. There are multiple ligamentous connections surrounding the SIJ, including the sacroiliac, sacrotuberous, and sacrospinal ligaments, which may contribute to pain. One double-blind, controlled study comparing periarticular corticosteroid injections with saline and lidocaine in those with and without spondyloarthropathy demonstrated significant short-term pain relief.[26] Another study using ultrasound guidance demonstrated positive outcomes with both intra-articular and periarticular corticosteroid injections, without any statistically significant difference between groups at 4 weeks.[27] Although the use of periarticular injections may be a cost-effective and safe alternative, the nonguided injection should be considered a soft tissue injection because of the inability to confirm presence of the injectate or needle in the intra-articular space.

LUMBAR ZYGAPOPHYSIAL JOINTS

The lumbar z-joints are paired synovial joints formed by the articulation of the superior articular process with the inferior articular processes of consecutive vertebrae, and they are commonly referred to by the nonspecific term of facet joints.[28] They are innervated by the medial branches of the dorsal rami of the lumbar nerve roots.[28] Studies have shown that the z-joint can be a source of back pain in healthy volunteers and that in certain cases back pain can be relieved by anesthetizing the joint.[4,29,30] Interventions directed at the z-joint and the medial branches innervating it include medial branch blocks and radiofrequency denervation as well as intra-articular corticosteroid injection. Collectively, interventions directed at the z-joint represent the most commonly used procedure code in interventional spine centers throughout the United States.[31]

Similar to the SIJ, studies using controlled diagnostic blocks of the z-joint have demonstrated no specific clinical features to be diagnostic of z-joint–mediated pain.[32,33] Likewise, studies have demonstrated that the radiographic appearance of the z-joint does not correlate with patients' symptoms.[34,35] The failure of multiple studies to identify any clinical features or radiographic findings that are indicative of lumbar z-joint pain leaves the diagnostic block as the only means of consistently diagnosing this entity with any certantity.[9] Diagnostic blocks should be controlled because single blocks have a demonstrated high false-positive rate.[36] In formal studies, the false-positive response and placebo response have been encountered in as many as 25% to 41% of patients tested.[36–38]

The pain relief required to label a block as positive is controversial. Most studies label a 50% reduction in pain as a positive block with clinical significance. There is, however, a vocal opposition to the use of a 50% pain reduction. Bogduk[14] and others have argued that using a 50% pain reduction may leave other potential pain generators undiscovered and also potentially generate a higher percentage of false-positive responses owing to the placebo effect.

The reported prevalence of z-joint–mediated pain is controversial because of the variable definition and degree of pain for a positive block. Using controlled blocks with 50% pain reduction as a positive block, the prevalence of z-joint–mediated pain has been reported at 15% in injured workers, 40% in older patients without trauma, and about 45% in a heterogeneous population in pain clinics.[32,37–40] Studies that required 90% or complete pain relief showed lower prevalence of 6% to 7% up to 34% in an elderly population.[39,41,42]

Similar to the SIJ, it is imperative to understand the methodology used to correctly identify the z-joint as the pain generator in each study. To date, there has not been a randomized controlled trial using dual comparative blocks as selection criteria for those receiving intra-articular corticosteroids. Currently, the published literature mostly consists of observational cohorts and descriptive studies that used back pain as the sole selection criterion. This has resulted in obviously varied results. Multiple observational studies with fewer than 100 subjects and follow-ups ranging from 6 weeks to 6 months have demonstrated significant variations in percentage of patients obtaining complete relief, ranging from 0% to 70%.[43–48] When pooled, the collective data show 47% have an initial positive response with a decay to 24% and 4 to 6 weeks, and stabilizing at 18% to 22% at 3 and 6 months.[14]

In addition to these observational cohorts, there have been a few controlled studies. Lilius and colleagues[49] compared 3 interventions in those with back pain: intra-articular corticosteroids, intramuscular corticosteroids, and intra-articular saline.[50] The groups did not differ significantly in their pain outcomes recorded at 2-month intervals out to 1-year follow-up. In a separate study, Marks and colleagues[51] showed that patients receiving intra-articular corticosteroid did not have a significantly greater proportion of those with either good or excellent results at up to 3 months when compared with those receiving only a medial branch block. The study by Carette and colleagues[42] is the only one to date to compare outcomes of intra-articular steroids with saline in patients with z-joint pain diagnosed by a single anesthetic block with 50% pain relief. At 1 and 3 months there was no difference in outcomes between the groups; however, at 6 months the steroid group had statistically better pain scores than those who received saline. The timing of this effect does not correspond with the known effect of corticosteroids and has thus led some to feel these data are spurious.[14]

Collectively, the literature is limited as to the benefit of intra-articular corticosteroids. This lack of literature has led some to state that they are ineffective in the treatment of z-joint–mediated back pain, especially when compared with techniques with more robust efficacy literature such as radiofrequency denervation.[9]

SUMMARY

Both the SIJ and the lumbar z-joint are synovial joints capable of producing pain. They are amenable to image-guided intra-articular injection with corticosteroids, a procedure that is commonly performed. The ability to correctly diagnose either as the source of pain relies on improving the diagnostic yield of the physical examination by anesthetizing the involved joint with an interventional procedure. To date, limited studies have been conducted with patients selected via comparative diagnostic blocks. Thus, despite their widespread use, the utility of intra-articular corticosteroid injections into either joint is still uncertain.

REFERENCES

1. Cohen SP, Stojanovic MP, Crooks M, et al. Lumbar zygapophysial (facet) joint radiofrequency denervation success as a function of pain relief during diagnostic medial branch blocks: a multicenter analysis. Spine J 2008;8(3):498–504.
2. Windsor RE, King FJ, Roman SJ, et al. Electrical stimulation induced lumbar medial branch referral patterns. Pain Physician 2002;5(4):347–53.
3. Cooper G, Bailey B, Bogduk N. Cervical zygapophysial joint pain maps. Pain Med 2007;8(4):344–53.
4. Mooney V, Robertson J. The facet syndrome. Clin Orthop Relat Res 1976;115:149–56.
5. Slipman CW, Jackson HB, Lipetz JS, et al. Sacroiliac joint pain referral zones. Arch Phys Med Rehabil 2000;81(3):334–8.
6. Bogduk N. Diagnosing lumbar zygapophysial joint pain. Pain Med 2005;6(2):139–42.
7. Dreyfuss P, Dreyer SJ, Cole A, et al. Sacroiliac joint pain. J Am Acad Orthop Surg 2004;12(4):255.
8. Bogduk N. Evidence-informed management of chronic low back pain with facet injections and radiofrequency neurotomy Spine J 8(1):56–64.
9. Bogduk N. Evidence-informed management of chronic low back pain with facet injections and radiofrequency neurotomy. Spine J 2008;8(1):56–64.
10. Weksler N, Velan GJ, Semionov M, et al. The role of sacroiliac joint dysfunction in the genesis of low back pain: the obvious is not always right. Arch Orthop Trauma Surg 2007;127(10):885–8.
11. Devor M, Govrin-Lippmann R, Raber P. Corticosteroids suppress ectopic neural discharge originating in experimental neuromas. Pain 1985;22(2):127–37.
12. Hall ED. Glucocorticoid effects on serotonergic and noradrenergic facilitation of spinal monosynaptic transmission. Psychiatry Res 1980;2(3):241–50.
13. Johansson A, Hao J, Sjölund B. Local corticosteroid application blocks transmission in normal nociceptive C-fibres. Acta Anaesthesiol Scand 1990;34(5):335–8.
14. Bogduk N. A narrative review of intra-articular corticosteroid injections for low back pain. Pain Med 2005;6(4):287–96.
15. Manchikanti L, Helm S, Singh V, et al. An algorithmic approach for clinical management of chronic spinal pain. Pain Physician 2009;12(4):E225–64.
16. Rupert MP, Lee M, Manchikanti L, et al. Evaluation of sacroiliac joint interventions: a systematic appraisal of the literature. Pain Physician 2009;12(2):399–418.
17. Maigne JY, Aivaliklis A, Pfefer F. Results of sacroiliac joint double block and value of sacroiliac pain provocation tests in 54 patients with low back pain. Spine 1996;21(16):1889–92.
18. Irwin RW, Watson T, Minick RP, et al. Age, body mass index, and gender differences in sacroiliac joint pathology. Am J Phys Med Rehabil 2007;86(1):37–44.
19. Fortin JD, Dwyer AP, West S, et al. Sacroiliac joint: pain referral maps upon applying a new injection/arthrography technique. Part I: asymptomatic volunteers. Spine 1994;19(13):1475–82.
20. Fortin JD, Aprill CN, Ponthieux B, et al. Sacroiliac joint: pain referral maps upon applying a new injection/arthrography technique. Part II: clinical evaluation. Spine 1994;19(13):1483–9.
21. Hancock MJ, Maher CG, Latimer J, et al. Systematic review of tests to identify the disc, SIJ or facet joint as the source of low back pain. Eur Spine J 2007;16(10):1539–50.
22. Dreyfuss PH, Dreyer SJ, Herring SA. Lumbar zygapophysial (facet) joint injections. Spine 1995;20(18):2040–7.

23. van der Wurff P, Buijs EJ, Groen GJ. A multitest regimen of pain provocation tests as an aid to reduce unnecessary minimally invasive sacroiliac joint procedures. Arch Phys Med Rehabil 2006;87(1):10–4.

24. Berthelot J, Labat J, Le Goff B, et al. Provocative sacroiliac joint maneuvers and sacroiliac joint block are unreliable for diagnosing sacroiliac joint pain. Joint Bone Spine 2006;73(1):17–23.

25. Slipman CW, Lipetz JS, Plastaras CT, et al. Fluoroscopically guided therapeutic sacroiliac joint injections for sacroiliac joint syndrome. Am J Phys Med Rehabil 2001;80(6):425–32.

26. Luukkainen RK, Wennerstrand PV, Kautiainen HH, et al. Efficacy of periarticular corticosteroid treatment of the sacroiliac joint in non-spondylarthropathic patients with chronic low back pain in the region of the sacroiliac joint. Clin Exp Rheumatol 2002;20(1):52–4.

27. Hartung W, Ross CJ, Straub R, et al. Ultrasound-guided sacroiliac joint injection in patients with established sacroiliitis: precise IA injection verified by MRI scanning does not predict clinical outcome. Rheumatology (Oxford) 2009. Available at: http://www.ncbi.nlm.nih.gov.ezproxy.galter.northwestern.edu/pubmed/20019067. Accessed May 10, 2010.

28. Bogduk N. Clinical anatomy of the lumbar spine and sacrum. 3rd edition. New York: Churchill Livingstone; 1997.

29. McCall IW, Park WM, O'Brien JP. Induced pain referral from posterior lumbar elements in normal subjects. Spine 1979;4(5):441–6.

30. Fairbank JC, Park WM, McCall IW, et al. Apophyseal injection of local anesthetic as a diagnostic aid in primary low-back pain syndromes. Spine 1981;6(6): 598–605.

31. Manchikanti L, Singh V. Interventional pain management: evolving issues for 2003. Pain Physician 2003;6(1):125–37.

32. Schwarzer AC, Aprill CN, Derby R, et al. Clinical features of patients with pain stemming from the lumbar zygapophysial joints. Is the lumbar facet syndrome a clinical entity? Spine 1994;19(10):1132–7.

33. Schwarzer AC, Derby R, Aprill CN, et al. Pain from the lumbar zygapophysial joints: a test of two models. J Spinal Disord 1994;7(4):331–6.

34. Schwarzer AC, Wang SC, O'Driscoll D, et al. The ability of computed tomography to identify a painful zygapophysial joint in patients with chronic low back pain. Spine 1995;20(8):907–12.

35. Lawrence JS, Bremner JM, Bier F. Osteo-arthrosis. Prevalence in the population and relationship between symptoms and x-ray changes. Ann Rheum Dis 1966; 25(1):1–24.

36. Schwarzer AC, Aprill CN, Derby R, et al. The false-positive rate of uncontrolled diagnostic blocks of the lumbar zygapophysial joints. Pain 1994;58(2): 195–200.

37. Manchikanti L, Pampati V, Fellows B, et al. The diagnostic validity and therapeutic value of lumbar facet joint nerve blocks with or without adjuvant agents. Curr Rev Pain 2000;4(5):337–44.

38. Manchikanti L, Pampati V, Fellows B, et al. Prevalence of lumbar facet joint pain in chronic low back pain. Pain Physician 1999;2(3):59–64.

39. Schwarzer AC, Wang SC, Bogduk N, et al. Prevalence and clinical features of lumbar zygapophysial joint pain: a study in an Australian population with chronic low back pain. Ann Rheum Dis 1995;54(2):100–6.

40. Manchikanti L, Pampati V, Fellows B, et al. The inability of the clinical picture to characterize pain from facet joints. Pain Physician 2000;3(2):158–66.

41. Jackson RP, Jacobs RR, Montesano PX. 1988 Volvo award in clinical sciences. Facet joint injection in low-back pain. A prospective statistical study. Spine 1988;13(9):966–71.

42. Carette S, Marcoux S, Truchon R, et al. A controlled trial of corticosteroid injections into facet joints for chronic low back pain. N Engl J Med 1991; 325(14):1002–7.

43. Carrera GF. Lumbar facet joint injection in low back pain and sciatica: preliminary results. Radiology 1980;137(3):665–7.

44. Destouet JM, Gilula LA, Murphy WA, et al. Lumbar facet joint injection: indication, technique, clinical correlation, and preliminary results. Radiology 1982; 145(2):321–5.

45. Carrera GF, Williams AL. Current concepts in evaluation of the lumbar facet joints. Crit Rev Diagn Imaging 1984;21(2):85–104.

46. Lippitt AB. The facet joint and its role in spine pain. Management with facet joint injections. Spine 1984;9(7):746–50.

47. Lau LS, Littlejohn GO, Miller MH. Clinical evaluation of intra-articular injections for lumbar facet joint pain. Med J Aust 1985;143(12-13):563–5.

48. Lynch MC, Taylor JF. Facet joint injection for low back pain. A clinical study. J Bone Joint Surg Br 1986;68(1):138–41.

49. Lilius G, Laasonen EM, Myllynen P, et al. [Lumbar facet joint syndrome. Significance of non-organic signs. A randomized placebo-controlled clinical study]. Rev Chir Orthop Reparatrice Appar Mot 1989;75(7):493–500 [in French].

50. Lilius G, Laasonen EM, Myllynen P, et al. Lumbar facet joint syndrome. A randomised clinical trial. J Bone Joint Surg Br 1989;71(4):681–4.

51. Marks RC, Houston T, Thulbourne T. Facet joint injection and facet nerve block: a randomised comparison in 86 patients with chronic low back pain. Pain 1992;49(3):325–8.

Lumbar and Sacral Radiofrequency Neurotomy

David A. Mazin, MD*, Joseph P. Sullivan, MD, PhD

KEYWORDS

• Radiofrequency • Neurotomy • Lumbar • Sacral • Sacroiliac

RADIOFREQUENCY NEUROTOMY OF THE LUMBAR ZYGAPOPHYSIAL JOINTS

Percutaneous radiofrequency (RF) medial branch neurotomy involves the use of an RF electrode to ablate the nerves that provide painful sensation in the lumbar zygapophysial (Z)-joints for long-term pain relief. RF neurotomy coagulates a length of the medial branch of a dorsal ramus or a dorsal ramus itself (L5), preventing sensation of the painful Z-joint until the nerve regenerates. An interventionist may use safe, valid, diagnostic medial branch blocks to confirm that low back pain is originating from the Z-joints before using RF neurotomy.[1–4]

Z-joints are the paired, posterior articulations between vertebrae composed of a synovial capsule, the articular cartilage, and the superior and inferior articular processes surrounded by a joint capsule. The lumbar Z-joints are pain generators with defined referral patterns.[5] Estimates vary regarding the prevalence of Z-joint pain in patients with chronic lower back pain: approximately 6% in a primary care setting,[6] 15% of younger patients, 40% of older patients seen for spine pain[7,8]; and 16% of patients with recurrent pain after spine surgery.[9]

A medial branch of a spinal nerve's dorsal primary ramus innervates the unilateral superior and inferior articular processes of a vertebra. Two unilateral medial branches, the one cephalad and the other caudad to a Z-joint, must be lesioned to provide relief to the Z-joint between them.

Bogduk and colleagues[10] performed a review of key historical and technical RF neurotomy developments, and this subsection refers specifically to percutaneous RF neurotomy as parallel placement of an RF electrode adjacent to a nerve supplying sensation to a Z-joint to achieve thermal ablation. The targeted nerve segment is the same in a diagnostic anesthetic block and a percutaneous RF neurotomy.

Department of Orthopedics & Physical Rehabilitation, UMass Memorial Medical Center, 119 Belmont Street, Worcester, MA 01605, USA
* Corresponding author.
E-mail address: david.mazin@umassmemorial.org

Phys Med Rehabil Clin N Am 21 (2010) 843–850
doi:10.1016/j.pmr.2010.06.010
1047-9651/10/$ – see front matter © 2010 Elsevier Inc. All rights reserved.

BACKGROUND OF RF NEUROTOMY

Medial branch neurotomy is a valid, safe, effective technique for long-term relief of pain to Z-joints.[10,11] Earlier techniques, such as rhizolysis with scalpel or facet denervation with RF electrodes, reportedly provided pain relief but lacked concept validity. It was not anatomically possible with either technique to lesion the medial branch nerves, the articular branches, or the L5 dorsal ramus that innervate the Z-joints.[12-14] Medial branch neurotomy emerged as an anatomically valid modification with the important technical aspect of parallel orientation of the tip of the RF electrode to the medial branch to reliably lesion the maximal length of this nerve.[15] Peripheral nerves regenerate in a proximal-to-distal direction at a certain distance per unit of time. Therefore, the longer the nerve that is completely lesioned, the longer the duration of denervation and pain relief. Dreyfuss and colleagues[11] (in 2000) demonstrated sustained effective relief of chronic lumbar Z-joint pain in a prospective study with patients selected after controlled diagnostic blocks. Lumbar RF neurotomy has an average duration of relief of 10.5 months and can be safely repeated with equal duration of relief and efficacy.[16]

To conduct RF neurotomy, a physician needs an alternating current voltage generator connected to the active and reference electrodes, an active electrode positioned approximately parallel to the nerve and a reference electrode, and an adhesive pad with a large surface area applied to the patient's skin.[17] The RF tissue lesion is produced in the immediate vicinity of the active electrode needle tip. The lesion extends approximately 1 to 2 electrode widths, a maximal effectiveness of 2 mm, away from the active needle tip in the shape of an oblate spheroid.[15,18] The active electrode needle is typically an insulated 22-gauge Sluijter-Mehta cannula 5, 10, or 15 cm long with an exposed metal tip to permit current flow. The rapidly alternating current fields oscillate charged molecules. Tissue electrical impedance to current flow produces heat in the tissue around the active electrode needle tip, which coagulates and destroys unmyelinated and myelinated fibers in the nearby nerve.[19] An oblate spheroid lesion is produced around the exposed needle. A physician can enlarge the size of the lesion by increasing the needle size (22, 20, or 18 gauge), exposed metal tip length (5, 10, or 15 mm), lesioning time (60 to 90 seconds), or number of needle placements or by repeated lesioning.

ANATOMY

A lumbar spinal nerve root gives rise to a dorsal and ventral primary ramus just lateral to the intervertebral foramen.[20] The dorsal ramus splits into a lateral and medial branch. The lateral branch innervates the longissimus and iliocostalis muscles and the overlying skin in the lower back. The medial branch innervates a superior articular process, an inferior articular process, the periosteum of the vertebral arch, the multifidus and interspinous muscles, and the interspinous ligament. The lumbar medial branch presents an anatomically consistent target for neurotomy, because it pierces the intervertebral ligament dorsally and runs inferomedially in a groove between the superior articular process and the root of the transverse process until covered by the mamillo-accessory ligament. Distal to the mamillo-accessory ligament, the multiple divisions of the medial branch are small and variable, making the specific division to the articular process a difficult target.

The L5 dorsal ramus itself is ablated for lesioning of the L5-S1 Z-joint, along with the L4 medial branch.

INDICATIONS, CONTRAINDICATIONS, AND COMPLICATIONS

The patient should have chronic back pain that is unresponsive to conservative care but has responded positively to controlled diagnostic blocks. Controlled diagnostic blocks of the nerve supply (medial branch, L5 dorsal ramus) to the Z-joints must produce significant, temporally concordant pain relief and functional gains in pain-limited activities before performing percutaneous RF neurotomy. Clinicians' views vary on thresholds indicating significant pain relief. Dreyfuss and colleagues[11] used a threshold of at least 80% relief, which is considered the gold standard. A history of spine surgery or prior RF neurotomy is not a contraindication; however, hardware or ossified scar tissue may prevent adequate access to the target nerve.

Generally, indications and contraindications of RF neurotomy are similar to those of the diagnostic medial branch blocks completed first (refer to article on diagnostic medial branch blocks by Dr Kennedy). RF is safe, with potential for standard percutaneous complications of infection or bleeding. A current infection, a history of bleeding, or a coagulopathy are contraindications. Localized back pain has been the only commonly observed complication in about 1% of patients.[21,22] Short-term painful neuritis for a few weeks is an uncommon complication.[23]

Dreyfuss and colleagues[24] studied 5 patients with lumbar spine magnetic resonance imaging (MRI) at an average of 21 months after medial branch neurotomy to determine the effects of deep paraspinal muscle denervation. These patients had diffuse multifidus atrophy that could not be reliably localized to the ablated levels by MRI, and patients had ongoing pain relief with no complications. Electrodiagnostic study may explain this phenomenon of diffuse atrophy because "lumbar multifidus muscle is polysegmentally innervated."[25] Therefore, multifidus muscle continues to support the lumbar spine despite selective denervation of the levels indicated by medial branch blocks.

TECHNIQUE

Key elements of the procedure technique are discussed in this section, with greater detail available in the reference texts.[5,17] The patient must be educated regarding the technique preprocedure, so that sensory and motor stimulation testing can be completed at the physician's discretion. The patient is placed in a prone position, sterile technique is used, and vital signs are monitored throughout the procedure. The reference electrode pad is applied to the patient's skin and attached to the RF generator. A sterile active RF electrode and cable is attached to the RF generator. A 3.5-in, 25-gauge spinal needle is used with local anesthetic to infiltrate the trajectory of the larger-gauge RF needle. The area closest to the target nerve is not anesthetized if the physician is to perform sensory and motor stimulation testing. Typically, intermittent fluoroscopy is used to guide the RF needle on a trajectory to achieve optimal parallel alignment of the target nerve and the RF needle tip. Needle tip placement is confirmed in anteroposterior, oblique, and lateral views. Some practitioners confirm proximity to the target nerve with the presence of a sensory response, and sufficient distance from the ventral ramus with the absence of peripheral motor activation or radicular pain. A positive sensory response is indicated by a tingling or pressure felt by the patient with 50 Hz stimulation at less than 0.5 V. A reassuring motor check is the absence of radicular pain and activation of muscles in the corresponding myotomal distribution at 2 Hz up to 3 V. If RF needle tip placement is satisfactory, a local anesthetic is injected through the RF needle cannula to prevent the sensation of the ablation. Typically, the ablation is conducted for 60 to 120 seconds at 80°C. The process of active electrode needle placement is repeated to ablate both nerves for each Z-joint. The needle is withdrawn and sterile dressings are applied. The patient is monitored after the procedure for any complications and is discharged with follow-up information.

SUMMARY

RF neurotomy is a safe, effective, repeatable interventional technique used to relieve chronic low back pain. The use of diagnostic medial branch blocks to confirm a Z-joint as the source of pain is essential before performing an RF neurotomy.

RF NEUROTOMY OF THE SACROILIAC JOINT

There are multiple techniques using RF neurotomy to lesion the dorsal innervation of the sacroiliac (SI) joint for long-term pain relief, but an optimal technique has yet to be determined. SI joint block is a mainstay for the diagnosis of SI joint pain refractive to conservative care. SI joint pain confirmed by repeated diagnostic injections may warrant a trial with RF neurotomy for longer-term pain relief. The prevalence of SI joint pain has been estimated by double diagnostic joint block at 19% of patients with lower back pain.[26] Study of the use of percutaneous RF neurotomy for SI joint pain is ongoing, reporting variability in technique and effectiveness.[27–32]

BACKGROUND AND ANATOMY

Debate over the role of the SI joint in low back pain in the twentieth century preceded systematic experiments using SI joint blocks to demonstrate that the joint is a pain generator.[33] The SI joint is an encapsulated joint surrounded by ligaments, which holds an average volume of 1.6 mL (0.8–2.5) normal saline in asymptomatic volunteers with reliable, inducible low back pain on capsular distion.[34,35]

The anatomy relevant to RF neurotomy is nerve supply to the SI joint. Anatomic studies have resulted in contention over SI joint innervation. Two studies conclude that sensation of the SI joint is predominantly, if not wholly, from dorsal innervation via the lateral branches of the sacral dorsi rami.[36,37] Ikeda[38] limits the lateral branches of the sacral dorsi rami to innervation of the inferior dorsal portion of the SI joint. Ikeda also found that the ventral ramus of L5 supplies the ventral superior portion, whereas the ramus of S2 and the sacral plexus combine to supply the ventral inferior portion of the SI joint. McGrath and Zhang[39] found that the long posterior sacroiliac ligament is innervated by the sacral dorsi rami. Therefore, RF neurotomy of the lateral branches of the sacral dorsi rami may ablate all or only the dorsal portion of SI joint innervation.

The correlate to medial branch blocks of Z-joints is lateral branch blocks of the SI joint. However, the lateral branches are more variable in anatomic position and tissue depth. Anesthetic block at multiple sites and depths of the L5 dorsal ramus and S1-4 lateral branches yielded greater anesthesia to painful provocative SI maneuvers than at a single site and depth.[40,41]

The perception of painful capsular distention may persist because of ventral innervation of the SI joint capsule that is not affected by the block of the lateral branches. The studies described earlier are consistent with Ikeda's findings. Block of the dorsal innervation limits sensation of the dorsum of the SI joint and, by extension, suggests that lateral branch neurotomy would affect pain in the dorsal portion of the SI joint.

Rupert and colleagues[42] found limited evidence (US Preventive Services Task Force [USPSTF] Level II-3) for RF neurotomy of the SI joint. Three studies were identified with selection of patients by controlled diagnostic blocks that eliminate the false-positive rate (ranging between 20% and 54% with a single SI joint block). Cohen and Abdi[28] completed a retrospective chart review of 18 patients, with 9 proceeding to RF neurotomy of the SI joint. Eight patients (89%) had more than 50% pain relief at 9 months. Burnham and Yasui[43] performed an uncontrolled, prospective, cohort study with 12 months of follow-up on 9 patients who underwent RF neurotomy of the SI joint. Eight of the 9 patients reported satisfaction, with reduced pain and analgesic use.

INDICATIONS, CONTRAINDICATIONS, AND COMPLICATIONS

There is no widespread consensus on the definitive diagnosis of SI joint pain. A controlled double diagnostic block composed of SI joint blocks or L5 dorsal ramus and lateral branch blocks of the SI dorsal rami with more than 50% pain attributable to the SI joint was used as a criterion for inclusion by Rupert and colleagues.[42] This block is analogous to controlled diagnostic blocks used to identify Z-joint pain before RF neurotomy. Contraindications and complications are also largely analogous to RF neurotomy of the medial branch nerves for Z-joint pain. However, the lateral branches of the dorsal sacral rami do innervate the skin overlying the sacrum, and transient feelings of "itchiness and numbness" within the respective dermatomes has been reported for 3 to 6 months after the procedure.[43]

TECHNIQUES

RF neurotomy of the SI joint is a direct extension of the same equipment (RF voltage generator and active needle electrode), preoperative education, use of fluoroscopic guidance with local anesthetic, and sterile procedural technique as RF neurotomy of the medial branches. However, the new anatomic target is the lateral branches of the L5 and sacral dorsal rami. RF neurotomy of the L5 dorsal ramus is performed at the junction of the sacral ala and the root of the superior articular process of S1. Next, the lateral branches of the dorsal rami of S1 through S3 are addressed. Practitioner-specific technique variation may address how to best complete the ablation in the face of anatomic variance of the lateral branches. Sensory stimulation (50 Hz with <0.6 V) testing and adjustment of the active needle tip reveals variability in the origin of the lateral branch, from 1:30 to 5:30 on the face of a clock lateral to a right sacral foramen and 7:00 to 10:00 on the left.[28]

Some practitioners use bipolar RF neurotomy to ablate between 2 needle tips generally less than 1 cm apart. The bipolar technique replaces the reference electrode pad with a second cannulated electrode needle, so that lesioning occurs primarily in the plane between the needle tips, thereby ablating any nerve that passes between them. A series of planar lesions can be created by successive leapfrog placements of the electrode needles. This technique has been used to ablate a semicircle around the lateral edge of each sacral foramen to capture the lateral branch as it originates from the foramen[43] or, going from the inferior to the superior SI joint line, to lesion all the distal sensory fibers as they enter the ligaments and dorsal joint capsule.[27]

SUMMARY

Research is ongoing regarding the optimal technique for RF neurotomy of the SI joint, aimed at reliable, efficacious, and long-term SI joint pain relief.

REFERENCES

1. Manchikanti L, Singh V, Pampati V. Are diagnostic lumbar medial branch blocks valid? Results of 2-year follow-up. Pain Physician 2003;6:147–53.

2. Manchikanti L, Manchikanti KN, Manchukonda R, et al. Evaluation of therapeutic thoracic medial branch block effectiveness in chronic thoracic pain: a prospective outcome study with minimum 1-year follow up. Pain Physician 2006;9: 97–105.

3. Manchikanti L, Singh V, Falco FJE, et al. Lumbar facet nerve blocks in managing chronic facet joint pain: One-year follow-up of a randomized, double-blind controlled trial: Clinical Trial NCT00355914. Pain Physician 2008;11:121–32.

4. Pampati S, Cash KA, Manchikanti L. Accuracy of diagnostic lumbar facet joint nerve blocks: a 2-year follow-up of 152 patients diagnosed with controlled diagnostic blocks. Pain Physician 2008;12:855–66.

5. Rathmell JP. Facet injection: intra-articular injection, medial branch block, and radiofrequency treatment. In: Rathmell JP, editor. Atlas of image-guided intervention in regional anesthesia and pain medicine. Philadelphia: Lippincott Williams & Wilkins; 2006. p. 65–92.

6. Newton W, Curtis P, Witt P, et al. Prevalence of subtypes of low back pain in a defined population. J Fam Pract 1997;45:331–5.

7. Schwarzer AC, Aprill CN, Derby R, et al. Clinical features of patients with pain stemming from the lumbar zygapophysial joints. Is the lumbar facet syndrome a clinical entity? Spine 1994;19:1132–7.

8. Schwarzer AC, Wang SC, Bogduk N, et al. The prevalence and clinical features of lumbar zygapophysial joint pain: a study in an Australian population with chronic low back pain. Ann Rheum Dis 1995;54:100–6.

9. Manchikanti L, Manchukonda R, Pampati V, et al. Prevalence of facet joint pain in chronic low back pain in postsurgical patients by controlled comparative local anesthetic blocks. Arch Phys Med Rehabil 2007;88:449–55.

10. Bogduk N, Dreyfuss P, Govind J. A narrative review of lumbar medial branch neurotomy for the treatment of back pain. Pain Med 2009;10:1035–45.

11. Dreyfuss P, Halbrook B, Pauza K, et al. Efficacy and validity of radiofrequency neurotomy for chronic lumbar zygapophysial joint pain. Spine 2000; 25:1270–7.

12. Bogduk N, Colman RRS, Winer CER. An anatomical assessment of the "percutaneous rhizolysis" procedure. Med J Aust 1977;1:397–9.

13. Bogduk N, Long DM. The anatomy of the so-called articular nerves and their relationship to facet denervation in the treatment of low back pain. J Neurosurg 1979; 51:172–7.

14. Bogduk N, Long DM. Percutaneous lumbar medial branch neurotomy. A modification of facet denervation. Spine 1980;5:193–200.

15. Lau P, Mercer S, Govind J, et al. The surgical anatomy of lumbar medial branch neurotomy (facet denervation). Pain Med 2004;5:289–98.

16. Schofferman J, Kine G. Effectiveness of repeated radiofrequency neurotomy for lumbar facet pain. Spine 2004;29:2471–3.

17. Standards Committee of ISIS. Percutaneous radiofrequency lumbar medial branch neurotomy. In: Bugduk N, editor. Practice guidelines for spinal diagnostic and treatment procedures. San Francisco (CA): International Spine Intervention Society; 2004. p. 189–218.

18. Bogduk N, Macintosh J, Marsland A. Technical limitations to the efficacy of radiofrequency of radiofrequency neurotomy for spinal pain. Neurosurgery 1987;20: 529–35.

19. Smith HP, McWhorter JM, Challa VR. Radiofrequency neurolysis in a clinical model. Neuropathological correlation. J Neurosurg 1981;55:246–53.

20. Bogduk N, Wilson AS, Tynan W. The human lumbar dorsal rami. J Anat 1982;134: 383–97.
21. Kornick C, Kramarich SS, Lamer TJ, et al. Complications of lumbar facet radiofrequency denervation. Spine 2004;29:1352–4.
22. Nath S, Nath CS, Pettersson K. Percutaneous lumbar zygapophysial (facet) joint neurotomy using radiofrequency current, in the management of chronic low back pain. Spine 2008;33:1291–7.
23. Royal MA, Bhakta B, Gunyea I, et al. Radiofrequency neurolysis for facet arthropathy: a retrospective case series and review of the literature. Pain Pract 2002;2: 47–52.
24. Dreyfuss P, Stout A, Aprill C, et al. The significance of multifidus atrophy after successful radiofrequency neurotomy for low back pain. PM&R 2009;1: 719–22.
25. Wu PB, Date ES, Kingery WS. The lumbar multifidus muscle in polysegmentally innervated. Electromyogr Clin Neurophysiol 2000;40:483–5.
26. Maigne JY, Aivaliklis A, Pfefer F. Results of sacroiliac joint double block and value of sacroiliac pain provocation tests in 54 patients with low back pain. Spine 1996; 21:1889–92.
27. Ferrante FM, King LF, Roche EA, et al. Radiofrequency sacroiliac joint denervation for sacroiliac syndrome. Reg Anesth Pain Med 2001;26:137–42.
28. Cohen SP, Abdi S. Lateral branch blocks as a treatment for sacroiliac joint pain: a pilot study. Reg Anesth Pain Med 2003;28:113–9.
29. Yin W, Willard F, Carreiro J, et al. Sensory stimulation-guided sacroiliac joint radiofrequency neurotomy: Technique based on neuroanatomy of the dorsal sacral plexus. Spine 2003;28:2419–25.
30. Olmez D, Ozturk AH. 520 Radiofrequency lesioning of lateral branches as a treatment for sacroiliac joint pain: a retrospective study. Eur J Pain 2006; 10:S137.
31. Cohen SP, Hurley RW, Buckenmaier CC III, et al. Randomized placebo-controlled study evaluating lateral branch radiofrequency denervation for sacroiliac joint pain. Anesthesiology 2008;109:279–88.
32. Cohen SP, Strassels SA, Kurihara C, et al. Outcome predictors for sacroiliac joint (lateral branch) radiofrequency denervation. Reg Anesth Pain Med 2009;34: 206–14.
33. Standards Committee of ISIS. Sacroiliac joint blocks. In: Bugduk N, editor. Practice guidelines for spinal diagnostic and treatment procedures. San Francisco (CA): International Spine Intervention Society; 2004. p. 66–86.
34. Fortin JD, Dwyer AD, West S, et al. Sacroiliac joint: pain referral maps upon applying a new injection/arthrography technique. Part I: asymptomatic volunteers. Spine 1994;19:1475–82.
35. Fortin JD, Tolchin RB. Sacroiliac provocation and arthrography. Arch Phys Med Rehabil 1993;74:125–9.
36. Grob KR, Neuhuber WL, Kissling RO. [Innervation of the sacroiliac joint of the human]. Z Rheumatol 1995;54:117–22 [in German].
37. Fortin JD, Kissling RO, O'Connor BL, et al. Sacroiliac joint innervation and pain. Am J Orthop (Belle Mead NJ) 1999;28:687–90
38. Ikeda R. [Innervation of the sacroiliac joint. Macroscopical and histological studies]. Nippon Ika Daigaku Zasshi 1991;58:587–96 [in Japanese].
39. McGrath MC, Zhang M. Lateral branches of dorsal sacral nerve plexus and the long posterior sacroiliac ligament. Surg Radiol Anat 2005;27:327–30.

40. Dreyfuss P, Snyder BD, Park K, et al. The ability of single site, single depth sacral lateral branch blocks to anesthetize the sacroiliac joint complex. Pain Med 2008; 9:844–50.

41. Dreyfuss P, Henning T, Malladi N, et al. The ability of multi-site, multi-depth sacral lateral branch blocks to anesthetize the sacroiliac joint complex. Pain Med 2009; 10:679–88.

42. Rupert MP, Lee M, Manchikanti L, et al. Evaluation of sacroiliac joint interventions: a systematic appraisal of the literature. Pain physician 2009;12:399–418.

43. Burnham RS, Yasui Y. An alternate method of radiofrequency neurotomy of the sacroiliac joint: a pilot study of the effect on pain, function, and satisfaction. Reg Anesth Pain Med 2007;32:12–9.

The Use of Spinal Cord Stimulation and Intrathecal Drug Delivery in the Treatment of Low Back-Related Pain

David Bagnall, MD

KEYWORDS

- Low back pain • Spinal cord stimulation
- Intrathecal drug delivery • Radiculopathy

Spinal cord stimulation (SCS) and intrathecal drug delivery (IDD) are forms of neuro-modulation. Neuromodulation attempts to alter the nervous system through augmentation rather than ablation, meaning that it is reversible and nondestructive. In terms of chronic pain treatment, SCS is primarily effective for neuropathic rather than nociceptive pain. Therefore, in low back-associated pain, it is generally limited to conditions such as radiculopathy and pain of CNS origin. IDD is primarily effective for nociceptive or mixed pain, and its usage is generally limited to conditions within that realm.

SPINAL CORD STIMULATION
History

In 1967, Shealy and colleagues[1] opened the door for a new intervention in pain treatment when they reported the ability to inhibit pain by subdural electrical stimulation of the dorsal columns of the spinal cord. Their surgical implantation of a unipolar stimulator directly on the spinal cord was based, in large part, on the theory of Melzack and Wall[2] proposed 2 years earlier. The gate control theory suggested that stimulation of large-diameter primary afferent (Aβ) cutaneous nerves in the spinal cord might inhibit pain transmission and therefore suppress pain perception.

SCS has since evolved at many levels. Perhaps the most important step occurred in 1975, when placement of an epidural stimulator[3] and the development of a system of ring electrodes on a flexible lead capable of percutaneous implantation[4] led to a notable change in the use of the systems. The ability to implant these units without

3980A Sheridan Drive, Suite 102, Amherst, NY 14226, USA
E-mail address: bagnall@rehabny.com

Phys Med Rehabil Clin N Am 21 (2010) 851–858
doi:10.1016/j.pmr.2010.06.004
1047-9651/10/$ – see front matter © 2010 Elsevier Inc. All rights reserved.

pmr.theclinics.com

the need for a laminotomy increased the number of practitioners with the technical expertise to permanently place SCS systems.

It became clear that focusing stimulation within a certain region of the spinal cord while avoiding stimulation of unintended spinal structures would improve effectiveness.[5] This notion has evolved in large part through computer modeling developed in the Netherlands in the early 1990s, and is based on electrode spacing, anatomic lead location, and the lead-cord cerebrospinal fluid (CSF) separation. The results of the work by Holsheimer and others helped illuminate several aspects of SCS: the relationship between dorsal column and dorsal root fiber stimulation thresholds; the effect of increasing CSF depth on decreasing the focal intensity of stimulation; and the value of narrow longitudinal fields and diminution in center-to-center contact separation in minimizing dorsal root fiber stimulation.[5]

Microtechnology has contributed significantly over the past decade to improving the efficacy of SCS. Multiple configurations of percutaneous and surgical leads are available. Pulse generators have evolved from external units transmitting via radio to self-contained, rechargeable, implanted units. Microcomputer technology has provided an opportunity for patient-controlled programming, allowing multiple programs to address postural changes, thereby increasing patient satisfaction.

Description

A spinal cord stimulator is essentially an electrical circuit opening at a battery source and closing at the tissues, and in its simplest form is based on Ohm's law ($I = V/R$). The current or voltage is converted into pulses and transmitted to the various electrodes of the SCS leads. The circuit is closed by the tissues in the spinal canal creating stimulation to nervous tissue. As low-threshold primary cutaneous afferents in the dorsal columns are stimulated, the perception of pain is reduced. Theoretically, stimulating the dorsal columns closes the gate over wide areas of the body. In fact, spinal cord stimulation is more complex. For example, SCS is effective for chronic but not acute pain, for neuropathic and sympathetically mediated pain but not nociceptive pain.

Primary afferent spinal neurons must be depolarized and must propagate an action potential to close the gate on peripheral painful input. This outcome occurs when the spinal neuron is made more electrically positive, which is achieved when a negatively charged external electrical stimulus called the *cathode* is applied and produces a *cathodal effect*.

Likewise, hyperpolarization occurs when a spinal neuron is made more electrically negative, which prevents propagation of an action potential; such a positively charged external stimulus is called an *anode* and produces an *anodal effect*.[6]

One can see that the ability to direct discrete electrical charges via electrodes placed close to the primary afferent spinal neurons allows focused depolarization and impedes the transmission of peripheral nociception and the perception of pain.

The dorsal column target for stimulation is typically several spinal levels higher than the exiting spinal nerves of the dermatome or dermatomes to be covered. This target is medial but in close proximity to the dorsal root structures, both running longitudinally. Because the propagation threshold of neurons in each of these regions is similar, the difference between producing pain-relieving paresthesia and unpleasant dorsal root stimulation is small. This hurdle is cleared by focusing the cathodal effect over the more midline dorsal columns, causing depolarization. Frequently, an anodal effect can be achieved over the dorsal root fibers, preventing their propagation and increasing the effect of the cathode at the dorsal columns.

A single SCS lead placed in the midline decreases the risk of stimulating lateral cord structures. Also, reduced center-to-center contact spacing diminishes the sphere of stimulation at the cathode. Conversely, lost paresthesia from lead migration and decreased ability to obtain bilateral and more complex pain patterns place limits on single midline leads.

Dual lead systems allow a greater amount of electronic steering that theoretically can focus stimulation more precisely at the target site and deeply into the cord structures. The concept of guarding the cathode by placing anodes on either side of it led to tripolar stimulation. Later, this evolved to transverse tripole stimulation using 3 parallel leads, 2 lateral anodes protecting a midline cathode from the dorsal root region and driving stimulation more deeply into the dorsal columns. Unfortunately, power consumption is increased using bi- or tripolar leads and closely spaced electrodes.[7] Current stimulation technology also achieves focused stimulation through interleaved[8] or multichannel stimulation. All these techniques were developed in the hope of increasing axial spine pain coverage, but its clinical effect remains unproven.

Paresthesia must successfully be superimposed over the area of pain for SCS to be an effective treatment.[9] However, even if paresthesia can be superimposed over the area of a patient's pain, that is not necessarily sufficient to elicit pain relief.[10] Furthermore, computer modeling predicts that the likelihood of achieving paresthesia over the low back is, at best, 45%.[5] This reflects the complicated nature of SCS and the clinical evidence of its greater effectiveness for neuropathic and sympathetic rather than nociceptive pain.

The most important limit to paresthesia seems to be the proximity of the stimulator electrodes to the spinal cord, which in turn is limited by the depth of CSF and epidural fat at any point along the cord. Physiologic impedance is suspected as a secondary effect. Within 3 weeks of implantation of percutaneous leads, the electrodes are generally encapsulated, theoretically stabilizing impedance. However, that is not consistently the case, and further understanding of this phenomenon is needed.[11]

Failed Back Surgery Syndrome

Perhaps the best studied use of SCS in low back-related pain occurs with failed back surgery syndrome (FBSS). FBSS represents a continuum of symptoms with a common genesis—the unfavorable response of lower back and/or radicular symptoms to surgical intervention. Patients with FBSS may have radicular or axial symptoms and commonly have both. Causes include recurrent pathology, surgical failure, postsurgical scarring, and instability. Furthermore, FBSS symptoms are not independent of emotional, psychological, and social influence. Evaluating the efficacy of SCS in FBSS from available literature is an elusive quest, because the definition of FBSS is imprecise.

Despite the obscure definition, many published studies reflect various experiences with SCS in patients with persistent spine-related pain after surgical intervention, and FBSS is a common indication for SCS.

As indicated previously, SCS has largely been effective for neuropathic pain but less so for nociceptive pain. One might suppose this premise would act as a guide for the use of SCS for patients falling under the generous umbrella of FBSS; however, the literature is difficult to interpret.

Several studies have focused primarily on patients with a greater radicular component to their FBSS. After long-term follow-up (mean range from 2.9 to 8 years), pain relief of 50% or greater ranged from 47% to 86%.[12–18]

In a retrospective study examining SCS for FBSS for predominately chronic axial lower back pain with follow-up ranging from 5 to 19 months, 70% of the patients were satisfied with the outcome.[19] Initial results using dual leads supported diminution in visual analog scale pain levels and narcotic usage, even in patients with significant axial pain complaints.[20] However, other studies reflect, at best, an inconsistent ability for SCS to reduce axial low back pain.[7,15,21–25]

Nevertheless, it remains very difficult to compare any of the studies, because patient selection criteria, rates of permanent implantation, outcome measurement, and follow-up are not equitable. Furthermore, rarely are these studies prospective, randomized, and controlled; they are more commonly retrospective. Duration of SCS trials also varies, extending from several days to 4 weeks. Rates of permanent implantation from these trials also vary from 65% to 96% of patients.

There have been several studies that have attempted to evaluate the relative cost-effectiveness of using SCS for FBSS. SCS is an expensive intervention; however, when compared with total health-care outlays and lost productivity, that cost is most often equivocated. One study reported a substantial improvement in health-care costs when comparing successful SCS for FBSS versus treatment with conventional medical management (CMM).[26] Others have found SCS to be cost-effective after 2.5 years[27] and 2.1 years[28] of use when compared with CMM. A systematic review found that SCS may increase quality of life and function, and it can be more cost-effective in the long term, despite the high initial device implantation costs.[29]

Technique

Perhaps the greatest benefit of SCS over other interventions is the ability to test the efficacy of the treatment before committing to permanent implantation. Because each trial is specific to the patient, success can more reliably be measured.

Percutaneous trials are straightforward and involve placing a lead or leads into the epidural space through a spinal needle and attaching the exposed leads to an external pulse generator. Permanent percutaneous lead placement is similar to the trial, with subcutaneous surgical placement of the leads and stimulator unit; it is beyond the scope of this chapter to provide greater detail.

Patient Selection and Risks

As with all pain-related interventions, SCS should only be considered after thorough and thoughtful evaluation. Perhaps the single most important aspect is patients accepting their responsibility in the rehabilitation process. Every intervention performed on a patient with low back-related disorders should be considered a rehabilitation process, intended to maximize the patient's function. Although achieving reduction of symptoms is a significant step in that rehabilitation process, it should not be the final goal.

Patients with major psychiatric disorders, inability to comprehend the goals of the procedure, substance abuse problems, and secondary gain issues are generally excluded from consideration for SCS. In appropriate cases that have not progressed despite conservative pharmacologic and percutaneous interventions, SCS may allow an opportunity for rehabilitation.[30]

Commonly, SCS trial success is defined as pain relief of 50% or greater following implantation. This arbitrary designation is used as a minimal threshold toward pursuing permanent implantation.

Unlikely but potential adverse events include hematoma, epidural hemorrhage, seroma, CSF leakage, infection, erosion, allergic response, lead migration, implant-site pain, loss of pain relief, chest wall stimulation, or paralysis.

Any sources of electromagnetic interference, such as defibrillators, diathermy, electrocautery, magnetic resonance imaging, radiofrequency ablation, and therapeutic ultrasonography, could interact with SCS systems causing damage or stimulation changes.

Patients should avoid aggressive activities that might place stress on spinal cord stimulator leads because they could cause fracture or migration, and postural changes might cause temporary changes in stimulation.

INTRATHECAL DRUG DELIVERY

For several decades, intrathecal drug delivery (IDD) has been available for the treatment of chronic pain. In 1973, opioid receptors were discovered in the central nervous system (CNS),[31] providing an alternative means for delivering opiates to the body. Since then, the ability of IDD to place opiates directly at the level of the CNS has evolved as a standard option for treatment of chronic pain.

Lower back-related pain is a generic concept that includes neuropathic, nociceptive, biomechanical, emotional, and psychological components, and treatment options must reflect that variability. The chronic radicular and neuropathic component of lower back-related pain has many treatment options. Conversely, the nociceptive component of lower back pain has been more difficult to treat.

Patients with chronic nociceptive pain recalcitrant to surgical intervention, exercise, percutaneous procedures, and activity modification frequently benefit from oral opioid administration. Unfortunately, there are several problems with opiates delivered via an oral route. Prominent physiologic effects include pruritus, nausea, vomiting, and altered cognition, and the potential for abuse and diversion cannot be ignored. Even when effective and trouble-free, orally administered opiates have significant cost, reflecting the pharmacokinetic inefficiency of delivering oral opiates to the CNS.

IDD may diminish the potential physiologic side effects, eliminate the risk of abuse and diversion, and reduce costs by maximizing the efficiency of opiates delivered directly to the target sites in the CNS.

An IDD system consists of 2 components: an intrathecal catheter and a nonprogrammable or programmable pump/reservoir. The catheter is implanted in the intrathecal space and carried subcutaneously to a pocket over the abdomen that contains the pump/reservoir system. The pump is generally placed over the abdominal wall to facilitate access to the catheter ports and for pump refills. Current reservoirs have volumes ranging from 10 mL to 60 mL and are filled percutaneously through a septum. Recent technological advances allow sophisticated programs, including constant or variable infusions and periodic boluses, depending on patient-specific diurnal and activity-based pain requirements. Furthermore, telemetric monitoring allows measurement of volume, rate of use, and performance.

As with SCS, patient selection is critical when considering IDD therapy. IDD has been used in patients with nociceptive, neuropathic, and mixed pain, but patients with greater axial than extremity pain may have more success with IDD trialing.[32] Also, patients who proceed with permanent IDD implantation must have objective evidence of pathology, exhausted treatments to reverse the source of pain, sufficient body size to accept implantation of a pump, no evidence of infection, and a favorable outcome to an IDD trial.

Typically, patients are excluded from consideration for IDD if they have a major psychiatric disorder, drug-abuse problems, or issues of secondary gain. Patients must have undergone a thorough assessment of previous diagnosis and treatment and of function and psychological stability. Nevertheless, the most important consideration before initiating IDD therapy is fully involving patients in the process. Shared decision-making is essential, whereby patients are fully educated in the risks, benefits, alternatives, goals, and especially, their responsibility to adhere to a goal-oriented plan. IDD, as with any therapy, is most effective when patients understand that the goal of treatment is to provide an opportunity to improve their function.

There are several options when considering an IDD trial. The drugs can be administered via an intrathecal or epidural route and include single or multiple injections and continuous infusion protocols. Nevertheless, trials should consistently be performed in a supervised environment with access to emergency intervention. Vital signs should be monitored and close observation maintained for other adverse effects including drug overdose. Morphine is the most commonly used analgesic when performing trials.[33]

Detail about analgesic options are beyond the scope of this article. Suffice to say that the Food and Drug Administration has approved only morphine and ziconotide for IDD use; however, in clinical practice, many other opioids and nonopiates have been used. Opioids, local anesthetics, adrenergic agonists, N-methyl-D-aspartate antagonists, and other agents, including but not limited to adenosine, baclofen, droperidol, ketorolac, and midazolam, have been considered, are being evaluated, or are in current use as adjuvant intrathecal components.[34]

Maintenance of an IDD system ranges from benign to potentially fatal. When the system is working appropriately, periodic refills and occasional pump replacements are all that is required. However, mechanical issues, including catheter migration, fracture and occlusion, and pump malfunction or rotation in the subcutaneous pocket, require attention, even emergently, depending on the pharmacologic amalgamation. Likewise, changes in analgesic efficacy, physiologic function, and psychomotor function require immediate evaluation to eliminate other potential problems, including but not limited to infection or neurologic compression related to a granuloma.

There have been several studies evaluating the effectiveness of IDD for generalized chronic pain, although most studies have focused on the application of IDD for chronic noncancer and cancer pain. The studies consistently indicate IDD as an effective means of controlling chronic pain in the right circumstances, noting decreased visual analog and numerical pain rating scales, improvement in function, decreased oral opioid use, and patient satisfaction.[32,35]

The most common complications of IDD are generally self-limiting and include nausea and vomiting, pruritus, constipation, hyperalgesia, and urinary retention. More serious complications, including meningitis and wound infection, are rare. Of most frequent concern is the development of a noninfectious granuloma associated with concentration-dependent opioid infusion, which can lead to neurologic injury and paralysis if not identified and treated appropriately.

SUMMARY

The capacity of SCS to positively affect patients with neuropathic pain is well-established, and its use in chronic radicular symptoms seems clear. However, studies in patients with axial lower back pain have failed to show consistent benefit from this type of treatment. Manufacturers have claimed the ability to target axial lower back pain using a more compact electrical field, directed stimulation, and unique means of delivering stimulation. However, to date, there is little convincing evidence establishing reliable indications for SCS in the treatment of axial low back pain.

IDD has consistently proven valuable for treatment of a subset of patients with chronic nociceptive and mixed low back pain complaints. Patients with irreversible painful conditions who respond favorably to but require high doses of narcotic analgesics may be candidates for this treatment option.

REFERENCES

1. Shealy CN, Mortimer JT, Reswick JB. Electrical inhibition of pain by stimulation of the dorsal columns: preliminary clinical report. Anesth Anal 1967;46:489–91.
2. Melzack R, Wall PD. Pain mechanisms: a new theory. Science 1965;150:971–9.
3. Burton C. Dorsal column stimulation: optimization of application. Surg Neurol 1975;4:171–6.
4. Hoppenstein R. Percutaneous implantation of chronic spinal cord electrodes for control of intractable pain: preliminary report. Surg Neurol 1975;4:195–8.
5. Aló KM, Holsheimer J. New trends in neuromodulation for the management of neuropathic pain. Neurosurgery 2002;50(4):690–704.
6. Oakley JC, Prager JP. Spinal cord stimulation: mechanism of action. Spine 2002; 27:2574–83.
7. Oakley JC, Espinosa F, Bothe H, et al. Transverse tripolar spinal cord stimulation: results of an international multicenter study. Neuromodulation 2006;9:192–203.
8. North RA, Kidd DH, Olin J, et al. Spinal cord stimulation with interleaved pulses: a randomized, controlled trial. Neuromodulation 2007;10:349–57.
9. North RB, Kidd DH, Zahurak M, et al. Spinal cord stimulation for chronic intractable pain. Experience over two decades. Neurosurgery 1993;32:384–95.
10. North RB, Ewend MG, Lawton MT, et al. Spinal cord stimulation for chronic intractable pain. Superiority of 'multi-channel' devices. Pain 1991;44:119–30.
11. Abejon D, Feler CA. Is impedance a parameter to be taken into account in spinal cord stimulation? Pain Physician 2007;10:533–40.
12. Rainov NG, Heidecke V, Burkert W. Spinal cord stimulation for failed back surgery syndrome. Minim Invasive Neurosurg 1996;39:41–4.
13. Fiume D, Sherkat S, Callovini GM, et al. Treatment of failed back syndrome due to lumbosacral epidural fibrosis. Acta Neurochir 1995;64(Suppl):116–8.
14. DeLa Porte C, Van de Kelft E. Spinal cord stimulation in failed back surgery syndrome. Pain 1993;52:55–61.
15. Kumar K, Taylor R, Jacques L, et al. Spinal cord stimulation versus conventional medical management for neuropathic pain: a multicentre randomized controlled trial in patients with failed back surgery syndrome. Pain 2007;132(1–2):179–88.
16. Kumar K, Hunter G, Demeria D. Spinal cord stimulation in treatment of chronic benign pain: challenges in treatment planning and present status, a 22-year experience. Neurosurgery 2006;58:481–96.
17. Leveque J-C, Villavicencio AT, Bulsara KR, et al. Spinal cord stimulation for failed lower back surgery syndrome. Neuromodulation 2001;4:1–9.
18. North RB, Ewend MG, Lawton MT, et al. Failed back surgery syndrome: five-year follow-up after spinal cord stimulator implantation. Neurosurgery 1991;28:692–9.
19. Ohnmeiss DD, Rashbaum RF. Patient satisfaction with spinal cord stimulation for predominant complaints of chronic, intractable low back pain. Spine J 2001;1:358–63.
20. Van Buyten J, Van Zundert J, Milbouw G. Treatment of failed back surgery syndrome patients with low back and leg pain: a pilot study of a new dual lead spinal cord stimulation system. Neuromodulation 1999;2(4):258–65.
21. Dario A. Treatment of failed back surgery syndrome. Neuromodulation 2001;4:105–10.
22. Chou R, Atlas SJ, Stanos SP, et al. Nonsurgical interventional therapies for low back pain: a review of the evidence for an American Pain Society clinical practice guideline. Spine 2009;34:1078–93.
23. North R, Shipley J, Prager J, et al. Practice parameters for the use of spinal cord stimulation in the treatment of chronic neuropathic pain. Pain Med 2007;8: S200–75.

24. North RB, Kidd DH, Farroki F, et al. Spinal cord stimulation versus repeated lumbosacral spine surgery for chronic pain; a randomized, controlled trial. Neurosurgery 2005;56:98–107.
25. Kumar K, Taylor RS, Jacques L, et al. The effects of spinal cord stimulation in neuropathic pain are sustained: a 24-month follow-up of the prospective randomized controlled multicenter trial of the effectiveness of spinal cord stimulation. Neurosurgery 2008;63:762–70.
26. Taylor RJ, Taylor RS. Spinal cord stimulation for failed back surgery syndrome: a decision-analytic model and cost-effective analysis. Int J Technol Assess Health Care 2005;21:351–8.
27. Kumar K, Malik S, Demeria D, et al. Treatment of chronic pain with spinal cord stimulation versus alternative therapies: cost-effectiveness analysis. Neurosurgery 2002;51:106–16.
28. Bell GK, Kidd D, North RB. Cost-effective analysis of spinal cord stimulation and treatment of failed back surgery syndrome. J Pain Symptom Manage 1997;13: 286–95.
29. Bala MM, Riemsma RP, Nixon J, et al. Systematic review of the cost-effectiveness of spinal cord stimulation for people with failed back surgery syndrome. Clin J Pain 2008;24:741–56.
30. Stanton-Hicks M. Spinal cord stimulation for the management of complex regional pain syndrome. Neuromodulation 1999;2:193–201.
31. Pert CB, Snyder SH. Opiate receptor: demonstration in nervous tissue. Science 1973;179:1011–104.
32. Deer T, Chapple I, Classen A, et al. Intrathecal drug delivery for treatment of chronic low back pain: report from the national outcomes registry for low back pain. Pain Med 2004;5:6–13.
33. Deer TR, Krames E, Levy RM, et al. Practice choices and challenges in the current intrathecal therapy environment: an online survey. Pain Med 2009;10:304–9.
34. Deer TR, Krames ES, Hassenbusch SJ, et al. Polyanalgesic consensus conference 2007: recommendations for the management of pain by intrathecal (intraspinal) drug delivery: report of an interdisciplinary expert panel. Neuromodulation 2007;10:300–28.
35. Doleys DM, Brown JL, Ness T. Multidimensional outcomes analysis of intrathecal, oral opioid and behavioral-functional restoration therapy for failed back surgery syndrome: a retrospective study with for years follow-up. Neuromodulation 2006;9:270–83.

Discography

Alison Stout, DO[a,b,*]

KEYWORDS

- Discography • Spine intervention • Lumbar disc
- Low back pain • Low back pain treatment

DISCOGRAPHY

Lumbar discography is a purely diagnostic procedure used to confirm or refute the hypothesis that a patient's low back pain is emanating from the intervertebral disc. It is generally reserved for patients with pain severe enough that they are considering surgery or other invasive treatments after adequate conservative management has failed. Discography is undertaken only when clinical evaluation suggests discogenic pain and other sources of lumbar pain have been ruled out. It should not be used as a stand-alone test. Practitioners often suspect discogenic pain on a clinical basis, but no physical examination finding can reliably diagnose discogenic pain, and trying to ascertain a specific level (eg, L4–L5 vs L5–S1) as the source is even more problematic. As discussed in the imaging article by Dr Maus, patients with disc degeneration and abnormal discs are often asymptomatic, leading to low reliability for imaging to precisely pinpoint a specific disc as a focal pain generator.[1–5] Lumbar provocation discography is the only technique available to diagnose whether a specific disc(s) is the cause of a patient's unremitting low back pain.

Discography involves fluoroscopically guided insertion of a needle into the nucleus pulposus of the target disc, followed by instillation of contrast dye to outline the morphology and evaluate for internal disruption. Manometry is used to measure opening pressure and intraprocedure pressure as it is increased. Disc provocation refers to the recording of a patient's response to the injection in a blinded manner in which the patient is not aware of the specific disc being injected or the pressure as it is increased. Additional information regarding the morphology of the disc can be obtained by fluoroscopy at the time of injection or with postinjection computed tomography.

The premise of the procedure is that if a disc is symptomatic, provocation should reproduce the patient's familiar or concordant pain. If stressing the disc does not cause pain or produces pain that is not concordant with the usual pain, then the cause

[a] Rehabilitation Care Services, Veterans Administration, Puget Sound HCS, 1660 South Columbian Way, Seattle, WA 98108, USA
[b] Department of Rehabilitation, University of Washington, 1959 NE Pacific Street, Seattle, WA 98195, USA
* Department of Rehabilitation, Veterans Affairs Puget Sound Health Care System, 117-RCS, 1660 South Columbian Way, Seattle, WA 98108.
E-mail address: stouta@uw.edu

Phys Med Rehabil Clin N Am 21 (2010) 859–867
doi:10.1016/j.pmr.2010.07.002
1047-9651/10/$ – see front matter © 2010 Published by Elsevier Inc.
pmr.theclinics.com

of the patient's pain cannot be attributed to that disc. However, even if stimulation of the disc results in concordant pain, it does not convey the pathoanatomic nature of that pain. The procedure is typically uncomfortable, if not painful. Patients are advised that their pain may be exacerbated for 1 to 3 weeks after discography.

According to the International Association for the Study of Pain (IASP) and the International Spine Intervention Society (ISIS), the diagnostic criteria for provocation discography to be determined to have a positive result include all of the following: (1) the provocation of the target disc reproduces the patient's typical pain, greater than or equal to 7/10 at a pressure less than 50 psi above opening pressure with less than or equal to 3.5 mL of injectate, (2) a grade III annular tear is seen, and (3) provocation of adjacent discs does not reproduce the patient's typical pain.[6] Pain provocation of greater than 6/10 at control levels yields an equivocal test, as does discordant pain. As with other provocation tests, there can be an inherent issue with false-positive results. To minimize this concern, strict adherence to a standardized protocol and the diagnostic criteria for the procedure is essential. The study of discography has been controversial and is complicated by the test being operator-dependent with varied diagnostic criteria and by the lack of a gold standard against which it can be tested.

Evidence

Discography was originally described by Lindblom to diagnose a herniated lumbar intervertebral disc and has been used clinically since the 1940s.[7] In early discography studies, patients were noted to commonly report reproduction of their typical pain[6] with stimulation, and abnormal discs were rarely painful in asymptomatic controls.[8] In 1968, Holt[9] found a high false-positive rate, but there were 16 ruptured discs, and there is conjecture that there could have been irritation of structures other than the disc.

The validity of discography has been more recently evaluated in several studies, but remains controversial. Discography has been performed in symptomatic and asymptomatic subjects to ascertain its reliability and validity. To determine the false-positive rate, the rate of positive lumbar discography in individuals asymptomatic of low back pain has been studied. In 1990, Walsh and colleagues[10] reported a false-positive rate of 0% in asymptomatic controls and a true-positive rate of 89% in symptomatic subjects. The study used pressures 58 to 72 psi above opening pressure. In 2000, Carragee and colleagues[11] performed lumbar discography on 10 volunteers who were asymptomatic of low back pain and without confounding factors, citing a false-positive rate of 10% per patient.[12] However, pressure manometry was up to 100 psi above opening pressure, and the sample size was small. In 2005, a study by Derby and colleagues[13] of lumbar discography on asymptomatic controls used more stringent criteria for a positive discogram including pain greater than or equal to 6/10 on pain scale, grade III annular tear, and pressure less than or equal to 50 psi above opening pressure. The investigators found a false-positive rate of 0% in 13 asymptomatic controls (including 6 with occasional low back pain, but <3 episodes per year). In asymptomatic patients without confounding factors and using standardized diagnostic criteria, lumbar discography has negligible false-positive rates.

Carragee and colleagues[14] also studied asymptomatic patients, but who had previously undergone discectomy. The investigators found a false-positive rate of 40% per patient and noted that 7 of 8 of the positive results were at the site of previous discectomy. Wolfer and colleagues[12] reviewed this study and noted that if ISIS/IASP standards were used, the false-positive rate decreased to 15% per patient and 9.1%

per disc. Previous surgical intervention at the disc increases the risk of a false-positive response for lumbar discography, especially if strict diagnostic criteria are not used.

In patients without low back pain but with chronic pain of other origin, higher false-positive rates are noted. Carragee and colleagues[15] studied the results of lumbar discography in patients without low back pain but with chronic pain at the iliac crest after bone graft harvest (for grafting at a site remote from the lumbar spine). False-positive discography results were found in 4 of 8 patients, with disc stimulation reproducing their usual iliac crest pain. However, pressures up to 100 psi above opening pressure were used, and on secondary analysis using ISIS/IASP standardized criteria, the false-positive rate dropped to 12.5% per patient and 7.1% (1/14) per disc.[12] The reproduction of pain at their iliac crest harvest site with provocation of normal discs was more pronounced at high pressures. These false-positive rates correlate to the overlapping nociceptive fields in the lumbosacral spine in which differentiation between pain generators is difficult (eg, sacroiliac joint vs zygapophyseal joint vs disc) and segmental sensitization can occur. In this study, it was not stated whether discography was done ipsilateral or contralateral to the side of the iliac crest pain. If injection was performed ipsilateral to the usual chronic pain, within the sensitized nociceptive field, it may have caused an increased false-positive rate. A lower false-positive rate would then have been possible if injection had been done on the side contralateral to the usual chronic pain, outside the sensitized nociceptive field.[12] The finding of increased false-positive rates in patients with pain from other structures within the lumbosacral region highlights the importance of considering other possible pain generators prior to discography.

In patients with chronic severe pain of the cervical spine, who had the poorest outcomes after cervical spine surgery but no significant low back pain, Carragee and colleagues[11] noted the false-positive rate for lumbar discography to be 40% per patient. Again, if the results are calculated using ISIS/IASP standardized diagnostic criteria, the false-positive rate drops to 0%.[12] This pool of patients had diagnoses of cervical degenerative disc changes and neck pain severe enough that they had undergone cervical surgery for their pain. Because cervical and lumbar disc disease coincide, it is possible that the lumbar discs of the patients also had some amount of disc disease. These mildly abnormal, albeit asymptomatic, discs could then test positive with less stringent diagnostic criteria.

In an extensive review by Wolfer and colleagues,[12] the results of lumbar discography in patients with chronic pain of nonlumbar origin were pooled. Including those with chronic cervical pain and chronic iliac crest pain, the original investigators cited a false-positive rate of 44%. By changing the diagnostic criteria as pain at less than 50 psi above opening pressure, the false-positive rate dropped to 33%, and by including all ISIS/IASP diagnostic standards, the false-positive rate was only 5.6% per patient and 3.85% per disc. Even in patients with chronic pain, lumbar discography has a low false-positive rate.

Carragee and colleagues[16] also studied lumbar discography false-positive rates in 4 patients with somatization disorder and no low back pain. The false-positive rate was high at 75% per patient with the investigators' analysis and 50% with ISIS/IASP standards.[12] However, this study had a small sample size and large confidence intervals (CIs) (0%–100%).[16] In contrast, another study of lumbar discography in 81 patients, 27 with abnormal psychometrics but without somatization disorder, showed no correlation between psychometric scores and positive discography.[17] It is unclear as to what degree psychological factors affect discography results. Nonetheless, the North American Spine Society position statement includes significant psychological overlay as a relative contraindication to discography. Especially in patients with somatization disorder, it should be considered that there is higher risk for iatrogenic illness and recurrent pain after any interventional or surgical procedure.

In another study, lumbar discography was performed on patients with chronic mild low back pain, and positive discography was cited as being false positive. A false-positive rate of 36% per patient was reported.[18] Secondary analysis applying ISIS/IASP standards found a false-positive rate of 16% per patient.[12] This increased false-positive rate is likely a result of some of these results actually being true-positives. Patients in this study with "low back pain every or almost every day" and a visual analogue scale (VAS) of 2.2 to 4.1 but not receiving medical care may still have discogenic pain for which a positive discography would be a true-positive rather than a false-positive result.[12] Discography is not designed to determine the severity of the discogenic pain but rather to determine whether provocation of the disc elicits the patient's typical pain.

Carragee reviewed the results of several of his own studies and evaluated for a change in the outcomes by changing from a threshold of 100 psi above opening pressure to the low-pressure standard of 22 psi. There was no statistical difference in false-positive rates, and therefore, it was concluded that there was no added value of using low-pressure criteria.[19] On further review, however, the somatization group and the chronic low back pain group were included in this analysis. The somatization group had a high incidence of false-positives at low pressures and the low back pain group most probably included true-positives. In an analysis of all studies, excluding these two populations, the false-positive rate (per patient) was found to be 16% using 22 psi above opening pressure, 10.7% using 15 psi, and 9.3% using ISIS/IASP standards.[12] The standardization of diagnostic criteria, including a low-pressure technique, does improve results.

In an extensive post hoc analysis of lumbar discography studies in asymptomatic patients without significant confounding factors, a total of 33 patients and 48 discs were included. Using ISIS/IASP standards across all studies, the false-positive rate is 3% per patient and 2.1% per disc.[12] In all subjects without low back pain, but excluding those who underwent prior discectomy and 2 subjects (because of incomplete data sets) with somatization disorder, the false-positive rate is 6% per disc and overall specificity is 94% (95% CI, 0.88–0.98).[12] This specificity is significantly improved over other studies because standardized ISIS/IASP diagnostic criteria were used. With these findings, lumbar discography remains a valid test to confirm or refute the hypothesis that a specific disc is the etiology of a patient's low back pain.

In 2006, Carragee and colleagues[20] measured the success of lumbar surgical fusion in subjects selected by positive lumbar discography in an effort to determine the positive predictive value of discography. The study followed 32 patients with single-level, low-pressure positive discography 2 years post-fusion. They were matched with 34 patients who underwent fusion for unstable spondylolisthesis (considered the best-case scenario for surgical fusion results and therefore chosen as the gold standard). Only 27% of the patients with positive discography had highly effective surgical success versus 72% of the spondylolisthesis cohort. The investigators reported a best-case positive predictive value for discography of 50% to 60%. The strengths of the study included stringent exclusion criteria for the discography group, including worker's compensation, abnormal psychometrics, other chronic pain, greater than 12 months of disability, and greater than 25% relief with zygapophysial or sacroiliac joint injections, thereby creating an uncomplicated population for discography with little in the way of confounding factors.

However, a major weakness of the study was the difference in inclusion criteria between the 2 groups. Although the discography group included chronic low back pain without sciatica, the spondylolisthesis group allowed patients with or without sciatica. Within the spondylolisthesis group, 6 patients were noted to have positive electromyography (EMG), 4 of whom had denervation.[20] It is not clear whether all patients underwent EMG, and it is possible that additional subjects could have had a positive EMG. With this discrepancy, it is not truly a matched cohort. The difference in surgical outcomes for those with radicular pain versus those without is widely accepted, and similar outcomes would not be expected.

Nonetheless, the finding that only 27% of patients with positive discography had highly effective surgical success is noteworthy. Discography was done with adequate diagnostic criteria: pain greater than or equal to 6/10, threshold less than or equal to 20 psi above opening pressure, annular fissure extending to the posterior annulus, and a control disc with less than 2/10 pain with pressurization up to 100 psi above opening pressure.[20] The criteria for highly effective surgical success, however, were stringent and included low back pain less than or equal to 2/10, Oswestry disability index (ODI) less than or equal to 15, full return to occupational duties, no narcotics, and no daily analgesics. These are not the typical criteria used to judge surgical success. A more favorable outcome of 43.2% success for patients who underwent discography was noted with the less stringent minimal acceptable outcome as judged by patients before interventions.[20] These are not exemplary outcomes but are favorable compared with surgical success rates for low back pain in other studies. Fritzell and colleagues[21] found that only 16% of patients reported excellent results, and Slosar and colleagues[22] concluded that only 10% of patients believed that surgery met their expectations. Discography may improve surgical results, especially in patients without confounding factors. Incomplete surgical success with discography may be caused by multiple factors aside from a low positive predictive value of the test, including nonmechanical pain emanating from the disc and surgical limitations for the treatment of axial low back pain.

ANESTHETIC DISCOGRAPHY

The purpose of anesthetic discography is to demonstrate relief of a patient's usual pain after injection of an anesthetic into the disc. A few different techniques exist; one, which has been studied, is referred to as discoblock. In a recent randomized controlled trial, the surgical outcomes of patients who had undergone standard discography were compared with the outcomes of those selected using discoblock for diagnosis.[23] Patients who underwent surgery after diagnosis with discoblock had statistically greater improvement in ODI and VAS scores at 3 years post-surgery. This study included 42 patients, 12 had negative discography and/or discoblock and 15 in each group went on to have surgery. The standard discography technique is not described clearly, and pressure manometry may not have been used. Volumes injected ranged from 0.4 to 3.2 mL and was described as "until severe pain or leak."[23] The discoblock group received 0.75 mL of bupivacaine 0.5% into the disc, and a positive block was one in which there was decreased pain. The investigators did not describe how much pain relief defined a positive response.[23] Despite the questionable methodology, both groups had statistically and clinically significant improvement in ODI and VAS scores at 3 years post-surgery. The investigators showed significantly better findings in the discoblock group, but this could be a result of false-positives in the standard discography group due to the use of a nonstandardized discography technique. It is unclear how these results should be interpreted.

Although anesthetic discography may have favorable results compared with standard discography, there may be side effects associated with intradiscal injection of bupivacaine. Bupivacaine has been shown to be toxic to cartilage in vivo, and recently it has also been shown to be toxic to the intervertebral disc in vitro.[24] In a time- and dose-dependent manner, human nucleus pulposus and annulus fibrosis cells showed necrosis. Bupivacaine 0.5% for 2 hours caused 40% cell death.[24] This in vitro study does not indicate clinical significance, but the possible implications need to be considered.

Side Effects

Immediate risks, contraindications, and potential complications are similar to those of all interventional spine procedures. Discography had, in the past, shown a slightly higher risk of infection than other intervention when antibiotic prophylaxis was not routinely used for lumbar discography. At that time, the rate of discitis was reported to be between 0.1% and 2.3% per patient, and 0.05% and 1.3% per disc.[25] Typically, infections were caused by *Staphylococcus aureus*, *Staphylococcus epidermidis*, and *Escherichia coli*. In current practice, intravenous and often intradiscal antibiotics are administered. Also, a change to a coaxial needle technique has likely decreased infections by skin flora. This technique uses an outer introducer needle, allowing an inner needle that has never contacted the skin to be inserted into the disc. Using current techniques, including routine prophylactic antibiotics, the rate of discitis is not greater than with other spine interventions.[26]

For long-term risk, a recent study has suggested that discography could be a cause of intervertebral disc disruption and degeneration. Carragee and colleagues[27] analyzed disc degeneration progression at 10 years in subjects who had undergone discography compared with a matched cohort. From their multiple studies of lumbar discography in patients without serious low back pain, 50 patients who had undergone discography and protocol magnetic resonance imaging (MRI) in 1997 had follow-up MRI 7 to 10 years later. From the same population, a matched cohort of patients who refused discography also underwent protocol MRI in 1997 and follow-up MRI 7 to 10 years later. MRI findings and changes over time were compared between the lumbar discography and the no discography groups to determine whether a difference could be detected. There was 21% greater progression to a higher grade of disc degeneration and a greater number of new disc herniations (55 vs 22, P = .0003) in the discography group compared with controls. In addition, new disc herniations were disproportionately found on the side of the annular puncture and in the region of usual disc entry.

Commendable effort was made to match the control cohort by enrolling patients for the control (no discography) group from the same pools of subjects as the discography group. Of the population studied, many patients had severe cervical spine disease or mild persistent low back pain. Those with more severe cervical or lumbar spine disease would be predicted to have more significant lumbar degeneration progression and new herniations because of heritability. Although the no discography group was from the same population, a difference in the extent of the cervical or lumbar disease between patients in the discography and the control groups could cause bias. This bias would be amplified by counting discs rather than patients with new findings (eg, 1 patient could have progression or new herniation at 2–3 discs), as was done in this study.

Needle size (25 vs 22 gauge) did not show a statistical difference, although there was a trend toward greater degeneration with larger needles. The laboratory method of reliably inducing disc injury in rabbits with comparatively much larger needles supports the theory that smaller needles would induce less injury. Comparing discography with other models of laboratory-induced disc injury causes concern regarding the amount of pressurization as well. In 2006, a gas pressurization model for inducing laboratory disc injury was described. The amount of gas pressurization of the annulus correlated to the degree of disruption of the disc tissue seen on MRI and on gross inspection.[28] Pressures studied included 69, 172, 345, and 690 kPa, correlating to 10, 25, 50, and 100 psi respectively. Carragee's discography protocols routinely used a threshold of 100 psi above opening pressure. If higher intradiscal pressure in vivo can cause increased disc disruption evident on MRI, then higher pressures with discography could also contribute to increased disc injury. Low-pressure discography may induce less internal disc disruption and, therefore, less degenerative progression and herniation.

Despite increased disc degeneration and herniation as seen on MRI 10 years after discography, the clinical significance is not clear. The poor correlation of clinical findings with disc degeneration on MRI is already accepted. Also, the size of the new herniations was not mentioned and may have included bulges and protrusions as small as 1 to 3 mm. If the findings of these new herniations and increased disc degeneration were causing clinical concern, one would expect new imaging utilization to be different between groups. Health care utilization was not determined in this study, but at 10-year follow-up, 13 discography and 8 control subjects had elective lumbar MRI (outside the study protocol) within the prior 3 years. This is not a considerable difference between groups, but it does not truly account for health care utilization. A complete study for potential difference in health care utilization and clinical implications from this study population is awaited.

Regardless of the limitations of this study, the findings draw attention to additional risks to consider for lumbar discography. Further modification of the technique may be considered, such as abandoning the use of a control disc, possibly using even smaller-gauge or noncutting needles for disc entry, and adhering to low-pressure thresholds. Although discography has diagnostic value in properly selected patients with standardized technique and diagnostic criteria, the potential risks must be weighed against the possible benefit and discussed with each patient.

SUMMARY

Discography is the only means available to diagnose a symptomatic lumbar disc, but the evidence of its validity and safety remains controversial. There is variability and subjectivity in technique and diagnostic criteria. This variability leads to the perception that results are not reproducible. In addition, results are variably reported as per disc or per patient. A false-positive rate reported per patient is typically higher than that reported per disc. There are arguments for reporting in either manner, and one must be cautious when comparing studies. Also, there is no gold standard against which discography can be compared and, therefore, no way to calculate the sensitivity or the likelihood ratio. Surgical results have been used to attempt to calculate positive predictive value, but this method is confounded by numerous extraneous variables. Despite its imperfections, lumbar discography remains a useful test when validated techniques and diagnostic criteria are used in patients when other etiologies of low back pain have been ruled out and conservative care has failed. It should be used in selected patients who have unremitting pain and are seeking further surgical or invasive treatment. Discography seems to increase disc degeneration and herniation detected on MRI. Although clinical significance of these findings is yet to be determined, it is an important consideration before performing discography and may justify modification of techniques and decreased frequency of its use. Overall, discography is the only means currently available to diagnose lumbar disc pain and remains a valid test when coupled with careful patient selection, strict adherence to standardized technique and diagnostic criteria, and careful consideration of possible long-term side effects.

REFERENCES

1. Boden SD, Davis DO, Dina TS, et al. Abnormal magnetic-resonance scans of the lumbar spine in asymptomatic subjects. A prospective investigation. J Bone Joint Surg Am 1990;72(3):403–8.
2. Jarvik JG, Deyo RA. Imaging of lumbar intervertebral disc degeneration and aging, excluding disc herniations. Radiol Clin North Am 2000;38(6):1255–66, vi.
3. Ashton IK, Walsh DA, Polak JM, et al. Substance P in intervertebral discs. Binding sites on vascular endothelium of the human annulus fibrosus. Acta Orthop Scand 1994;65(6):635–9.
4. Freemont AJ, Peacock TE, Goupille P, et al. Nerve ingrowth into diseased intervertebral disc in chronic back pain. Lancet 1997;350(9072):178–81.
5. Guyer RD, Ohnmeiss DD. Lumbar discography. Position statement from the North American Spine Society Diagnostic and Therapeutic Committee. Spine (Phila Pa 1976) 1995;20(18):2048–59.
6. Bogduk N. Lumbar disc stimulation. In: International Spine Intervention Society practice guidelines for spinal diagnostic and treatment procedures. San Francisco (CA): International Spine Intervention Society; 2004. p. 20–46.
7. Lindblom K. Diagnostic disc puncture of intervertebral discs in sciatica. Acta Orthop Scandinav 1948;17:231–9.
8. Massey WK, Stevens DB. A critical evaluation of discography. J Bone Joint Surg Am 1967;49:1243–4.
9. Holt EP Jr. The question of lumbar discography. J Bone Joint Surg Am 1968; 50(4):720–6.
10. Walsh TR, Weinstein JN, Spratt KF, et al. Lumbar discography in normal subjects. A controlled, prospective study. J Bone Joint Surg Am 1990;72(7):1081–8.
11. Carragee EJ, Tanner CM, Khurana S, et al. The rates of false-positive lumbar discography in select patients without low back symptoms. Spine (Phila Pa 1976) 2000;25(11):1373–80 [discussion: 1381].
12. Wolfer LR, Derby R, Lee JE, et al. Systematic review of lumbar provocation discography in asymptomatic subjects with a meta-analysis of false-positive rates. Pain Physician 2008;11(4):513–38.
13. Derby R, Lee SH, Kim BJ, et al. Pressure-controlled lumbar discography in volunteers without low back symptoms. Pain Med 2005;6(3):213–21 [discussion: 222–4].
14. Carragee EJ, Chen Y, Tanner CM, et al. Provocative discography in patients after limited lumbar discectomy: a controlled, randomized study of pain response in symptomatic and asymptomatic subjects. Spine (Phila Pa 1976) 2000;25(23): 3065–71.
15. Carragee EJ, Tanner CM, Yang B, et al. False-positive findings on lumbar discography. Reliability of subjective concordance assessment during provocative disc injection. Spine (Phila Pa 1976) 1999;24(23):2542–7.
16. Carragee EJ, Chen Y, Tanner CM, et al. Can discography cause long-term back symptoms in previously asymptomatic subjects? Spine (Phila Pa 1976) 2000; 25(14):1803–8.
17. Derby R, Lee SH, Chen Y, et al. The influence of psychologic factors on discography in patients with chronic axial low back pain. Arch Phys Med Rehabil 2008;89(7):1300–4.

18. Carragee EJ, Alamin TF, Miller J, et al. Provocative discography in volunteer subjects with mild persistent low back pain. Spine J 2002;2(1):25–34.
19. Carragee EJ, Alamin TF, Carragee JM. Low-pressure positive discography in subjects asymptomatic of significant low back pain illness. Spine (Phila Pa 1976) 2006;31(5):505–9.
20. Carragee EJ, Lincoln T, Parmar VS, et al. A gold standard evaluation of the "discogenic pain" diagnosis as determined by provocative discography. Spine (Phila Pa 1976) 2006;31(18):2115–23.
21. Fritzell P, Hagg O, Wessberg P, et al. Chronic low back pain and fusion: a comparison of three surgical techniques: a prospective multicenter randomized study from the Swedish Lumbar Spine Study Group. Spine (Phila Pa 1976) 2002; 27(11):1131–41.
22. Slosar PJ, Reynolds JB, Schofferman J, et al. Patient satisfaction after circumferential lumbar fusion. Spine (Phila Pa 1976) 2000;25(6):722–6.
23. Ohtori S, Kinoshita T, Yamashita M, et al. Results of surgery for discogenic low back pain: a randomized study using discography versus discoblock for diagnosis. Spine (Phila Pa 1976) 2009;34(13):1345–8.
24. Lee H, Sowa G, Vo N, et al. Effect of bupivacaine on intervertebral disc cell viability. Spine J 2010;10(2):159–66.
25. Bogduk N, Aprill C, Derby R. Discography. St Louis (MO): Mosby; 1995.
26. Fraser RD, Osti OL, Vernon-Roberts B. Discitis after discography. J Bone Joint Surg Br 1987;69(1):26–35.
27. Carragee EJ, Don AS, Hurwitz EL, et al. 2009 ISSLS Prize Winner: does discography cause accelerated progression of degeneration changes in the lumbar disc: a ten-year matched cohort study. Spine (Phila Pa 1976) 2009;34(21): 2338–45.
28. Oliphant D, Frayne R, Kawchuk G. A new method of creating intervertebral disc disruption of various grades. Clin Biomech (Bristol, Avon) 2006;21(1):21–5.

Percutaneous Vertebroplasty: Role in Treatment of Vertebral Compression Fractures

Nayna Patel, MD*

KEYWORDS

- Osteoporosis • Vertebral compression fractures
- Percutaneous vertebroplasty • PMMA

OSTEOPOROSIS

Osteoporosis is the most common metabolic bone disorder in the world and is a considerable source of morbidity and mortality in the United States.[1] Osteoporosis is defined as a decrease in bone mineral density (BMD) that is 2.5 standard deviations less than the mean peak value in young adults of the same race and sex (World Health Organization). However, a decrease in BMD by only 1 standard deviation increases the risk of vertebral compression fractures (VCFs) by nearly 2-fold.[2] In the United States alone, nearly 700,000 patients are affected with VCFs each year. Patients with symptomatic VCFs suffer a significant amount of back pain and disability. Quality of life is affected, as activities of daily living and ambulation are often gravely affected. Patients with VCFs have an increased likelihood of falls and are 5 times more likely to sustain additional fractures than patients without VCFs.[3] Long-term disability can ensue, as can depression and anxiety.[1] Patients with VCFs have a 6.4 times greater mortality.[3] Economic implications of VCFs are significant. The United States spends nearly $15 million on the treatment of osteoporotic fractures, and VCFs account for more than 150,000 hospital admissions each year.[1]

PATHOLOGY

VCFs are a significant cause of back pain. Pain after VCF can be attributed to incomplete healing and progressive collapse of the bone. Incomplete healing causes motion of the fractured vertebral body, which stresses the interosseous and periosteal nerves. The irritated nerves generate substance P, a known factor of nociception. Progressive

Core Orthopaedic, Encinitas, CA 92024, USA
* 634 Pacific View Drive, San Diego, CA 92109.
E-mail address: napatel@coreorthopaedic.co

Phys Med Rehabil Clin N Am 21 (2010) 869–876
doi:10.1016/j.pmr.2010.07.001
1047-9651/10/$ – see front matter © 2010 Published by Elsevier Inc.

pmr.theclinics.com

vertebral collapse can result in spinal deformity, altering individual biomechanics. Kyphotic deformity associated with VCFs shifts the patient's center of gravity anteriorly, increasing the lever arm and flexion moment at the apex of the kyphosis. The altered biomechanics can lead to progressive kyphosis and future VCFs.[4]

STANDARD TREATMENT OF VCFs

Historical treatment options for patients with painful VCFs have been conservative management. Bed rest, acetaminophen, nonsteroidal antiinflammatory drugs, narcotic medications, bracing, and physical therapy have been used to decrease pain and increase functionality. Although seemingly harmless, conservative treatment can be risky for elderly patients suffering VCFs. Bed rest and inactivity can lead to pneumonia, decubital ulcers, deep vein thrombosis, and pulmonary emboli. More recently, injection of polymethylmethacrylate (PMMA) directly into the VCF, or vertebroplasty, has been used to hasten pain relief and return to function.

HISTORY OF PERCUTANEOUS VERTEBROPLASTY

For many decades, open vertebroplasty has been performed to augment pedicle purchase of surgical instrumentation in spinal fusion cases. Percutaneous vertebroplasty (PV) was first introduced in France in 1984[5] as an alternative to open vertebroplasty. Galibert and Deramond[6] from the Department of Radiology of the University Hospital of Amiens in France first performed the procedure on a 54-year-old woman with a chief complaint of severe cervical pain with a C2 radiculopathy. Plain radiographs showed a large vertebral hemangioma involving the entire C2 vertebral body, and computerized axial tomographic (CAT) scan confirmed epidural extension. A C2 laminectomy was performed to excise the epidural component of the hemangioma. PMMA was injected percutaneously to obtain reinforcement of the C2 vertebral body. The patient experienced complete pain relief of not only the radicular symptoms but also the axial neck symptoms. The results of the procedure were so impressive that PV was subsequently performed on 6 other patients. In 1987, the first patient with painful VCF was treated with PV, and the procedure was first introduced in the United States in 1988 at the Annual Meeting of the Radiological Society of North America.[6]

PHYSIOLOGY OF PV

The exact mechanism of pain relief via vertebroplasty is not understood completely. Initially, pain relief was believed to be secondary to thermal energy.[7] Studies have now shown that in vivo temperatures after vertebroplasty are not high enough to cause thermal necrosis of sensory nerves.[7] Alternatively, pain relief from vertebroplasty likely arises from improved vertebral body strength and stiffness and decreased motion of the vertebral body and periosteal and interosseous nerves.[7–9] Cadaveric studies have suggested that there is also new bone formation after PV.[8]

TECHNIQUE

PV is performed under strict sterile conditions using C-arm fluoroscopy or CAT for guidance of needle placement. The C-arm is turned obliquely from the anteroposterior (AP) position to maximize the ovoid appearance of the pedicle, known as "looking down the barrel." Once this view is achieved, the skin, subcutaneous tissues, and periosteum are anesthetized with a local anesthetic. A small incision is made. A large-bore needle (10–13 gauge) is directed under intermittent fluoroscopic guidance to the midpoint of the pedicle and advanced until the osseum is reached. At this point, lateral fluoroscopy helps to place the tip of the needle at the upper to midpoint of the pedicle. It is imperative that frequent monitoring of the needle position is performed in both planes.[10,11]

The AP view should demonstrate that the needle is proceeding parallel to the x-ray beam as in a hub view. Lateral projections show the needle moving either parallel to or slightly downwards to the superior and inferior edges of the pedicle.

As the needle tip enters the soft bone marrow, less pressure is required to advance the needle. Frequent AP and lateral views are required to monitor needle positioning and ensure that the needle does not breech either the anterior vertebral wall or vertebral end plates. The needle is advanced until the stylet tip is located near the junction of the anterior and middle thirds of the vertebral body.

Venography can be performed before injection of the cement.[12] For immunocompromised patients, gentamicin or tobramycin can be added to the PMMA mixture.[11] Commercially available PMMA must be mixed with a radiopaque substance before injection. Injection is then completed under continuous lateral fluoroscopy to confirm that the cement does not extravasate during the procedure into the epidural space or inferior vena cava. The amount of pressure required to inject the cement increases as the vertebral body is filled and settling of the PMMA cement occurs. If venous uptake occurs, the injection is halted until the cement thickens. End points include holovertebral filling, hemivertebral filling, extravasation of PMMA into either veins or disk space, or until no more cement can be injected.

After the procedure is completed, the patient should remain supine for several hours to ensure curing of the PMMA before axial loading.

EFFICACY

Current standard of care for VCFs without neurologic compromise is nonoperative. Treatment includes rest, analgesic medications, physical therapy, and bracing. However, this treatment modality is not without risk. Prolonged bed rest and immobility can lead to further compression fractures, decubital ulcers, pneumonia, deep venous thrombosis, and pulmonary emboli.[13]

Many retrospective studies have found that PV gives immediate[14–21] and long-term[14–16,22,23] pain relief to patients suffering from VCFs. Decreased analgesic use has been reported.[17,19,24] Improvement in the quality of life, activities of daily living,[19] and mobility[16–19,24,25] has also been demonstrated after PV. Although patients with VCFs as old as 24 months have been shown to have improvement in pain scores,[25,26] subacute VCFs seem to be associated with the best outcomes and least adverse outcomes.[22]

Similar results have been found in prospective case series. Decreased pain,[6,24,27–35] improved function and mobility,[3,6,24,30] decreased usage of pain medications,[24,33] and improved quality of life[30,36,37] have all been demonstrated. In addition, PV has been shown to stabilize VCFs and prevent further vertebral body collapse.[3,27,29,30]

For 2 years, Diamond and colleagues[13] prospectively studied 88 patients who underwent PV and 38 patients who were treated with conservative therapy. Lower pain scores were found in the PV group at 6 weeks, but at 6 to 12 months and 2 years, there was no statistical difference in pain scores between the 2 treatment groups. Favorable natural history of VCFs and possible regression to the mean of PV are possible reasons that no long-term clinical or statistical difference was present between the 2 groups.

In addition to osteoporotic compression fractures, PV has also been shown to be efficacious for the treatment of pathologic compression fractures. Both primary and metastatic lesions of the spine can cause substantial pain, instability, and kyphotic deformity in the spine. PV has been shown to decrease pain,[35,38] stabilize the vertebral body,[15,38] and improve the quality of life[37,39] in patients with lesions of the vertebral body.

PV was first used for the treatment of painful hemangioma. Several studies have also demonstrated efficacy of PV in decreasing pain caused by hemangioma.[40,41]

Although the studies mentioned earlier have documented that vertebroplasty is often associated with an immediate dramatic pain reduction in patients with VCFs, recent randomized controlled trials (RCTs) have failed to show any difference in the outcomes of patients treated with PV versus sham procedure or conservative care.[42–45] Voormolen and colleagues[42] initiated an RCT, the VERTOS study, comparing PV with optimized pain medication (OPM). Patients were randomized to a treatment group of PV or OPM, and at 2 weeks, the patients randomized to the OPM group were allowed to cross over to PV. Most patients in the OPM group elected to undergo PV after only 2 weeks, and the study was terminated early. The primary clinical outcome was measured using the visual analog scale (VAS). Follow-up occurred at 1 day and 2 weeks after initiation of either PV or OPM treatment. Intention-to-treat analysis was used. On day 1, both groups were found to have a statistically significant decrease in VAS and analgesic use. Two weeks after the initiation of treatment, the difference on the VAS between PV and OPM groups was not statistically significant.

Kallmes and colleagues[44] studied PV versus a simulated noncemented procedure in 131 patients. At 1 month, although there was a trend toward a higher rate of clinically meaningful improvement in pain (30% decrease from baseline), there was no statistical difference between the treatment and control groups in regard to pain scores, quality of life, and physical disability related to back pain.

Buchbinder and colleagues[45] failed to find any significant difference in patients treated with PV versus sham procedure. Seventy-eight patients with 1- or 2-level VCFs were randomized into treatment and sham groups and followed up for 6 months. After the procedure, both groups had a significant decrease in pain and use of narcotics, with no difference between groups at 1 week, 1 month, 3 months, and 6 months.

COMPLICATIONS

Although PV is a safe procedure in experienced hands, several serious complications have been reported. Refractures, largely at adjacent levels, are related to kyphotic deformity associated with compression fractures. Kyphotic deformity anteriorly shifts the patient's center of gravity, increasing the lever arm and flexion moment at the apex of the kyphosis. Because vertebroplasty does not correct the kyphotic deformity, cementing a vertebral body may increase stress at the adjacent vertebral segments.[46] Refracture rates have been estimated to be between 10% to 53%.[13,18,22,24,36,37,47]

Self-limited adverse events include radiculitis, infection, diskitis, and rib fracture.[24] More serious complications can arise as well. Case reports of fatal fat embolism,[48] pulmonary embolism,[49–52] inferior vena cava syndrome,[53] paraplegia,[54–56] renal embolism,[57] paradoxic cerebral artery embolism,[20] and cardiac tamponade[50] following PV exist, most of which are related to cement leakage. The risk of cement leakage increases in acute VCFs, as the bony cortex has cracks without hematoma or callus formation to stop cement leakage.[20,22]

DISCUSSION

VCFs are a significant cause of morbidity in the United States. Historically, VCFs have been managed conservatively, but PV is an effective treatment for VCFs in some patients. The exact mechanism by which PV decreases pain caused by VCFs is unknown, but the decrease is speculated to be secondary to decreased motion of interosseous and periosteal nerves. Because of rare, but serious, complications that can arise, PV should be performed only by experienced spine interventionalists with excellent knowledge of spinal anatomy. At present, only level 2 to 5 data exist to support the use of PV as a treatment for painful VCFs. There are no published level 1 data demonstrating superiority of PV with that of conservative methods for the treatment of painful VCFs. Conservative methods should therefore be considered as first-line treatments in most patients unless contraindications exist. Until further studies show that PV is superior to conservative treatment, with an equivalent complications profile, PV should be reserved for patients who have failed conservative treatment.

REFERENCES

1. Gardner MJ, Demetrakopoulos D, Shindle MK, et al. Osteoporosis and skeletal fractures. HSS J 2006;2:62–9.
2. Lane JM, Johnson CE, Khan SN, et al. Minimally invasive options for the treatment of osteoporotic vertebral compression fractures. Orthop Clin North Am 2002;33: 431–8.
3. Lau E, Ong K, Kurtz S, et al. Mortality following the diagnosis of a vertebral compression fracture in the Medicare population. J Bone Joint Surg Am 2008; 90(7):1479–86.
4. White AA, Panjabi MM, Thomas CL. The clinical biomechanics of kyphotic deformities. Clin Orthop Relat Res 1977;128:8–17.
5. Mathis JM, Belkoff SM, Deramond H. Percutaneous vertebroplasty and kyphoplasty, vol. 2. China: Springer; 2006. p. 1–5.
6. Zoarski GH, Snow P, Olan WJ, et al. Percutaneous vertebroplasty for osteoporotic compression fractures: quantitative prospective evaluation of long-term outcomes. J Vasc Interv Radiol 2002;13:139–48.
7. Anselmetti GC, Manca A, Kanika K, et al. Temperature measurement during polymerization of bone cement in percutaneous vertebroplasty: an in vivo study in humans. Cardiovasc Intervent Radiol 2009;3:491–8.
8. Braunstein V, Sprecher CM, Gisep A, et al. Long-term reaction to bone cement in osteoporotic bone: new bone formation in vertebral bodies after vertebroplasty. J Anat 2008;212:697–701.
9. Belkoff SM, Mathis JM, Jasper LE, et al. The biomechanics of vertebroplasty: the effect of cement volume on mechanical behavior. Spine (Phila Pa 1976) 2001;26: 1537–41.
10. Mathis JM, Barr JD, Belkoff SM, et al. Percutaneous vertebroplasty: a developing standard of care for vertebral compression fractures. AJNR Am J Neuroradiol 2001;22:373–81.
11. Jensen ME, Evans AJ, Mathis JM, et al. Percutaneous polymethylmethacrylate vertebroplasty in the treatment of osteoporotic vertebral body compression fractures: technical aspects. AJNR Am J Neuroradiol 1997;18(10):1897–904.

12. Peh WC, Gilula LA. Additional value of a modified method of intraosseous venography during percutaneous vertebroplasty. AJR Am J Roentgenol 2003;180:87–91.

13. Diamond TH, Champion B, Clark WA. Management of acute osteoporotic vertebral fractures: a nonrandomized trial comparing percutaneous vertebroplasty with conservative therapy. Am J Med 2003;114:257–65.

14. Grados F, Depriester C, Cayrolle G, et al. Long-term observations of vertebral osteoporotic fractures treated by percutaneous vertebroplasty. Rheumatology (Oxford) 2000;39:1410–4.

15. Barr JD, Barr MS, Lemley TJ, et al. Percutaneous vertebroplasty for pain relief and spinal stabilization. Spine (Phila Pa 1976) 2000;25:923–8.

16. Serra L, Kermani M, Panagiotopoulos K, et al. Vertebroplasty in the treatment of osteoporotic vertebral fractures: results and functional outcome in a series of 175 consecutive patients. Minim Invasive Neurosurg 2007;50:12–7.

17. Kallmes DF, Schweickert PA, Marx WF, et al. Vertebroplasty in the mid and upper thoracic spine. AJNR Am J Neuroradiol 2002;23:1117–20.

18. Kobayashi K, Shimoyama K, Nakamura K, et al. Percutaneous vertebroplasty immediately relieves pain of osteoporotic vertebral compression fractures and prevents prolonged immobilization of patients. Eur Radiol 2005;15:360–7.

19. Evans AJ, Jensen ME, Kip KE, et al. Vertebral compression fractures: pain reduction and improvement in functional mobility after percutaneous polymethylmethacrylate vertebroplasty retrospective report of 245 cases. Radiology 2003;226: 366–72.

20. Hodler J, Peck D, Gilula LA. Midterm outcome after vertebroplasty: predictive value of technical and patient-related factors. Radiology 2003;227:662–8.

21. Costa F, Ortolina A, Cardia A, et al. Efficacy of treatment with percutaneous vertebroplasty and kyphoplasty for traumatic fracture of thoracolumbar junction. J Neurosurg Sci 2009;53:13–7.

22. Yu SW, Lee PC, Ma CH, et al. Vertebroplasty for the treatment of osteoporotic compression spinal fracture: comparison of remedial action at different stages of injury. J Trauma 2004;56:629–32.

23. Peh WC, Gelbart MS, Gilula LA, et al. Percutaneous vertebroplasty: treatment of painful vertebral compression fractures with intraosseous vacuum phenomena. AJR Am J Roentgenol 2003;180:1411–7.

24. Layton KF, Thielen KR, Koch CA, et al. Vertebroplasty, first 1000 levels of a single center: evaluation of the outcomes and complications. AJNR Am J Neuroradiol 2007;28:683–9.

25. Brown DB, Gilula LA, Sehgal M, et al. Treatment of chronic symptomatic vertebral compression fractures with percutaneous vertebroplasty. AJR Am J Roentgenol 2004;182:319–22.

26. Kaufmann TJ, Jensen ME, Schweickert PA, et al. Age of fracture and clinical outcomes of percutaneous vertebroplasty. AJNR Am J Neuroradiol 2001;22: 1860–3.

27. Heini PF, Orler R. Kyphoplasty for treatment of osteoporotic vertebral fractures. Eur Spine J 2004;13:184–92.

28. Nirala AP, Vatsal DK, Husain M, et al. Percutaneous vertebroplasty: an experience of 31 procedures. Neurol India 2003;51:490–2.

29. Perez-Higueras A, Alvarez L, Rossi RE, et al. Percutaneous vertebroplasty: long-term clinical and radiological outcome. Neuroradiology 2002;44:950–4.

30. Legroux-Gérot I, Lormeau C, Boutry N, et al. Long-term follow-up of vertebral osteoporotic fractures treated by percutaneous vertebroplasty. Clin Rheumatol 2004;23:310–7.

31. Cortet B, Cotten A, Boutry N, et al. Percutaneous vertebroplasty in the treatment of osteoporotic vertebral compression fractures: an open prospective study. J Rheumatol 1999;26:2222–8.

32. McGraw JK, Lippert JA, Minkus KD, et al. Prospective evaluation of pain relief in 100 patients undergoing percutaneous vertebroplasty: results and follow-up. J Vasc Interv Radiol 2002;13:883–6.

33. Afzal S, Dhar S, Vasavada NB, et al. Percutaneous vertebroplasty for osteoporotic fractures. Pain Physician 2007;10(4):559–63.

34. Muijis SJ, Nieuwenhuijse MJ, Van Erkel AR, et al. Percutaneous vertebroplasty for the treatment of osteoporotic vertebral compression fractures. J Bone Joint Surg Br 2009;91:379–84.

35. Purkayastha S, Gupta AK, Kapilamoorthy TR, et al. Percutaneous vertebroplasty in the management of vertebral lesions. Neurol India 2005;53(2):167–72.

36. McKiernan F, Faciszewski T, Jensen R. Quality of life following vertebroplasty. J Bone Joint Surg Am 2004;86:2600–6.

37. Alvarez LA, Alcaraz M, Perez-Higueras A, et al. Percutaneous vertebroplasty: functional improvement in patients with osteoporotic compression fractures. Spine (Phila Pa 1976) 2006;31:1113–8.

38. Weill A, Chiras J, Simon JM, et al. Spinal metastases: indications for and results of percutaneous injection of acrylic surgical cement. Radiology 1996;199: 241–7.

39. Wegner M. Vertebroplasty for metastasis. Med Oncol 2003;20:203–9.

40. Guarnieri G, Ambrosanio G, Vassallo P, et al. Vertebroplasty as treatment of aggressive and symptomatic vertebral hemangiomas: up to 4 years of follow-up. Neuroradiology 2009;51(7):471–6.

41. Chen L, Zhang C, Tang T. Cement vertebroplasty combined with ethanol injection in the treatment of vertebral hemangioma. Chin Med J 2007;120:1136–9.

42. Voormolen MH, Mali WP, Lohle PN, et al. Percutaneous vertebroplasty compared with optimal pain medication treatment: short-term clinical outcome of patients with subacute or chronic painful osteoporotic vertebral compression fractures. The VERTOS study. AJNR Am J Neuroradiol 2007;28:555–60.

43. Gray LA, Jarvik JG, Heagerty PF, et al. Investigational vertebroplasty efficacy and safety trial (INVEST): a randomized controlled trial of percutaneous vertebroplasty. BMC Musculoskelet Disord 2007;8:126.

44. Kallmes DF, Comstock BA, Gray LA, et al. Baseline pain and disability in the investigational vertebroplasty efficacy and safety trial. AJNR Am J Neuroradiol 2009;30(6):1203–5.

45. Buchbinder R, Osborne PR, Wark JD, et al. Efficacy and safety of vertebroplasty for treatment of painful osteoporotic vertebral fractures: a randomised controlled trial. BMC Musculoskelet Disord 2008;156:1–29.

46. Chevalier Y, Pahr D, Charlebois M, et al. Cement distribution, volume, and compliance in vertebroplasty: some answers from an anatomy-based nonlinear finite element study. Spine (Phila Pa 1976) 2008;33:1722–30.

47. Cyteval C, Sarrabere MP, Roux JO, et al. Acute osteoporotic vertebral collapse: open study on percutaneous injection of acrylic surgical cement in 20 patients. AJR Am J Roentgenol 1999;173:1685–90.

48. Syed MI, Jan S, Patel NA, et al. Fatal fat embolism after vertebroplasty: identification of the high-risk patient. AJNR Am J Neuroradiol 2006;27:343–5.

49. Scroop R, Eskridge J, Britz GW. Paradoxical cerebral arterial embolization of cement during intraoperative vertebroplasty: case report. AJNR Am J Neuroradiol 2002;23:868–70.

50. Canyak B, Onan B, Sagbas E, et al. Cardiac tamponade and pulmonary embolism as a complication of percutaneous vertebroplasty. Ann Thorac Surg 2009; 87:299–301.

51. Padovani B, Kasriel O, Brunner P, et al. Pulmonary embolism caused by acrylic cement: a rare complication of percutaneous vertebroplasty. AJNR Am J Neuroradiol 1999;20:375–7.

52. Bernhard J, Heini PF, Villiger PM. Asymptomatic diffuse pulmonary embolism caused by acrylic cement: an unusual complication of percutaneous vertebroplasty. Ann Rheum Dis 2003;62:85–6.

53. Kao FC, Tu YK, Lai PL, et al. Inferior vena cava syndrome following percutaneous vertebroplasty with polymethylmethacrylate. Spine (Phila Pa 1976) 2008;10: 329–33.

54. Birkenmaier C, Seitz S, Wegener B, et al. Acute paraplegia after vertebroplasty caused by epidural hemorrhage. A case report. J Bone Joint Surg Am 2007; 89(8):1827–31.

55. Lopes N, Lopes V. Paraplegia complicating percutaneous vertebroplasty for osteoporotic vertebral fracture. Arq Neuropsiquiatr 2004;62(3-B):879–81.

56. Lee BJ, Lee SR, Yoo TY. Paraplegia as a complication of percutaneous vertebroplasty with polymethylmethacrylate. Spine (Phila Pa 1976) 2002;27:E419–22.

57. Chung SE, Lee SH, Kim TH, et al. Renal cement embolism during percutaneous vertebroplasty. Eur Spine J 2006;15:S590–4.

Index

Note: Page numbers of article titles are in **boldface** type.

A

Abuse, history of, chronic low back pain related to, 803
Acetaminophen, in low back pain management, 794
Acupuncture, in low back pain management, 782–783
Allergy(ies), low back pain treatment and, 820
Anesthetic discography, 863–865
Annular fissure, imaging of, 738
Antidepressant(s), in low back pain management, 795
Antiepileptic medications, in low back pain management, 795
Anti-inflammatory drugs, nonsteroidal, in low back pain management, 794

B

Baastrup syndrome, imaging of, 750
Back pain
  dilemma of, **659–677**
  imaging of, **725–766**
    Baastrup syndrome, 750
    Bertolotti syndrome, 750–751
    CT in, 733–734
    CT myelography in, 734
    degenerative spondylolisthesis, 749–750
    described, 725–727
    early, 727–728
    herniation, 739–744
    modalities in, 733–734
    MRI in, 733–734
    nuclear medicine studies in, 734
    of degenerative phenomena, 734–739. See also *Degenerative phenomena, imaging of.*
    radiography in, 733
    reliability in, 729–733
    risk/benefit analysis in, 728–729
    sacroiliac, coccygeal degenerative disease, 751
    sensitivity in, 729–733
    specificity in, 729–733
    spinal stenosis, 744–745
    spine neoplasm, 758–760
    synovial cysts, 748–749
    zygapophysial joints, 745–748
  low. See *Low back pain.*
  systemic disease presenting as, 751–760

Phys Med Rehabil Clin N Am 21 (2010) 877–885
doi:10.1016/S1047-9651(10)00078-1
1047-9651/10/$ – see front matter © 2010 Elsevier Inc. All rights reserved.
pmr.theclinics.com

Moving?

Make sure your subscription moves with you!

To notify us of your new address, find your **Clinics Account Number** (located on your mailing label above your name), and contact customer service at:

Email: journalscustomerservice-usa@elsevier.com

800-654-2452 (subscribers in the U.S. & Canada)
314-447-8871 (subscribers outside of the U.S. & Canada)

Fax number: 314-447-8029

Elsevier Health Sciences Division
Subscription Customer Service
3251 Riverport Lane
Maryland Heights, MO 63043

*To ensure uninterrupted delivery of your subscription, please notify us at least 4 weeks in advance of move.

ELSEVIER

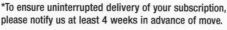

United States Postal Service

Statement of Ownership, Management, and Circulation
(All Periodicals Publications Except Requestor Publications)

1. Publication Title	2. Publication Number	3. Filing Date
Physical Medicine and Rehabilitation Clinics of North America	0 0 9 - 2 4 3	9/15/10

4. Issue Frequency	5. Number of Issues Published Annually	6. Annual Subscription Price
Feb, May, Aug, Nov	4	$230.00

7. Complete Mailing Address of Known Office of Publication (Not printer) (Street, city, county, state, and ZIP+4®)

Elsevier Inc.
360 Park Avenue South
New York, NY 10010-1710

Contact Person
Stephen Bushing

Telephone (Include area code)
215-239-3688

8. Complete Mailing Address of Headquarters or General Business Office of Publisher (Not printer)

Elsevier Inc., 360 Park Avenue South, New York, NY 10010-1710

9. Full Names and Complete Mailing Addresses of Publisher, Editor, and Managing Editor (Do not leave blank)

Publisher (Name and complete mailing address)

Kim Murphy, Elsevier, Inc., 1600 John F. Kennedy Blvd. Suite 1800, Philadelphia, PA 19103-2899

Editor (Name and complete mailing address)

Deb Dellapena, Elsevier, Inc., 1600 John F. Kennedy Blvd. Suite 1800, Philadelphia, PA 19103-2899

Managing Editor (Name and complete mailing address)

Barbara Cohen-Kligerman, Elsevier, Inc., 1600 John F. Kennedy Blvd. Suite 1800, Philadelphia, PA 19103-2899

10. Owner (Do not leave blank. If the publication is owned by a corporation, give the name and address of the corporation immediately followed by the names and addresses of all stockholders owning or holding 1 percent or more of the total amount of stock. If not owned by a corporation, give the names and addresses of the individual owners. If owned by a partnership or other unincorporated firm, give its name and address as well as those of each individual owner. If the publication is published by a nonprofit organization, give its name and address.)

Full Name	Complete Mailing Address
Wholly owned subsidiary of	4520 East-West Highway
Reed/Elsevier, US holdings	Bethesda, MD 20814

11. Known Bondholders, Mortgagees, and Other Security Holders Owning or Holding 1 Percent or More of Total Amount of Bonds, Mortgages, or Other Securities. If none, check box ☐ None

Full Name	Complete Mailing Address
N/A	

12. Tax Status (For completion by nonprofit organizations authorized to mail at nonprofit rates) (Check one)
The purpose, function, and nonprofit status of this organization and the exempt status for federal income tax purposes:
☐ Has Not Changed During Preceding 12 Months
☐ Has Changed During Preceding 12 Months (Publisher must submit explanation of change with this statement)

PS Form 3526, September 2007 (Page 1 of 3 Instructions Page 3)) PSN 7530-01-000-9931 PRIVACY NOTICE: See our Privacy policy in www.usps.com

---

13. Publication Title	14. Issue Date for Circulation Data Below
Physical Medicine and Rehabilitation Clinics of North America	August 2010

15. Extent and Nature of Circulation		Average No. Copies Each Issue During Preceding 12 Months	No. Copies of Single Issue Published Nearest to Filing Date
a. Total Number of Copies (Net press run)		1410	1400
b. Paid Circulation (By Mail and Outside the Mail)	(1) Mailed Outside-County Paid Subscriptions Stated on PS Form 3541. (Include paid distribution above nominal rate, advertiser's proof copies, and exchange copies)	612	663
	(2) Mailed In-County Paid Subscriptions Stated on PS Form 3541 (Include paid distribution above nominal rate, advertiser's proof copies, and exchange copies)		
	(3) Paid Distribution Outside the Mails Including Sales Through Dealers and Carriers, Street Vendors, Counter Sales, and Other Paid Distribution Outside USPS®	185	223
	(4) Paid Distribution by Other Classes Mailed Through the USPS (e.g. First-Class Mail®)		
c. Total Paid Distribution (Sum of 15b (1), (2), (3), and (4))		797	886
d. Free or Nominal Rate Distribution (By Mail and Outside the Mail)	(1) Free or Nominal Rate Outside-County Copies Included on PS Form 3541	68	39
	(2) Free or Nominal Rate In-County Copies Included on PS Form 3541		
	(3) Free or Nominal Rate Copies Mailed at Other Classes Through the USPS (e.g. First-Class Mail)		
	(4) Free or Nominal Rate Distribution Outside the Mail (Carriers or other means)		
e. Total Free or Nominal Rate Distribution (Sum of 15d (1), (2), (3) and (4)		68	39
f. Total Distribution (Sum of 15c and 15e)		865	925
g. Copies not Distributed (See instructions to publishers #4 (page 6))		545	475
h. Total (Sum of 15f and g)		1410	1400
i. Percent Paid (15c divided by 15f times 100)		92.14%	95.78%

16. Publication of Statement of Ownership
☐ If the publication is a general publication, publication of this statement is required. Will be printed in the November 2010 issue of this publication. ☐ Publication not required.

17. Signature and Title of Editor, Publisher, Business Manager, or Owner

Stephen R. Bushing

Stephen R. Bushing – Fulfillment/Inventory Specialist

Date September 15, 2010

I certify that all information furnished on this form is true and complete. I understand that anyone who furnishes false or misleading information on this form or who omits material or information requested on the form may be subject to criminal sanctions (including fines and imprisonment) and/or civil sanctions (including civil penalties).

PS Form 3526, September 2007 (Page 2 of 3)

Printed and bound by CPI Group (UK) Ltd, Croydon, CR0 4YY

03/10/2024

01040448-0003